The Politics of Fear

The Politics of Fear

Médecins Sans Frontières and the West African Ebola Epidemic

EDITED BY MICHIEL HOFMAN
and
SOKHIENG AU

OXFORD
UNIVERSITY PRESS

OXFORD
UNIVERSITY PRESS

Oxford University Press is a department of the University of Oxford. It furthers
the University's objective of excellence in research, scholarship, and education
by publishing worldwide. Oxford is a registered trade mark of Oxford University
Press in the UK and certain other countries.

Published in the United States of America by Oxford University Press
198 Madison Avenue, New York, NY 10016, United States of America.

© Oxford University Press 2017

Library of Congress Cataloging-in-Publication Data
Names: Hofman, Michiel, editor. | Au, Sokhieng, editor.
Title: The politics of fear : Médecins Sans Frontières and the West African
Ebola epidemic / edited by Michiel Hofman and Sokhieng Au. Description: Oxford : Oxford University
Press, [2016] | Includes bibliographical references and index.
Identifiers: LCCN 2016027983 (print) | LCCN 2016042202 (ebook) |
ISBN 9780190624477 (hardcover : alk. paper) | ISBN 9780190624484 (ebook) |
ISBN 9780190624491 (ebook) Subjects: LCSH: Ebola virus disease—Africa, West. | Ebola virus
disease—Social aspects—Africa, West. | Ebola virus disease—Political aspects—Africa, West. |
Epidemics—Social aspects—Africa, West. | Epidemics—Political aspects—Africa, West. |
Médecins Sans frontières (Association) | Africa, West—Social conditions.
Classification: LCC RC140.5 .P65 2016 (print) | LCC RC140.5 (ebook) |
DDC 362.196/92—dc23
LC record available at https://lccn.loc.gov/2016027983

3 5 7 9 8 6 4 2

Printed by Sheridan Books, Inc., United States of America

CONTENTS

PREFACE

With the clarity of hindsight, the word "unprecedented" is now firmly associated with the West African Ebola epidemic of 2014 and 2015. The figures speak for themselves: 25,213 cases were confirmed in the first year of the outbreak and 10,460 patients died. Health professionals deployed by MSF were not immune to the disease either: in the same period, 28 MSF staff were diagnosed with Ebola and 14 of them died. However, these cold figures do not show the tremendous impact this epidemic had, not only on those directly infected by the virus, but also on the societies through which the disease spread and on those who responded to the crisis. The world, including MSF, was slow to respond. All of us, without exception, underestimated how rapidly and how far the virus would spread. We also underestimated the scale of the efforts that would be needed to assist those affected and to control the epidemic.

Prior to the West African outbreak, Ebola was a relatively rare disease that had limited local impact and that burned out fairly quickly. MSF, as one of the few agencies with direct experience responding to Ebola outbreaks in the past, had built up a level of expertise. As a result, from the first days of the epidemic, MSF found itself at the center of the response in West Africa. Nothing, however, had prepared MSF for what happened next in Guinea, Sierra Leone, and Liberia. The disease not only spread over a wide geographic region, but also, for the first time ever recorded, reached densely populated areas such as Monrovia and Conakry.

MSF was severely challenged in recognizing the scale of this epidemic, and subsequently in scaling up the medical and human resources necessary to respond. The impact was profound. Not only did this epidemic push the medical and logistical infrastructure of MSF to the limit, driving personnel at all levels to exhaustion, but it also severely strained MSF's own ethical values, forcing staff into making daily decisions between poor, bad, and even worse options while lives were at stake.

Under these circumstances the usual cost/benefit evaluations are worse than inadequate. This epidemic tested the political resolve and operational choices both inside and outside of MSF. It has left a legacy of lessons to be learned in terms of much-needed technical improvements but also forces us all to reconsider how the world at large deals with transnational health emergencies. A pervasive factor influencing the decisions made during this crisis was fear. To examine this theme, MSF has sponsored this book and made the unprecedented step of allowing the authors full access to the internal archives of MSF's Ebola response in 2014 and 2015. The majority of the authors are external to MSF, providing a unique insight into the processes of fear that informed many of the decisions made by the politicians and the responders such as MSF.

Not all aspects of the outbreak are covered in the 10 chapters. The authors made their own choices regarding which aspects they wanted to highlight, and most of the chapters will elaborate on the wider response, going beyond the specific role played by MSF. This can give the impression that fear affected only others, while the fearless MSF "heroes" ventured into the epidemic with iron resolve. Nothing could be further from the truth; fear "infected" and partially paralyzed MSF as well. Not only did MSF fail to realize that the epidemic was unprecedented even as it was spreading across multiple, frequently heavily populated locations, but MSF had difficulty scaling up its response once the disease was recognized as being out of control. As described powerfully in the eyewitness account by Lindis Hurum, the moment the first health staffer from a partner organization in Monrovia was infected with the Ebola virus, MSF itself was on the verge of deciding the risk was too great and pulling out.

On a more institutional level, some of the MSF resources were also paralyzed by fear. MSF is organized as an international conglomeration of five semiautonomous "operational centers," each with its own medical, logistical, and human resource capacity to respond to emergencies. As the majority of the Ebola experts were located in the Brussels operational center, the coordination for the response was allocated there. It quickly became apparent, however, that the scale of the epidemic required resources from the other centers as well, but this was slow in coming. Fear was a clear internal factor in this delayed response: fear of staff contamination, fear of lack of expertise, and fear of lack of resources. Finally, the fear of being literally as well as figuratively overwhelmed by the epidemic when it was at its peak in the summer of 2014 pushed MSF to take yet another unprecedented step: to make the first call in the history of MSF for a military intervention in an epidemic response.

Yet these unimaginable numbers of deaths, the rapid spread of the virus over three countries, the vast number of people working to respond, and MSF's first-ever appeal for the deployment of militarily trained biological warfare experts are not what constitute the lasting memory of this crisis. What remains is the perpetual doubt about the impossible choices everyone involved, patients and responders alike, had to make throughout this epidemic:

- Do I report to a hospital when I feel sick, and risk death in quarantine? Or do I stay home and risk infecting my family?
- Do I allow everyone in need access to the Ebola center, even though it means the lack of resources will force me to compromise on the levels of care? Or, do I shut the gates and give the very best available treatment to a privileged few?
- Do I use experimental drugs never tested on human patients and risk making their condition worse? Do I offer the patient this choice?
- Do I evacuate all infected foreign health staff to enjoy higher-quality care abroad, but leave my locally based infected colleagues to be treated with the lower standard of care available in country?

These are all profound questions putting the ethics of MSF and other responders under immense pressure. They are very real questions that have all occurred during this crisis. Impossible environments make for impossible choices. Very few would envy those who made the choices, or would want to pass judgement. The main accountability is surely to be found in the future, and in helping those who will confront similar hard ethical choices to learn from the past. We hope this book will help inform future health responders who will have to ask themselves these same questions in the years to come.

Christopher Stokes
General Director
MSF Operational Center Brussels

CONTRIBUTORS

Editors

Michiel Hofman works as senior humanitarian specialist for MSF, based in Belfast, Northern Ireland, involved in training, research, and publications in the humanitarian sector. First working with MSF in 1993, he has served as MSF Country Director in many countries, most recently in Russia and Afghanistan, and as Operations Director for MSF in Amsterdam. He co-founded the Antares Foundation, a Dutch nonprofit organization that supports local NGOs in providing psychosocial support for staff working in high-stress environments.

Sokhieng Au is a member of the program staff with the Advocacy and Analysis Unit, MSF. Also an independent research fellow at Katholieke University Leuven, she has done research on a wide range of topics on colonial and post-colonial health, history, and society. She is the author of *Mixed Medicines: Health and Culture in French Colonial Cambodia* (University of Chicago Press, 2011). She most recently co-edited *Bodies Beyond Borders: Moving Anatomies Between 1750 and 1950*, KU Leuven Press (in press).

Authors

Annick Antierens is an anesthesiologist and emergency doctor with a degree in public health. She has been working with MSF since 1995 in a variety of contexts and medical problematics. She coordinated the medical referents and research for four years and from 2014 she has been the leader of the MSF platform around Ebola experimental products and Ebola survivors.

Adia Benton is an assistant professor of anthropology and African studies at Northwestern University. She has written extensively about the cultural politics of global health and humanitarianism. Her first book, *HIV Exceptionalism: Development Through Disease in Sierra Leone*, was published by the University of Minnesota Press in 2015.

Jean-Francois Caremel is a socio-anthropologist and postdoctoral researcher at CERMES3 (INSERM-CNRS) (Paris) and associate researcher at LASDEL (Niger). His research focuses on the dynamics of medical innovations in humanitarian medicine and how they feed into the politics of global health.

Patricia Carrick is a family nurse practitioner who has worked intermittently with MSF since 2007. She comes from a ranching family in the Rocky Mountains of southwestern Montana in the United States, where her husband, David Hagenbarth, holds her world together when she is away.

Alice Desclaux is a medical anthropologist and a senior researcher in the Institut de Recherche pour le Développement based in Dakar, where she has done extensive work on anthropology and the ethics of HIV, pharmaceuticals, medical research, and women and health, before turning to Ebola in Senegal and Guinea.

Moustapha Diop is professor of anthropology in Université Général Lansana Conté-Sonfonia at Conakry and scientific director of Laboratoire d'Analyse Socio-Anthropologique de Guinée. He has done extensive work on the juridical and anthropological aspects of the land property system and other aspects of contemporary Guinea. He was involved in several social research studies on Ebola during the outbreak.

Stéphane Doyon has been head of the Dakar Regional Unit for MSF OCBA since April 2013. He has been involved in representation tasks for MSF in Dakar related to this regional Ebola outbreak and led the MSF response in Senegal when a case emerged in August 2014.

Sylvain Landry B. Faye is a socio-anthropologist and a researcher/lecturer in the sociology department of the Université Cheikh Anta DIOP (Dakar Sénégal). Having received his PhD in social and cultural anthropology from the Université Victor Segalen de Bordeaux, he specializes in the anthropology of health. His current research focuses on sociocultural and historical aspects of the Ebola epidemic in West Africa and community engagement practices in the framework of humanitarian crisis management.

Lindis Hurum has been with MSF since 2006, working in more than 15 different humanitarian crises. In 2014 she was part of the Emergency Unit in OCB, and during the West African Ebola epidemic, she was the emergency coordinator in Monrovia during the first two months of the MSF intervention. She has a communication background and holds a master's degree in disaster management from Copenhagen University.

Thomas Kratz is a physician with field experience with MSF in treating Lassa fever and Ebola virus disease. He is currently working as a research associate in the Federal Information Centre for Biological Threats and Special Pathogens at Robert Koch Institut, Berlin, Germany.

Prince Lahai is a trained certificate nurse who worked throughout the Ebola epidemic in an Ebola treatment center in Kailahun, Sierra Leone. He is an Ebola survivor. He lives with his mother, his partner, and their three children. He is a leader in his District Survivors' Group and is seeking work in his profession as a nurse.

Allie Tua Lappia graduated as a brand-new community health officer from Njala University in Bo, Sierra Leone, in June 2014, shortly after the Ebola epidemic surged across the border from Guinea into Sierra Leone. His first job as a health worker was in an MSF-run Ebola treatment center, where he worked until it closed. He plans to begin medical school in fall 2016.

Duncan McLean holds a PhD in history and divides his time between humanitarian work and academia. He has managed operations within MSF in both field and headquarters starting in 2002. He has also contributed to various publications, including the International Crisis Group, and currently lectures in the history of disease and colonialism at Charles University and the Anglo-American University in Prague.

João Nunes is a lecturer in international relations at the University of York, United Kingdom. His research interests are health security, neglected diseases, and Brazilian health policy. He is the author of *Security, Emancipation and the Politics of Health* (Routledge) and of articles in the journals *Third World Quarterly, Review of International Studies, Security Dialogue*, and *Contemporary Politics*. He has a PhD from Aberystwyth University and was a research fellow at the University of Gothenburg and the University of Warwick.

Tim O'Dempsey is a senior clinical lecturer in tropical medicine at the Liverpool School of Tropical Medicine, United Kingdom. He worked as a clinician in various locations and for a variety of organizations in Sierra Leone during the Ebola epidemic between July 2014 and December 2015. At the time of the account in this book, he was on secondment from LSTM to WHO as WHO clinical lead at the Ebola treatment center in Kenema.

Ramatou Ouedraogo is an anthropologist who holds a postdoctoral position at the Fondation des Maisons des Sciences de l'Homme de Paris. She is also associate researcher in the laboratory Les Afriques dans le Monde at IEP-Bordeaux. Her research focuses on reproductive health, young people in Africa, infectious diseases (HIV, Ebola), gender, and intergenerational relationships.

Mit Philips is the health policy and medical advocacy advisor in the Analysis and Advocacy Unit at MSF. Her work focuses on HIV/AIDS, health financing and financial barriers to health care, and global health and health systems policies. She was a medical doctor and coordinator with MSF in the field for 15 years, serving later as director of operations in Brussels.

Annette Rid is senior lecturer in bioethics and society at King's College London. She works in a variety of areas in bioethics, including research ethics, clinical ethics, justice in health and health care, and ethics in transplantation medicine. Her publications on the West African Ebola epidemic include "Ethical considerations of experimental interventions in the Ebola outbreak" (with Ezekiel Emanuel; *Lancet*, 2014) and "Ethical rationale for the Ebola 'ring vaccination' trial design" (with Franklin Miller; *American Journal of Public Health*, 2015).

Maud Santantonio is a clinical doctor working with Samusocial, a Belgian association that provides social services, including medical care, to the homeless. After receiving her MD in 2011, she worked for five months in a primary health-care center in Mayotte before joining MSF. She worked from 2013 to 2015 on various missions with MSF. She remains committed to working with disadvantaged populations both in Europe and abroad.

Armand Sprecher is an emergency physician and epidemiologist who has worked with MSF since 1997. He has been involved with filovirus outbreak response since 2000, including the outbreaks in Uganda in 2000, Angola in 2005, and the Democratic Republic of the Congo in 2007, and the outbreak in West Africa. Alongside filovirus disease issues, he also works on health informatics. He has also worked with the International Medical Corps and the U.S. Center for Disease Control and Prevention's Epidemic Intelligence Service.

INTRODUCTION

MICHIEL HOFMAN AND SOKHIENG AU

The West African Ebola epidemic is familiar in its broad strokes to most of the news-reading public. A small boy in the remote forested Gueckedou region of Guinea died quickly following a short, undiagnosed illness in December 2013. This toddler's mysterious death was the beginning of a two-year Ebola epidemic that would grip the world, threatening to draw the distant nations wealthy and poor alike into its expanding narrative. In brief outline, the story continues as follows. The epidemic smoldered undetected until mid-March 2014, when the international medical aid organization Médecins Sans Frontières (MSF) first confirmed the diagnosis in Guinea and the World Health Organization (WHO) published a formal notification of the disease (WHO 2014). Ebola epidemics prior to this had occurred in remote, sparsely populated regions and had quickly burned themselves out. This initial notice elicited little interest by the international health authorities, and the epidemic continued to spread. The first victim of this epidemic had died in a forested region of Guinea that bordered Sierra Leone and Liberia. The path of the epidemic would serve as a reminder that manmade borders have little meaning in the natural world, as the virus quickly spread within the region to other countries. The epidemic was officially recognized on March 23 in Guinea, March 30 in Liberia, and May 25 in Sierra Leone.

By early April, MSF staff in Guinea and, by then, neighboring Liberia were very uneasy. The organization had had experience with numerous Ebola epidemics and had never seen the geographic reach or the numbers of this one. Worldwide, Ebola experts numbered in the dozens, many of those were MSF staff, and limits in expertise were being reached. On March 31, MSF warned that the epidemic was unprecedented, and two months later, on June 23, 2014, tried to alert the international health authorities that it was "out of control." Both alarms resulted in little more than a berating of MSF staff on the ground by national governments for their interference and politicking (Pagano and Poncin, in press). WHO finally declared the epidemic a "public health emergency of international concern" on August 8, 2014. Finally, when the epidemic was in full swing through the countries of Guinea, Sierra Leone, and Liberia, and, crucially, a case had been diagnosed in Texas in a traveler from Liberia on September 24, most of the world turned its attention to these three small West African countries.

Media coverage of the epidemic dramatically intensified in August and September, and Ebola became a cultural phenomenon worldwide. Western media churned out doomsday scenarios, people in the U.S. Midwest bought Ebola survival kits, flight routes from some cities in Europe were canceled, travelers' temperatures were screened at airports, and returning humanitarian workers were reviled for being selfish (Anderson 2014; Cordery 2014). Money and resources began pouring into the region in August 2014. The epidemic began to recede in the following months, declining steadily if not dramatically into 2015. By the time the epidemic was declared over (which, by late April 2016, has been done repeatedly in the three countries[1]) or, to put it more technically, person-to-person transmission had ended, 28,646 people had been confirmed infected, with 11,308 deaths (WHO 2016b). On March 29, 2016, WHO officially declared the "public health emergency of international concern" over (WHO 2016c).

Fear was the catchword of this epidemic. In some cases, it was a genuine reaction to an uncertain situation involving a deadly disease. In other cases, fear was stoked by those in power in a calculated manner for political gain. It was also an unintended consequence of dramatic, noncontextualized public health messages in the region, such as "Ebola kills," that inadvertently emphasized the futility in seeking treatment (Bianchi 2015). And certainly those seeking to draw attention and aid to West Africans suffering in the epidemic were not innocent of using fear to invoke action for their cause. Narratives of danger generated both positive and negative interest. Unfortunately, the undercurrent of fear, rather than rational consideration, would drive many of the responses within West Africa and from involved wealthy nations.

But just as there were several stages to the epidemic, one could also categorize the stages of fear. Initially Guineans, Sierra Leoneans, and Liberians were largely left alone in their own fright, as they suffered and died suddenly from often nonspecific, generic ailments. In poor countries with weak or nonexistent health systems, these initial victims of strange fevers and diarrhea were little different than others dying from malaria or dysentery or typhus in the region. But these mundane symptoms were tragically lethal, as the Ebola virus attacked a wide range of cells in the human body, insidiously hijacking the cells of the immune system to spread from the point of entry throughout the body. Although its mechanisms of action are still poorly understood, what is known about this virus is that it causes widespread metabolic havoc, expressed like other viruses at times as fevers, diarrhea, vomiting, headaches, muscle pains, and joint pains (Schieffelin et al. 2014; Singh et al. 2016). Ebola symptoms are not, by and large, the bleeding orifices and instant collapse dramatized by Hollywood, but they are as lethal. Unlike most other viruses, Ebola Zaire, the particular strain causing this epidemic, was ruthlessly efficient, more often than not killing its host as its presence (or viral load) increased to levels the body could no longer combat. Even with improved clinical care, the case-fatality rate by the end of the epidemic was 40% (WHO 2016a). Severe acute respiratory syndrome (SARS), perhaps the only other comparable major international epidemic in recent history, had a case-fatality rate of just under 10% (U.S. Centers for Disease Control and Prevention [CDC] 2003).

There was another peculiarity of Ebola that separated it from other notable epidemics such as H1N1 ("swine flu") or SARS: it is not particularly contagious in the early stages. Whereas epidemics like SARS were spread by airborne droplets emitted by individuals who could be only mildly symptomatic, Ebola is a disease spread by intimate contact with the fluid and excreta of a visibly diseased body. The more the body was showing the ravages of the virus—when the person was visibly sick and expressing, in his or her blood or vomit or diarrhea, the virus—the more contagious the person was. Thus, caregivers, medical staff, and those giving funerary rites were most at risk. The dead body in particular was soaked in contagion. However, Ebola quickly became associated with even casual social contact. In the three countries, touching became something to be feared. But fear was also linked to uncertainty and bad information.

As authorities tried to organize against the spreading epidemic, questions of sovereignty and international guidance continued to be muddled, and the response reflected this lack of clarity. Much blame has been placed on WHO for its lack of strong guidance, but, as some have argued, global governance of public health emergencies is more an ideal than a reality. As the epidemic clearly became an emergency, it seems that its particularities, or exceptionalities, were still little taken into account. According to Chapter 3 in this volume, by Jean-François Caremel and colleagues, the response would become the "standard" emergency response, whose lack of flexibility itself highlights deep systemic problems with the international global health structure. Local authorities had to juggle national sovereignty with international guidance. International or national, the authorities had to act through, with, and upon its populations. Public health is always political; medical priorities and political priorities clashed. For example, the institution of quarantine was as much political as medical. It showed that the authorities were doing something, providing a theater of state power to both cow and reassure the general population. It was heavy-handed, but that was sometimes the point. Local communities could react with violence to such impositions of power or perceived coercive measures (AFP 2014; Phillips 2014; Anonymous 2015). Other reactions could be more nuanced, as Chapter 9, by Alice Desclaux and colleagues, reveals. Adia Benton's analysis in Chapter 2 further casts light on how such reactions cannot be understood if uncoupled from the recent history of conflict in the region.

The fear of social contact on the ground was paralleled on the global scale in the international reaction to the disease, a stage of fear that began in August 2014. In much of the media from a distance, the intense spotlight on Ebola did not lead so much to an outpouring of sympathy and support for those threatened and suffering as it did a deluge of self-protective, "securitizing" actions against this threat, as João Nunes discusses in Chapter 1. To be sure, resources were pledged from around the globe to fight the epidemic, in large part driven by the argument that the security threat must be neutralized at its source. The fear "from a distance" that Ebola evoked in policymakers on other continents led to controversial quarantines of returning humanitarian workers, restricted and sometimes banned flights to and from the region, and forced screening of travelers (Miles 2015). As Duncan McLean discusses in Chapter 10, this urge to isolate the problem rather than addressing it led to unwillingness of states to accept the return and care of their own citizens who were afflicted in the course of fighting the disease. In general populations on distant continents, reactions expanded into the absurd. In the United States, public pressure mounted to fight this extremely low local threat. In November 2014, a Gallup poll found that one in six Americans believed that Ebola was the country's top health problem (Saad 2014). To put this into perspective, in 2014 the United States had more cases of bubonic plague than Ebola (CDC: Maps and Statistics, Plague in the United States). Nonetheless, several how-to books on surviving Ebola were published and doomsday scenarios were aired in the media, leading one expert to coin the term "fear-bola" for this disproportionate reaction (Robbins 2014). Anthony Fauci, director of the U.S. National Institute of Allergy and Infectious Diseases, would observe at the height of the crisis, "What we're seeing is a catastrophic health crisis in West Africa, and an epidemic of fear here" (CSPAN-2 2014). Further, fear of the disease and fear of the diseased became one, as Ebola became the poor, sick, black African, further conflated with the continent of Africa itself, continuing "the long and ugly tradition of treating Africa as a dirty, diseased place."[2] Europe and Asia were not immune from this irrationality as schools in France, Belgium, and England denied entry to students of West African origin, a bar in South Korea refused to serve black patrons, and Chinese taxi drivers took the precaution of not shaking hands with black riders (Anonymous 2014a, 2014b; Fadoul 2014; Higgins 2014; Nadeau 2014; Waldmeir and Hornby 2014). Global hysteria

spread much further than actual cases as "Africa" and "African" became syn-
onymous with "Ebola."

Although these distant reactions would have an impact on the epidemic,
this volume maintains its focus on the epicenter of the catastrophic health crisis, where resource-poor national governments initially tried to protect their
sovereignty and economies by denying the effect of the disease on the population's health and well-being, a case of putting the cart before the horse. In
West Africa, where 99.9% of the total cases occurred, the epidemic changed
everything—and nothing. While, a year later, most of the world has comfortably turned its attention away, most of the population there still lives in grind-
ing poverty, quality healthcare continues to be a luxury few can find or afford,
and the population still continues to die of easily treatable diseases. Ministries
of Health, often the lowest-priority ministries in low-income countries, are still
low priority. Healthcare workers, already insufficient before this epidemic, have
been decimated. On the other hand, WHO has pledged assistance in monitoring
survivors of Ebola, and funds are reserved for medical and psychosocial care for
them. This is a mixed blessing, as Prince's story reveals in Vignette 2, since the
offer of care cannot be unbound from the difficult economic and political situation that each survivor negotiates. It also neglects the battering that the general
health systems (already extremely fragile) of these three countries suffered from
the epidemic, as Mit Philips shows in Chapter 5, and does little to aid in their
recovery.

The book is organized into four thematic sections. The first section, "The
Response," examines the role of different actors in an international public health
emergency. In Chapter 1, João Nunes untangles the threads between security
and health as he examines the growing association between global health and
fear. As he observes, disease is increasingly perceived as an international security threat, as a result of post-9/11 concerns about bioterrorism and anxieties
about possible social and political turmoil caused by disease epidemics. While
public health has always been political, its growing links to securitization add
another dimension to its political configuration. The concept of risk—and its
focus on potential threat rather than actual problems—facilitates preemptive
political reordering of society. Health emergencies such as Ebola are framed as
existential threats demanding exceptional measures. As Nunes spells out, fear
as an animating principle for action privileges containing and managing "crises"
rather than addressing the deep-seated problems that give rise to these events
in the first place. He further highlights the specific example of the rhetorical
and aspirational positioning of MSF in relation to global health responses, and
this changing security landscape. MSF, he observes, is at a crossroads in this
post-Ebola moment: it could choose to continue on the path taken by much of
the global health community, or it could work further to break down borders,

delegitimizing the underlying "us versus them" mentality of the securitization framework.

Turning toward an institution with an increasing presence in health emergencies, in Chapter 2 Adia Benton examines the role of foreign and national militaries in the Ebola crisis. She uses MSF's uncharacteristic call for a military response to the Ebola crisis to examine the dynamics of army and police involvement in humanitarian emergencies. The MSF recommendation for military involvement was unexpected, given MSF's default policy against such interventions. It was also somewhat paradoxical, as it called for this involvement to exclude quarantine, crowd control, and containment—essentially the delivery of military medicine without military might. Nonetheless, the inclusion of the military meant that certain responses to the epidemic were implicitly undertaken with the threat of force, begging the question of who was deemed worthy of protection and from what. In the context of West Africa, colonial occupation, independence, and civil war were all recent brutal episodes of armed forces policing civilians. A military response invoked this history, an unpleasant association for most of the population. Ultimately, Ebola incidence began to decline quite early in the military involvement, making it unclear how or to what extent it contributed to a decline in cases. The military's role in public health emergencies is a vexing issue that continues to be pertinent in the increasingly complex world of global public health.

The first section of our book ends with a vignette about a personal experience at a watershed moment in the epidemic. Lindis Hurum provides an evocative account of a few crucial days in Liberia when she and her staff had to decide whether to continue working against what seemed to be insurmountable obstacles. Her story highlights that true engagement in this crisis involved more than simply a commitment of material goods or money. The needs of the community and the nature of the struggle against Ebola were not neatly contained within the mandate of providing medical care. For those face to face with the sick and dying, the fight against Ebola was also a psychological and social commitment to stand in solidarity with those in need.

As these chapters reveal, the global health community is a community in evolution. The Ebola epidemic revealed some of the strengths and some of the weaknesses in this fluctuating community, and the need to rethink some of these relationships. If we are to use the military to deliver medical relief, it must be decoupled from the security ethos of the military but also, and certainly more difficult to achieve, the cultural understandings of an armed state force (police or military). Global health governance needs to be more inclusive but also more transparent. The security mindset must also incorporate solidarity. How can these various goals be aligned? How does commitment on an individual level engage with systemic governance structures, or larger institutional apparatus? These chapters reveal that we must discuss how we choose to engage with the increasingly complex and interlinked health problems of the 21st century, rather than simply continuing to operate with the systems we have inherited, with their unquestioned frameworks and underlying biases.

The second section, "The System," takes a closer look at the individuals and organizations fighting against Ebola on the ground. In Chapter 3 Jean-François Caremel and his colleagues examine the epidemic management response in Guinea to illuminate the complicated dynamics and politics between international and national actors, as well as the routinized international response to exceptional events. They fruitfully explore the contradictions found in the mundane and standardized reaction to what are labeled unique and complicated emergencies. Local populations have specific readings of the disease and the disease response drawn from autochthonous medical knowledge, experience, and a historical distrust of state and foreign actors. International actors, the authors observe, constructed the notion of Ebola "risk" around conventional tropes of an epidemic and humanitarian moralism. This construction ignored the rich local readings of the disease and justified a large, inefficient, bureaucratic international response. In the end, was there much exceptional about the Ebola response in West Africa? They suggest not. Transformations in aid and the effective reinforcement of health systems expected after Ebola remain largely illusory.

Bringing the lens even closer to the epidemic response, Thomas Kratz in Chapter 4 relates the early response to the epidemic, with a reflection on the actions and actors (or lack thereof) during different stages of the epidemic. Drawing on his personal experience as one of the first international doctors on the ground, he relates some of the dysfunction among various public health figures in the summer of 2014. He provides an experiential lens on the problems discussed on the policy or systemic level by other authors in this volume. Neglect, mismanagement, or lack of staff is contextualized through his experience in the early and later stages of the epidemic. His account makes explicit the real effects of the late and inadequate international response to the epidemic, as well as continuing problems with aid response even as it became "normalized."

In Chapter 5 Mit Philips turns to the question of death, and life, beyond Ebola in West Africa. As she observes, most deaths in West Africa in 2014 and 2015 were not from Ebola. However, the evidence reveals the volume of these "mundane" deaths considerably increased as a result of the epidemic. Coordination of the Ebola response did not consider the overall functioning of the health system; rather, it monopolized health-coordinating structures on all levels. The amplitude of the epidemic pulled in vital resources that were funnelled away from other health programs, reducing the already limited capacity to handle existing health issues. Both healthcare workers and patients found novel ways to manage their fear and navigate this weakened healthcare environment. Still, vulnerabilities increased. In this context, the outcome for those suffering from obstructed labor, respiratory illnesses, malaria, and many common diseases in Sierra Leone, Guinea, and Liberia worsened. Recently, as these health systems are slowly resuming, governments and aid organizations have increasingly focused on building "resilient" systems for the future, a move, she argues, that may take attention away from the pressing needs of today.

In Vignette 2, the story of Prince, as told to Patricia Carrick, reveals how these systemic problems impact the individual sufferer. Prince worked in an Ebola treatment center, where he was infected with the disease and became a patient. After his recovery, he returned to continue working against the disease and for his community in the same treatment center. As a survivor of Ebola, a caregiver for other Ebola victims, and a health worker in Sierra Leone, Prince represents the successes of the fight against Ebola as well as the failures that continue to haunt the health system. His story and continued struggle remind us that the end of the epidemic is not the end of the tragedy that surrounds it.

Taken together, the three chapters and the vignette in this section link the global to the local. They reveal the dysfunction built into the response system from different perspectives. The actors and systems that structured the immediate response to the epidemic suffered from shortcomings that were both structural and personal. Nonetheless, in defiance of any structural determinism, these authors highlight these faults in part to suggest solutions. Specific programmatic goals should be designed that move these countries in the direction of a "healthy health system," as Philips phrases it. Individuals are constrained but not contained by the systems they work in, and the systems can be adapted for the good of its users and beneficiaries. These essays suggest that global governance, operational practices, and the health structures can all be rethought, improved, and strengthened for future emergencies.

The third section, "Patients," looks at care for the sick. Chapter 6, by Annette Rid and Annick Antierens, examines the ethically charged question of the use of experimental therapeutic and vaccine treatments during the epidemic. The epidemic began with no proven vaccines or targeted treatments for the disease. Moreover, infection with Ebola was largely mortal in the affected countries due to a lack of adequate health infrastructure. These grim prospects quickly prompted proposals to use unproven vaccines and treatments for Ebola, some of which were in the earliest phases of testing. When two U.S. citizens received experimental treatment after they had contracted Ebola in Liberia, extensive controversy arose as to how unproven vaccines and treatments should be used in this epidemic. A crux in the controversy was whether the unproven interventions should be used in clinical trials or as part of experimental clinical care or prevention, which is more conventionally called "compassionate use." Furthermore, the design of trials was problematic. MSF took a clear stance on these issues, agreeing to collaborate on clinical trials but excluding the use of individually randomized controlled trial designs on both ethical and practical grounds. By examining the values and beliefs that informed MSF's position on clinical trials in the ongoing epidemic, Rid and Antierens explore how MSF made decisions about the trials and draw some lessons learned for how unproven vaccines and treatments should be used and how priorities should be established for experimental designs, data collection, and therapeutic trials in future epidemics.

Chapter 7 concerns a topic that was perhaps one of the most troubling and sensitive for health staff working in the Sierra Leone Ebola response: the death of Dr. Sheik Humarr Khan. Tim O'Dempsey attempts to unravel some of the complicated politics and ethics around experimental drug protocols. The chapter, written from a deeply personal perspective, hovers around the unfortunate truism that all lives are not equal. In the case of Dr. Khan, the valuation of life is central, but the process is profoundly complex. Decisions around treatments were driven by many factors beyond the individual patients, resulting in different levels of care and mortality outcomes for different types of patients. Tracing the events surrounding Dr. Khan's infection and failed treatment, this chapter seeks to understand how and why the decision was made to deny this highly experimental treatment to one of the most prominent Sierra Leonean doctors treating Ebola during the height of the epidemic. Did fear of public perceptions during a time of extremely fragile public trust in the health system unduly impact the treatment regimen for the doctor? Were the unknown risks of ZMapp reasonably weighed against the potential benefit? Should the patient have been given the choice to decide for himself? Ultimately, the death of Dr. Khan colors the final analysis, and we are left with the unresolved question of not just how to value all life, but how to treat all human life *equally*.

The final chapter in this section is also driven by a highly charged episode in the Ebola response. Armand Sprecher, in Chapter 8, examines the care provided at an Ebola treatment center during the height of the epidemic against the charges that containment was prioritized over patient care. He observes that, during a stage in the epidemic when patients vastly outnumbered available beds, Ebola treatment centers were terribly understaffed, and the sick were waiting and dying outside the gates, an impossible compromise was demanded between volume of care and quality of care. Observers would lay charges of substandard care, driven they believed by a prioritizing of a sort of catchment of the sick over provision of best care. Sprecher, an MSF clinical doctor, defends against these charges, arguing that care is defined far beyond prevention of dying. Rather, care also encompasses alleviation of suffering and offering a dignified shelter during illness. This belief, that care should be offered to the most even if certain standardized procedures must be abandoned, is at odds with the idea that therapeutics must be at the highest standards, even if it can only be offered to a few.

The "Patients" section is closed out with a heart-wrenching vignette by Allie Tua Lappia and Patricia Carrick on the children in the Ebola treatment centers. In this essay, we see clearly that the virus deformed the idea of care, forcing it to become something less than what any caregiver would deem ideal, as human contact—the most basic human need—became an unacceptable risk. Parents, sick and contagious, were separated from their small children. Children sought out but were denied their parents, not understanding the implications of their positive or negative Ebola tests. Caregivers in their cumbersome protective gear and their limited resources were at a loss as to how to comfort infants or small children, even at the moment of death. As the authors poignantly reveal through their story of a handful of children who ended up in these centers, both the patients and caregivers suffered from this loss of care and human contact.

Where should the line be drawn when resources are few and needs are many? When and how should an individual's role in the epidemic, in an organization, or indeed in society more generally, be considered when allotting treatments? When is it is right and when is it wrong to provide an unproven therapy to a patient, and what sort of patient is the most appropriate? Ebola brought these questions starkly to the fore and, in many cases, flipped them around. For example, while much ink has been spilled on the wrongness of clinical experimentation on minorities and marginalized groups, here the *withholding* of experimentation from such groups is the troubling wrong.[3] Social inequality is reflected in complicated ways in the politics of therapeutics, and in the decisions around treatment, as this section reveals. Financial inequality is inextricable from this. Poverty, if little discussed directly, is central to these analyses. An elderly cancer patient in Western society will have resources and money to extend his or her life a few years, resources that, if redistributed in West Africa, could treat thousands of young people, extending their lives for decades. This sort of global redistribution is currently unachievable; it also still poses an ethical dilemma. Indeed, as Sprecher has shown, even the shared resource distribution among a few extra patients can be seen as a crime against the individual patient. The calculus of risk, resource, and responsibility in therapeutics represents insolvable equations, although we continue to try to puzzle out the solutions.

The two chapters and vignette in the final section, "Containment," look at forms of confinement, quarantine, and medical evacuations, examining what movement (or lack thereof) meant to those involved, and how keeping people in place or refusing to bring people out were integral parts of the Ebola experience. Epidemics create fear, and fear creates distance. In many instances, social distancing was spontaneous (as hinted at by Caremel and colleagues in Chapter 3) until it became bureaucratized. During the Ebola response, quarantine came into full force in various incarnations from individual quarantines to the cordoning off of huge geographic areas to movement, such as the *cordon sanitaire* attempted as a cooperative measure between Guinea, Sierra Leone, and Liberia to block off the "triangle" of infection near the Mano River Union in August 2014 (RFI 2014). Movement into and out of West Africa also became controlled, with many airlines canceling or severely restricting flights to the region. Medevac of sick individuals back to their home countries, even those sick of a disease other than Ebola, became difficult, as Duncan McLean reports in Chapter 10. On a smaller scale, sick individuals moving into and out of medical care were also controlled according to their perceived risk of being contaminated. The chapters in this section look more closely at the consequences of controlling movements as a proxy for controlling the disease.

Through in-depth anthropological interviews, Alice Desclaux and her coauthors in Chapter 9 relate how official containment measures were perceived by the individuals who lived through these measures. Examining different sorts of containment (or quarantine) in two countries (Senegal and Guinea) and different epidemic periods, they illustrate the concrete effects of such strategies on those on either side of the barriers as well as how individuals understood these measures. Through a careful analysis of four case studies, the authors discuss the relevance of these containment efforts, as well as organizational frames for confinement. The analysis illuminates the dynamics of the evolving relationships between quarantined individuals and caregivers, while also speaking to the varieties of containment and some of the official reasoning behind them. Importantly, this chapter contextualizes the experience of quarantine and the social sequelae that continue long after confinement has been removed.

Duncan McLean turns an analytical lens to the complicated politics of medical evacuation. At the start of the epidemic, medical evacuation seemed relatively straightforward and the need self-evident—but they weren't. International medical evacuations are expensive and logistically complicated in the best of circumstances, and the context of Ebola added further complications related to the reluctance of air crews unwilling to transport potential cases, nations unwilling to allow such planes in their airspace, and technical issues with post-evacuation plane decontamination. The inability to guarantee the evacuation of sick staff members heightened already severe recruitment difficulties for an unprecedented epidemic response. Still, the most significant obstacle to finding a means to ensure international evacuation was neither the availability of cash nor technical difficulties, but the lack of political will. The failure of cooperation among EU member states reflected a broader fear of political backlash from constituent populations. No one wanted to be blamed for "importing" Ebola into their home country. This infighting and deferral of responsibility succeeded only in further isolating the affected countries. These issues are traced through a history of MSF's efforts to arrange medevac during the crisis, its lobbying for pooled medevac services by the EU member states, and its late success in finding a solution that it would ultimately not use.

Maud Santantonio's vignette on triage in the ETC in Conakry, Guinea, provides a snapshot of how, at the moment of diagnosis, Ebola also created ethical dilemmas relating to confinement and isolation. Sick individuals entering the ETC who were deemed suspect cases were held apart until their status could be confirmed by a blood test. What would seem to be a sound epidemiological and medical measure is in fact a deeply unnatural act when considered in the context of families and friends admitted together, advised to keep their distance from their sick and dying loved ones. As she illustrates from one particular incident, sometimes the stark contrast between the medically sound and the socially acceptable led to reactions of violence and incomprehension from family members. Denying the virus routes of transmission by isolating human beings also meant denying the living access to the dying.

Social distancing can be both self-imposed and society-imposed as a protective measure against a perceived danger. The measures discussed by Desclaux, McLean, and Santantonio were, ostensibly, to limit contagion and contain the virus. However, a sick person flying 10,000 feet overhead in a nation's airspace cannot infect that nation. Confining a noncontagious person in a home did not stop the person-to-person spread of the disease, while it did seem to encourage the sick to go underground rather than to seek care, and thus increase spread of the epidemic. The epidemiological arguments against such confinement often fall on deaf ears, as these acts frequently served symbolic and political goals rather than medical goals. They provided a sense of security to those on the "protected" side of the divide and could be offered to an uneasy public as concrete measures of defense. Even at the level of the individual patient, separation of one human being from his or her community for the good of all is a rational argument that can often seem devoid of compassion. At times, the fight to stop the spread of the epidemic through control of human movements lost sight of the fact that these potential "Ebola spreaders" were more than disease vectors: they remained human beings, suffering and in need of care.

The chapters in *Politics of Fear* are an eclectic mix ranging from policy discussions to personal stories. This is a reflection of the topic and the aspirations of the book. Health policy should not be separated from suffering patients. In the end, all drama is human drama, and the human perspective should remain at the fore. Thus, within each of the sections of the book, we also have included a vignette, a personal account of the epidemic. A conceit of this book is that it must remain focused on the victims, and on West Africa. All the chapters, even those on policy, are framed in some way around this region.

This book began in part from a desire by some at MSF to have a more political reading of what happened during the epidemic, and the role MSF had in this political landscape. Thus, the decision was made to open up the organization's internal documentation to outside scholars, but also to invest in a collection that encompasses much more than what MSF did, as, of course, many facets of the epidemic fall well outside of the MSF experience. Dozens of organizations would ultimately work in the fight against Ebola. Myriad topics not included in this book should and will be discussed elsewhere, such as Ebola survivors' syndrome, Ebola deniers, legal frameworks for epidemic measures, economic consequences, Ebola and the West, Ebola orphans, and so forth. Further, many of the consequences have yet to be written. Of course, no one book on Ebola can be comprehensive. This book brings together many disparate strands to contribute to this complicated story.

Ultimately, the human response to the West African Ebola epidemic was messy and inadequate. The disease harshly revealed the fragility of the human body, society, and the body politic. It was a disaster, but—as the steep decline of the epidemic toward the beginning of 2015, in defiance of mathematical projections, reveals—human will and action, albeit imperfect, seem to have been effective in averting an even greater disaster. The chapters here tell some of this story by examining this disease through various disciplinary lenses (political science, anthropology, clinical medicine, bioethics, history) but also through individual perspectives. No one owns Ebola. Ebola can rightly claim to be a disease that was the most widely experienced (perhaps only through fear) across the globe in recent history. We hope that this book has captured some of this experience and engenders discussions that will ultimately improve the lives of future epidemic victims.

Notes

1. Lingering cases are labeled flare-ups, and a countdown of a flare-up in Guinea is currently ongoing as of April 28, 2016.
2. See Seay and Yi Dionne 2015, in response to the article in *Newsweek* claiming illegally smuggled African bushmeat would sneak Ebola into the United States (Flynn and Scutti 2014).
3. See, for example, Epstein 2007.

References

AFP. 2014. "Ebola patients flee as armed men raid Liberia clinic." *The Telegraph*, Aug. 17. Accessed April 10, 2016, from http://www.telegraph.co.uk/news/worldnews/africaandindianocean/liberia/11039693/Ebola-patients-flee-as-armed-men-raid-Liberia-clinic.html.

Anderson, Marc. 2014. "Ebola: Airlines cancel more flights to affected countries." *The Guardian*, August 22.

Anonymous. 2014a. "Ebola fears prompt Stockport school to cancel Sierra Leone charity worker visit," October 8, Press Association. Accessed April 12, 2016, from http://www.theguardian.com/world/2014/oct/08/ebola-fears-stockport-school-cancel-charity-visit.

Anonymous. 2014b. "Par peur d'Ebola, ils retirent leurs enfants de l'école," Oct. 8. Accessed April 10, 2016, from http://www.europe1.fr/sante/ils-retirent-leurs-enfants-de-l-ecole-par-crainte-d-ebola-2252169.

Anonymous. 2015. "Ebola crisis: Red Cross says Guinea aid workers face attacks." *BBC News*, Feb. 12. Accessed April 10, 2016 from http://www.bbc.com/news/world-africa-31444059.

Bianchi, Sergio. 2015. "Determinants of Ebola health-seeking behaviors: Reflections from Freetown." UREPH, Unpublished Internal Report, MSF OCG, May.

Centers for Disease Control and Prevention. 2003. "Revised U.S. surveillance case definition for severe acute respiratory syndrome (SARS) and update on SARS cases—United States and worldwide, December 2003." *Morbidity and Mortality Weekly Report* 52: 1202–206. Accessed March 7, 2016, from http://www.cdc.gov/mmwr/preview/mmwrhtml/mm5249a2.htm.

Centers for Disease Control and Prevention. *Maps and Statistics: Plague in the United States.* Accessed April 19, 2016, from http://www.cdc.gov/plague/maps/index.html.

Cordery, Amy. 2014. "Aid workers creating Ebola risk in Australia, Bob Katter claims." *Sydney Morning Herald*, October 9. Accessed April 16, 2016, from http://www.smh.com.au/federal-politics/political-news/aid-workers-creating-ebola-risk-in-australia-bob-katter-claims-20141009-113x3z.html#ixzz43uxY4DtM.

C-SPAN2. 2014. Dr. Anthony Fauci on Ebola [Video file]. Accessed February 20, 2016, from http://www.c-span.org/video/?322439-6/dr-anthony-fauci-ebola

Epstein, Steven. 2007. *Inclusion: The politics of difference in medical research.* Chicago, University of Chicago Press.

Fadoul, Karim. 2014. "Ebola: panique à l'école 6 de Schaerbeek à l'inscription d'un petit Guinéen," *La Capitale*. Oct. 20. Accessed April 12, 2016, from http://www.lacapitale.be/1128276/article/2014-10-19/ebola-panique-a-l-ecole-6-de-schaerbeek-a-l-inscription-d-un-petit-guineen

Flynn, Gerald, and Susan Scutti. 2014. "Smuggled bushmeat is Ebola's backdoor." *Newsweek*, Aug. 21.

Higgins, Andrew. 2014. "In Europe, fear of Ebola exceeds the actual risks." *New York Times*, Oct. 17. Accessed April 12, 2016, from http://www.nytimes.com/2014/10/18/world/europe/in-europe-fear-of-ebola-far-outweighs-the-true-risks.html?_r=0.

Miles, Steven H. 2015. "Kaci Hickox: Public health and the politics of fear." *American Journal of Bioethics* 15: 17–19. doi:10.1080/15265161.2015.1010994.

Nadeau, Barbie Latza. 2014. "Ebola-fueled racism is on the rise in Europe." *Daily Beast*, Aug. 21. Accessed April 10, 2016, from http://www.thedailybeast.com/articles/2014/08/20/ebola-fueled-racism-is-on-the-rise-in-europe.html.

Pagano, Heather, and Marc Poncin (in press). "Treating, containing, mobilizing: The role of Médecins Sans Frontières in the West Africa Ebola epidemic response. In *Global infectious disease threats after Ebola*, ed. Sam Halabi et al. (Oxford University Press).

Phillips, Abby. 2014. "Eight dead in attack on Ebola team in Guinea. 'Killed in cold blood.'" *Washington Post*, Sept. 18. https://www.washingtonpost.com/news/to-your-health/wp/2014/09/18/missing-health-workers-in-guinea-were-educating-villagers-about-ebola-when-they-were-attacked/?tid=a_inl.

RFI. 2014. «Ebola: un cordon sanitaire pour stopper la propagation du virus», August 1. Accessed April 10, 2016, at http://www.rfi.fr/afrique/20140801-ebola-cordon-sanitaire-stopper-propagation-virus-oms-margaret-chan-epidemie/.

Robbins, M. 2014. "'Fear-bola' hits epidemic proportions." CNN. Accessed March 31, 2016, from http://www.cnn.com/2014/10/15/opinion/robbins-ebola-fear/.

Saad, Lydia. 2014. "Ebola ranks among Americans' top three healthcare concerns." Nov. 17. Accessed April 10, 2016, from http://www.gallup.com/poll/179429/ebola-ranks-among-americans-top-three-healthcare-concerns.aspx.

Schieffelin, John S., et al. 2014. "Clinical illness and outcomes in patients with Ebola in Sierra Leone." *New England Journal of Medicine* 371: 2092–100.

Seay, Laura, and Kim Yi Dionne. 2015. "The long and ugly tradition of treating Africa as a dirty, diseased place." *Washington Post*, Aug. 25.

Singh, Gurpeet, et al. 2016. "Ebola virus: An introduction and its pathology." *Reviews in Medical Virology* 26: 49–56.

Waldemir, Patti, and Lucy Hornby. 2014. "Africans in China feel the brunt of Ebola panic." *Financial Times*, Nov. 3. Accessed on April 12, 2016, from http://www.cnbc.com/2014/11/03/africans-in-china-feel-the-brunt-of-ebola-panic.html.

WHO. 2014. "Ebola virus disease in Guinea." Accessed February 15, 2016, from http://www.afro.who.int/en/clusters-a-programmes/dpc/epidemic-a-pandemic-alert-and-response/outbreak-news/4063-ebola-virus-disease-in-guinea.html.

WHO. 2016a. Ebola Situation Report, March 2, 2016. Accessed March 7, 2016, from http://apps.who.int/iris/bitstream/10665/204521/1/ebolasitrep_2Mar2016_eng.pdf?ua=1.

WHO. 2016b. Ebola Situation Report, March 31, 2016. Accessed April 2, 2016, from http://apps.who.int/iris/bitstream/10665/204714/1/ebolasitrep_30mar2016_eng.pdf?ua=1.

WHO. 2016c. "Statement on the 9th meeting of the IHR Emergency Committee regarding the Ebola outbreak in West Africa," March 29. Accessed April 2, 2016, from http://www.who.int/mediacentre/news/statements/2016/end-of-ebola-pheic/en/.

THE RESPONSE

1

Doctors Against Borders

Médecins Sans Frontières and Global Health Security

JOÃO NUNES

In 2016, the international context is much different from the one Doctors without Borders (Médecins Sans Frontiéres, henceforth MSF) encountered in 1971, the year of its creation. Security concerns are part of the day-to-day of politics, seeping into the design and justification of policies in many areas ranging from the environment and the Internet to the economy and health. Contrary to what is often assumed, the novelty of this context is not simply a matter of "new" threats having emerged. More fundamentally, we are witnessing a novel configuration of the place of security in contemporary political life. MSF is now operating in an environment that is prone to the securitization of issues hitherto kept outside the realm of security—that is, to their framing as existential threats demanding exceptional measures. This is happening not only explicitly through political discourse, but also in implicit ways within a deep-seated imaginary ruled by fear.

In this chapter, I suggest that this security- and fear-based environment presents a challenge for MSF. It exacerbates a tension that has shaped the trajectory of the organization since its inception: between, on the one hand, its self-professed role as a humanitarian action and emergency response organization and, on the other hand, its position as an advocate for global public health and health justice. This tension is at the heart of the uneasiness with which MSF engages with other health actors. Being at the frontline in the fight against health emergencies, MSF has become one of the most vocal critics of global health governance—but this position has arguably precluded more fruitful collaboration and learning. I argue that the 2014-15 Ebola virus disease outbreak in West Africa powerfully illustrates this quandary. The MSF response to this outbreak was conditioned by the challenges of the security environment and serves as an illustration of longstanding tensions in this organization's self-perceptions and relations with other global health actors.

At the same time, however, the security landscape offers an opportunity to move forward. I offer a reflection about the present and future role of MSF focused on its role as a global health security actor. Specifically, I suggest three ways in which MSF can tackle the aforementioned tension. First, it should embrace its security actorness without reservations, firmly embedding its emergency response role within a conception of health security that looks toward the alleviation of longstanding harm and systematic vulnerability. Second, MSF can move forward by acknowledging the broad transformative potentialities of health interventions. Finally, MSF should revisit its approach to borderlessness in a global health arena that is still strongly determined by multiple borders, pertaining not just to territorial divisions but also to inequalities of gender, race, class, and sexual orientation.

Security, Risk, and the Politics of Fear

As a pluralistic organization committed to reflecting in a critical way about its own activities, MSF has been involved in debates about humanitarianism, sovereignty, and the responsibility to protect—among other themes. Surprisingly, however, MSF has so far remained largely absent from discussions about security. It has overlooked a reflection about the ways in which security concerns impact upon its work, and also about its own contribution to promoting particular ideas and practices of security. This is an important omission given the importance that security has assumed in our political climate.

The present centrality of security can be traced back to the end of the Cold War, when space was opened for a consideration of "new" threats—"novel" forms of war, for example, but also threats to the environment, to the economy, and to health (Garrett 1995; Kaldor 1999; Kaplan 2002). It can be questioned to what extent these threats were new at all. Nonetheless, this awareness led scholars to reconsider the concept of security in order to include sectors other than the military and referents other than the state (Buzan and Hansen 2009, pp. 187–225). It became common to speak of environmental security, economic security, energy security, human security, and health security among others—even if the meanings often remained unclear. In the wake of the terrorist attacks of September 11, 2001, security became an unavoidable presence in public life, being regularly invoked in political discourse to justify the curbing of individual freedoms and rights. The October 2001 U.S. PATRIOT Act is a good example of this.

Parallel to the recognition of nonmilitary threats there was an emerging interest in the relationship between security and the political sphere. Politics began to be recognized as intrinsically connected to security. On the one hand, scholars argued that security was "intensely political" (Buzan 1991, p. 12) because our understanding of what it means depends upon ideological assumptions about what in our societies should be secured and how. At the same time, security is also political insofar as ideas and practices of security help to change political process, justifying or enabling certain policy responses (Krause and Williams, 1997). In other words, security can be considered a form of politics because it does things or allows things to be done at the political level.

The notion of securitization captures these political dimensions. According to securitization theory, a threat is a social construct—the felicitous result of a securitizing move through which an actor invokes an existential danger and calls for exceptional measures to deal with it (Buzan, Wæver, and de Wilde, 1998). At the heart of this theory is the recognition that "security" is not a description of reality but a tool for shaping reality. Security involves a transformation in the political procedure, namely the circumvention of normal processes of deliberation and the adoption of fast and unchecked measures. The notion of securitization helps to explain the current tendency to use security to make sense of events (for example, using a rhetoric of "national security" when talking about refugees) and the resulting ability to create or expand areas of exception where normal rules do not apply (Guantanamo, for instance). Even when there is no explicit invocation of "threat," a security rationality is often present in the surreptitious creation of a climate of suspicion and unease around certain issues or groups—such as migrants, for example (Huysmans and Buonfino 2008).

Another noteworthy element in the security environment is the tendency to perceive and deal with reality in terms of risk (Beck 1992). The standpoint of risk implies a different conception of the place of security in politics. The concern is not primarily with clear and present threats but with events (normally located in the future) that may become hazardous. Thinking in terms of risk means calculating uncertain possibilities and preempting probable dangers. As with securitization, it is not simply about identifying or responding to an empirical situation (that is, an identifiable threat) but rather about enabling a change in the political procedure. Risk has been recognized as a technique of government, a tool for "ordering our world through managing social problems and surveying populations" (Aradau and Van Munster 2007, p. 97). Scholars have since shown how security permeates political life not simply by way of exceptional measures, but also via the minute bureaucratic practices of security professionals that attempt to calculate the future and manage unease around certain issues (Bigo 2002).

Taken together, securitization and risk help us to understand how health issues are now being framed and tackled in the international arena. For example, since the 1990s there has been a strong association between HIV/AIDS and both national and international security (Fourie and Schönteich 2001; McInnes

2006). In 2000, the United Nations Security Council recognized in its resolution 1308 the impact of AIDS on peacekeeping operations and security in Africa. By highlighting the potential impact of disease incidence upon a country's military preparedness and social cohesion and upon international stability, this and other documents revealed the close connection between security and health policies. The tools of securitization theory have been applied to understand how diseases are now being framed as threats, and how security concerns have conditioned response to health issues (Elbe 2006; Curley and Herington 2011). In particular, securitization has been used to explain the tendency to approach epidemic outbreaks as existential threats, and to deploy a range of extraordinary measures (like curfews, travel restrictions, or sanitary cordons).

The idea of risk has also been mobilized in the analysis of health issues (Nettleton 1997; Elbe 2008; Wolff 2009). Significantly, global health norms—namely the International Health Regulations (2005)—now reflect the shift toward risk. A prime example of this is the legal status of the "public health emergency of international concern," recently declared by the World Health Organization (WHO) in the wake of the 2014 Ebola outbreak in West Africa and the 2015 Zika virus disease outbreak. For Lorna Weir and Eric Mykhalovskiy (2010, p. 126), this status signifies a "fundamental shift from surveillance of the certain to vigilance of public health risk" in the form of uncertain and unexpected events.

Instances of securitization and the concern with risks do not occur in a vacuum. They have been supported by a longstanding cultural context that makes them possible. This cultural context can be understood by drawing on the notion of the "imaginary." Charles Taylor has defined a social imaginary as incorporating

> the ways people imagine their social existence, how they fit together with others, how things go on between them and their fellows, the expectations that are normally met, and the deeper normative notions and images that underlie these expectations. (Taylor 2004, p. 23)

The imaginary consists of the ways in which people imagine their surroundings, often by use of images, stories, and myths. It comprises a shared set of meanings, expectations, and assumptions regarding what is natural, necessary, and legitimate in a society. These meanings help to define the boundaries of political imagination—that is, the conditions of possibility of thought and action in a given context.

In the context of health, the imaginary is one decisively influenced by fear. One of the reasons for this is the fact that throughout history perceptions of health problems have been intertwined with narratives of social crisis—from the plague in ancient Athens to the Black Death in 14th-century Europe, from

HIV/AIDS to H1N1. This is particularly true of infectious disease outbreaks but can also be observed in contemporary responses to issues such as obesity, autism, addiction, or attention-deficit disorder. As Philip Alcabes (2009) has argued, the fears that surround health issues do not just relate to their specific physical or clinical dimensions. Rather, disease functions as a catalyst of other fears in society—the fear of strangers, of technological development, of racial difference, and so on. The dread of disease is never just about a specific disease; it is also about the political fate of a society.

These are the terms in which it is possible to speak of a politics of fear in contemporary political practice—and, specifically, in global health practice. This security- and fear-based context is the background against which the work of MSF should be understood. MSF is not immune to the securitizing tendencies and the encroachment of risk in global health policymaking. The security environment presents critical challenges for MSF as it shapes itself in its unavoidable role as a security actor.

MSF and the West African Ebola Crisis

In many respects, the 2014-15 Ebola outbreak epitomizes the role of security and fear in global health. As Colin McInnes (2016, p. 387) has argued, the emergence of Ebola as a "crisis" was the result of a specific process of framing in which security played a key role; crucial to this was the embedding of the Ebola outbreak within a narrative that "emphasised the shared risk from infectious disease." McInnes (2016, p. 388) notes that this narrative comprised three key concerns: "that disease outbreaks risked state failure, posed a risk to regional and global security, and threatened to spread beyond the region concerned creating fears for the lives of citizens elsewhere." Fear played a key role in the emergence of Ebola as a crisis—and it also shaped the nature of this crisis.

The outbreak began in December 2013 in Guinea, with MSF teams being the first to react to what was then an unnamed "mysterious disease." After laboratory tests in Europe, the Guinean Ministry of Health officially declared the Ebola outbreak on March 21, 2014. Ten days later, MSF warned that this outbreak was "unprecedented" because of the geographic spread of the cases—an assessment that was then considered exaggerated and alarmist. On the same day, cases were confirmed in Liberia; meanwhile, newly discovered cases in Guinea were reported to come from Sierra Leone—the first case from this country was only confirmed in May. By the end of June, according to MSF (2015a), Ebola was "actively transmitting in more than 60 locations in Guinea, Liberia and Sierra Leone" and local healthcare workers were "dying by the dozens." It was only in August—after Western nationals had become infected—that WHO (2014) declared Ebola a "public health emergency of international concern." This was followed by an MSF appeal for a robust civilian and military intervention to help tackle the epidemic (MSF 2014a). The framing of Ebola drew from the politics of fear insofar as what "tipped the scale" in allowing for a resolute response was ultimately the specter of a catastrophic global pandemic—and not exactly the suffering of populations in West Africa. Ebola received attention not because West Africans were suffering from it, but because it supposedly presented a risk to the world and, specifically, to countries in the North.

Global health governance mechanisms—most explicitly visible in the International Health Regulations (2005) that enabled the declaration of a "public health emergency of international concern"—revealed their predominantly reactive nature. They responded to a problem already under way instead of working proactively to address the conditions that allow problems such as these to emerge. The world sought to "respond" to Ebola—when it should have responded to the deep-seated problems that gave rise to it. Framing Ebola as an emergency and a crisis happened to the detriment of seeing the outbreak from a broader perspective—that is, as the result of a series of events and conditions that stretch out into past choices and inactions. What of the social and economic conditions that have turned Ebola into an endemic problem in parts of the African continent? And the weak and inefficient health systems that have rendered some West African countries unable to survey the health status of their populations and respond in an adequate manner? And the low levels of trust between the populations and public authorities, which, as MSF recognized, considerably weakened the ability of health actors to influence individual behavior? Finally, what about the global context in which the outbreak emerged, and the structural inequalities therein? These questions were not given sufficient attention as global governance mechanisms were almost entirely directed toward containing the spread of the virus and managing the crisis—a short-termist and myopic agenda.

The reduction of Ebola to a discrete crisis event—and a risk potentially leading to a catastrophic scenario—was heightened by the underlying process of securitization visible in deployment of militaries. The securitized modality of response was also present in the imposition of curfews, sanitary cordons, and quarantines, as well as in the circumvention of traditional burial rites. Securitization and the crisis narrative interacted in fruitful ways. Whereas securitization relies upon the externalization of threat (disease is something foreign to the political body that must be contained and kept at bay), the crisis narrative is more strongly focused on internal elements. Narratives of internal decay, degeneracy, or vulnerability—and the anxiety they create—are an intrinsic element of the crisis narrative. In the case of Ebola, this took the form of an anxiety about the uncontrollable nature of existing social and economic processes.

The threat was not simply Ebola, but also the inherent vulnerabilities in the globalized world—particularly in its more developed regions—with complex networks in which humans, non-humans, goods, and information circulate at great speed. Both narratives were markedly solipsistic: while in the securitization frame the primary concern was the protection of the (Western) self vis-à-vis external others, in the crisis frame the emphasis was also laid on the inherent vulnerability of the self, which left it exposed to disruption. The regions, populations, and individuals that were most affected by the disease became merely the background in a narrative about the West and its travails. This narrative was visible in Western media representations of Ebola, which overwhelmingly presented it as "an issue around which public fears could be harnessed and mobilised as an avenue for domestic politics" (Abeysinghe 2016, p. 464).

When assessing the role of MSF in this context, it is important to recognize that MSF was the first responder and the most vocal voice for a resolute international intervention. It also played an essential role in the humanitarian response, contributing to the alleviation of the suffering of those most in need. The failures in this context cannot be directly attributed to MSF because they are connected with a misguided view of global health governance as an apolitical and technical endeavor, which results in the systematic neglect of health determinants, but also of more fundamental debates about inequality and justice—all of which are deeply political. Thus, if Ebola was certainly a problem of humanitarian response, it was also a problem pertaining to political, social, economic, and cultural structures. The misrecognition of Ebola meant that MSF was effectively working in an environment that was inhospitable to addressing the underlying issues that gave rise to the outbreak and that facilitated the uncontrolled spread of the disease. The constraints faced by MSF were, on the one hand, ideational: a mindset that privileged containment, crisis management, and the biomedically inspired faith in "magic bullets" in the form of pharmacological or technical fixes (such as vaccines, surveillance mechanisms, or information-sharing procedures). On the other hand, these constraints were very practical: they influenced agenda setting and issue prioritization, manifesting themselves in a lack of interest or support for sustained policies that would address the social and economic determinants of Ebola (Leach 2015). MSF's failed attempt to contain the militarization of the Ebola response by insisting that military assets and personnel not be used for quarantine, containment, or crowd-control measures—but only for their expertise in biowarfare—illustrates the inability of this organization to fully control the securitized environment in which much of this response took place (MSF 2015a, p. 14).

MSF certainly cannot be put at fault for focusing on humanitarian relief to vulnerable individuals—after all, the organization's resources were put under immense strain and it can hardly be blamed for devoting its full attention to saving lives, even if this meant neglecting broader aspects of the problem. Understandably, MSF had to focus on six key activities throughout the outbreak: isolation and care for patients; providing for safe burials; raising awareness with the objective of countering misinformation and fear; disease surveillance; and tracing contacts—and this while doing other non-Ebola activities that were nonetheless important in the context of the outbreak, such as anti-malaria work (MSF 2015b).

However, the Ebola epidemic presents important questions for MSF and its responsibilities in global health. The Ebola crisis illustrates, and has arguably exacerbated, a fundamental tension at the heart of MSF, its self-understandings, and its work. Since its inception, the way in which this organization sees itself and its work has been traversed by a tension between, on the one hand, an understanding of MSF as a humanitarian aid and emergency response actor and, on the other hand, a vision of MSF as an advocate for global health justice. As a plural organization, it is no surprise that the two visions are present—but, at the same time, it is now becoming clear that this tension is hindering the engagement of MSF with other global health actors.

MSF is, at its core, a humanitarian assistance organization, but its visibility and popularity have meant that it is also much more than that. In the 2014 International Activity Report, Joanne Liu and Jérôme Oberreit, International President and Secretary General of MSF respectively, felt the need to reaffirm the identity of MSF in light of the ongoing response to the Ebola outbreak. They argued that in spite of being vocal about the failings of the global Ebola response, MSF had humanitarian assistance as its primary concern. They wrote:

> MSF is a patient-focused organisation and our attention remains primarily on those in need of medical care and not on overhauling global systems. MSF concentrates on individuals and we are constantly striving to provide assistance to those who need it most. Our role is to save patients' lives, today, and we respond to crises with that at the forefront of our minds. (MSF 2014b)

This statement highlighted once again an uneasy relationship between "saving patients' lives today" and "overhauling global systems" that has been present throughout the history of MSF (Leebaw 2007; Givoni 2011a).

This tension has been recognized by Rony Brauman, president of MSF from 1982 to 1994. For Brauman, in its charter MSF affirmed its independence and its commitment to not interfere in the internal affairs of the countries where it conducts its work, thereby aligning itself with the tradition of a "silent humanitarian agency, wholly focused on medical aid" (Brauman 2012, p. 1526). Nonetheless, as Brauman notes, MSF gradually came to avail itself of "the 'right' to speak out publicly against repeated abuses of which its members are the sole witnesses" (Brauman 2012, p. 1528). This right emerged out of the need to prevent MSF from becoming a "medical enabler of oppression, whether it involves torture, forced population displacement, or famine." (Brauman 2012, 1528; see also Givoni 2011b). This right is being exercised at the time of writing this chapter, as MSF finds itself in the position of victim in the wake of a series of bombing attacks to its hospitals—including the October 2015 airstrike in Kunduz, Afghanistan, in which at least 42 people were killed, and more recently the April 2016 airstrike in Aleppo, Syria, which killed 14 patients and staff members.

While it seems uncontroversial how MSF is an emergency response actor, the question of exactly how far it should go in a more explicitly political role of global health advocacy has been the target of much debate. On the one hand, MSF has at times suggested a willingness to assume such a political role. This can be seen in its critical stance toward the failings and insufficiencies of other health actors. The Ebola crisis is a telling example of this. In its scathing report *Pushed to the Limit and Beyond*, MSF (2015a, p. 8) spoke about a "global coalition of inaction." For MSF, the Ebola outbreak shed light on the flaws of global health governance: the weakness of health systems, the lack of global leadership, and the "reticence of those in power to engage in the Ebola response" (MSF 2014b, p. 7). Its main target was the WHO. In addition to not recognizing early enough the severity of the outbreak and being unwilling to assume responsibility for a hands-on deployment, the WHO had other failings according to MSF. They argued that "decisions on setting priorities, attributing roles and responsibilities, ensuring accountability for the quality of activities, and mobilising the resources necessary were not taken on the necessary scale" (MSF 2015a, p. 9).

The other way in which MSF has assumed a political role of advocacy is through programs that seek to raise awareness of, and help to tackle, some underlying issues in global health. Examples are the Access Campaign, launched in 1999 by MSF with the objective of pushing for the development of and access to medicines, diagnostic tests, and vaccines. Another example is MSF's ongoing support for the Drugs for Neglected Diseases Initiative (DNDi). In these initiatives, MSF veers closer to the role of an advocacy group. It is also in this spirit that MSF has published reports on neglected tropical diseases, like the 2012 report *Fighting Neglect*.

While these critical positions and initiatives would seem to signal an attempt by MSF to cast itself as more overtly political, at the same time the organization has a track record of going in the opposite direction and seeking to reaffirm its "purely humanitarian" stance. For example, MSF members have taken extremely cautious positions in debates surrounding conflict, the protection of civilians, and international law. Discussing the doctrine of the responsibility to protect, for example, Brauman highlighted the "unintended, unintentional and unexpected consequences of wars" before arguing that "if we believe in the responsibility to protect we should also be prepared to wage an endless war" (MSF 2009). Discussing the notion of civilian protection in 2007, Marc DuBois, then Head of Humanitarian Affairs of MSF-Holland, decried the "delusion of grandeur" in the humanitarian community, arguing that the belief that humanitarian actors could protect civilians was "diminishing the luster of aid itself" and providing a "humanitarian fig-leaf" behind which governments could hide their failures (MSF 2007). A similar concern is present in recent statements by MSF in which it sought to distance itself from the "incorporation of humanitarian assistance into a broader development and resilience agenda"—this "fig-leaf of good intentions" being one of the reasons why MSF decided to pull out of the May 2016 World Humanitarian Summit (MSF 2016).

Cautious positions are certainly welcome, particularly given that the concepts criticized by MSF have often been instrumentalized to justify violence and to cast a shadow over responsibilities and inactions. MSF's cautious approach is presented as a radical critique of an assumed establishment—the "industries" of development, resilience, protection, and human rights, among others. Nonetheless, it paradoxically runs the risk of becoming an entrenched and conservative stance, as the organization displays either its unwillingness or inability to collaborate in long-term processes of political transformation. An illustration of this risk is the uneasy relationship of MSF with the International Criminal Court. In 2010, in a debate about international justice, Fabrice Weissman, then Research Director at MSF-France, argued that MSF should focus on its humanitarian task of containing the violence of war instead of advocating for a new "global moral order" (MSF 2010, p. 9). In response, his colleague Kate Mackintosh, then Head of Humanitarian Affairs with MSF-Holland, maintained that ideas of justice should be part of humanitarian action and that the work of MSF is intrinsically confrontational in the sense that it seeks to help "the vulnerable and the excluded, those who are not on the side of the powerful, or those in control of a particular territory" (MSF 2010, p. 10). This is revealing of a tension within the very ranks of MSF as to how far beyond the strict humanitarian remit the organization should go in order to fulfill its purpose—not only to respond to emergencies in the strictest sense, but also to contribute to a sustained improvement of the health of its patients.

This tension in MSF's self-understanding matters because it determines how this organization relates with other health actors. Here, MSF faces a predicament. Because of its important frontline role, MSF is well placed to deliver a powerful critique of global health governance mechanisms. It also has the moral legitimacy to do so, given that it faces and alleviates human suffering on a daily basis, often in extremely risky circumstances. Moreover, because of its popularity, MSF has the clout to highlight the failings of other actors. As was clear in relation to the Ebola outbreak, MSF has often expressed a disenchantment with other actors in the health and humanitarian sectors. In this respect, it is symptomatic that MSF's reflection about its "internal challenges" in the aftermath of the Ebola response was less a reflection about its own failings and more an explanation as to how it was prevented from doing better by the force of circumstances. Given the unprecedented challenge it was facing, its capacities were stretched to the limit and workers "were trying to do everything everywhere"— while others, as Joanne Liu remarked, were reluctant to "jump in and care for patients" and "do anything risky" (MSF 2015a, pp. 19, 14).

Thus, while MSF collaborates routinely with other actors in many different situations (including in the Ebola response, in which it partnered with research institutions, the WHO, ministries of health, and pharmaceutical companies to trial experimental treatments and vaccines), there are also times in which MSF seems to see itself as occupying a "higher ground," with its own desire for independence veering close to the temptation to "do it alone." In a news piece published in *Nature*, Liu acknowledged that in the Ebola response the organization could have done better communicating with others on the ground, namely local leaders and communities (Hayden 2015). This is, in fact, an issue that MSF had recognized as crucial in an earlier report (MSF 2014c). However, at the same time that MSF was inviting partners for an open discussion about the Ebola epidemic in Dakar, Senegal, Liu expressed doubts about the possibility of MSF having something to learn from others. She is quoted as saying, "We're going to get a lot of people who haven't treated a patient who are now the world experts, and who are going to give us lessons . . . We can only smile at this" (Hayden 2015, p. 19).

In sum, there is at the heart of MSF an important tension that the Ebola outbreak has brought once again to the fore. MSF sees itself as a humanitarian actor while criticizing the global emergency response system—to the point of pulling out of a high-profile humanitarian summit in protest against the supposed hijacking of the humanitarian effort by "development, peace-building and political agendas" (MSF 2016). At the same time, MSF signals toward a broader political role—thereby accepting that the success of humanitarian work hinges upon broader political struggles. This is done somewhat hesitantly, however: MSF sponsors health justice initiatives like the Access Campaign while reaffirming that discussions about international law and the International Health Regulations are of lesser importance than the "practical concern of how to get treatment to people who need it" (Hayden 2015, p. 19).

This tension would not be a problem in a pluralistic organization like MSF were it not for two adverse consequences. First, these conflicting identities lead to difficulties when engaging with other actors and present obstacles to learning—as MSF seeks to be simultaneously apolitical and a champion of health justice, detached from "murky politics" and at the same time heavily engaged in political debates pertaining to health justice and (in the wake of Kunduz and Aleppo) to the laws of war. Second, in the current security environment, which as mentioned has contributed to reproducing a myopic, crisis-management approach to health governance, MSF needs to consider whether its reluctance to assume an overtly political role is complicit with the short-termist approach that is now prevalent in the global agenda.

From Health Security to Political Transformation

The aftermath of the Ebola crisis presents an opportunity for MSF to re-envision its position and responsibilities within the global health landscape. The remainder of this chapter suggests ways in which MSF can begin to resolve the tension described above. The starting point should be a recognition that the two "identities"—that of an emergency responder and an advocate for health justice—can be combined in a newly defined role of health security actor.

Arguing that MSF should embrace its role as a health security actor is not the same as saying that it should join the securitization bandwagon. In fact, by neglecting a reflection about its own role as a security actor, MSF can unwittingly contribute to the securitization of health issues—MSF seemed to suspect this when it recognized that its call for a military intervention during the Ebola outbreak was "risky" (MSF 2015a, p. 14). Securitization is ultimately undesirable. While it may in some circumstances have immediate benefits—raising awareness, garnering resources, and breaking political deadlocks—if left unquestioned it can do long-term harm. This is because it helps to reproduce a political imaginary in which health issues are conceived as emerging crises requiring quick fixes (often through exceptional and undemocratic measures) instead of structural problems pertaining to inequalities, injustice, and inadequate health infrastructure. Moreover, privileging those issues that are successfully securitized runs the risk of reproducing the neglect of other important issues that have not been framed as security problems (Hansen 2000). By playing into the politics of fear currently shaping global health governance, securitization opens the door for the instrumentalization of emotions that has often resulted in exclusionary and repressive measures against groups like migrants or ethnic minorities, historically associated with health risks (Markel and Stern 2002).

The notion of health security suggested here focuses instead on individual experiences of insecurity. It assumes that achieving security entails opening up space for individuals to make decisions and act in matters pertaining to their own lives—an idea that is already close to MSF's commitments. Individuals who are more secure are generally more able to influence in a meaningful way the course of their lives—free from social constraints like physical aggression, political persecution, poverty, or ill health (Booth 2007; Nunes 2014). Health issues can be considered matters of security if they restrict in a decisive way the "space" necessary for individuals, families, and/or groups to live autonomously.

This approach to health security is underpinned by the identification of the multiple forms of harm and vulnerability that prevent individuals from freely deciding and acting. Harm is more than physical: it also encompasses indirect or insidious injuries that may be economic, social, or psychological, and not necessarily intended. In addition to the physical injury of disease an individual might suffer from the psychological harm of being stigmatized and segregated because of prevalent ideas and prejudices. The harm he or she suffers may be the result of a deliberate action (as in the release of a toxic agent) or inadvertent (the unintended transmission of a disease). Sometimes, this harm may be the result of negligence or omission on the part of those responsible for avoiding it (as in the case of industrial accidents stemming from unsafe conditions). Harm to health can also result from social relations that systematically place certain groups in harm's way so that others can benefit (for example, the case of miners exposed to fumes and radiation). Harm can also be indirect, as when damage is done to public health services, or when rules and paywalls condition access to healthcare (Linklater 2011).

Vulnerability refers in turn to a group's or an individual's susceptibility to harm (Goodin 1985). In its most basic sense—that is, as the possibility of being harmed—vulnerability is an intrinsic part of being human. Vulnerability becomes a matter of security when it assumes a systematic character—that is, when certain groups are structurally positioned so that they are more prone or likely to be harmed. In addition to being a condition of susceptibility, vulnerability also encompasses a relative lack of capacity to "bounce back" and overcome harm. This is because harm can reinforce vulnerability—for example, when individuals with long-term illnesses end up unemployed or even homeless as a result.

Admittedly, this is a broad understanding of health security that goes well beyond the remit of MSF. This organization cannot be expected to assume the functions of a health system, and it does not have the capacity to single-handedly tackle the determinants of health and disease in the places where it provides its assistance. Nonetheless, this conception of health security speaks to the core of the MSF mission. This was recognized by the Norwegian Nobel Committee when it awarded MSF the Nobel Peace Prize in 1999. The Committee argued that in addition to providing assistance in emergency situations MSF also seeks to draw attention to the causes of these emergencies. In fact, for the Committee this was the distinctive feature of MSF:

> more clearly than anyone else, they combine in their work the two criteria . . . humanitarian work and work for human rights. They achieve this by insisting on their right to arouse public opinion and to point to the causes of the man-made catastrophes, namely systematic breaches of the most fundamental rights. (Norwegian Nobel Committee 1999)

The Committee praised MSF for remaining "pervaded by idealism" and for its "willingness to take great risks." Presumably, these pertained not only to the concrete risks MSF workers faced in their day-to-day activity, but also the political risk of drawing attention to human rights violations and distress. In a nutshell, MSF was awarded the Nobel Peace Prize because, according to the Committee, it epitomized the idea that "to alleviate distress one must also get to its roots" (Norwegian Nobel Committee 1999).

The notion of health security advanced in this chapter dovetails with this idea. Embracing health security actorness for MSF means conceiving humanitarian work and emergency response efforts as components of a broader proactive strategy that includes systematic and long-term efforts "upstream" (in the identification of existing vulnerabilities and forms of harm) and "downstream" (working to reduce vulnerability and develop local capacity to "bounce back" from harm). In concrete terms, this means working to address the multiple political, social, economic, cultural, and infrastructural determinants of health. It also means identifying, and seeking to tackle, the broader political structures and relations at the global level that systematically place certain groups in harm's way, or in positions of vulnerability. This is because health security is also about global relations of inequality and injustice. These go a long way in determining who is vulnerable to or harmed by disease, how systematically, and what opportunities and resources there are with which to deal with the occurrence of disease.

Part of the work of MSF already contributes to raising awareness of, and ultimately tackling, these global structures and relations. But there is still scope for MSF to have a more decisive influence. The health work of MSF should be more explicitly linked with broader political transformation, in light of the recognition that the struggle over the right to health is always about broader political struggles pertaining to the recognition of rights to citizenship, dignity, equality, and justice (Hayden 2012). In this context, MSF has much to gain from furthering its connections with health social movements and patient and caregiver organizations that recognize the deeply political character of health struggles.

Seeing health as a stepping stone to broader political transformation is not new. MSF, a Nobel Peace Prize laureate, could take inspiration from the "Health as a Bridge for Peace" (HBP) agenda. In the 1980s, the Pan-American Health Organization (PAHO) sought to bring together nations and factions in conflict to plan and implement joint health activities. The underlying rationale was that health constituted a superordinate goal—that is, one that transcends political and ethnic divisions—and that cooperation in the field of health could in turn promote solidarity and further dialogue. Bringing together governments, international institutions, and civil society actors, PAHO brokered the implementation of several health initiatives, most notably a series of humanitarian ceasefires for immunization purposes ("Days of Tranquility") between 1985 and 1991 in El Salvador. Ceasefires for immunization campaigns and other humanitarian reasons have since been successfully implemented in other countries.

The capacity of health initiatives to bring about political transformation in the form of lasting peace has been the subject of debate, with some authors arguing that health measures cannot replace broader political processes and that health intervention should be kept within its "technical" medical remit (Beigbeder 1998; Garber 2002). Nonetheless, there are reasons to be optimistic about the peace-building impact of health initiatives. For example, there have been several instances of public health cooperation in the Middle East (Skinner and Sriharan 2007; Horton 2009). While so far these initiatives have not succeeded in ending the conflict, it would be reductionist to claim that their peace-building role is a complete failure. Analyzing the Middle East Consortium on Infectious Disease Surveillance (MECIDS), William J. Long (2011) found some reasons to be optimistic. In his view, MECIDS succeeded in establishing a real-time communication network for emergency response; this has allowed the consortium to become a channel for quick communication across the region. Long has not been able to identify significant functional spillover into other policy areas. He argues, however, that optimism is justified because this is an unlikely case of international cooperation. The question for him is not so much why cooperation has not spread to other areas, but rather how cooperation happened in the first place—in a highly sensitive issue area, in conditions of extreme resource scarcity, and despite historical and present tensions. By providing the opportunity for successful instances of cooperation in unfavorable environments, health holds the potential to have a positive impact in situations of enmity and tension. While this may not be peace, it constitutes change and thus demonstrates the transformative potential of health.

According to the HBP idea, in situations of conflict medical interventions can become privileged avenues for peace-building. Graeme MacQueen and Joanna Santa Barbara have identified five main mechanisms through which health may contribute to peace. The first is conflict management: conflicts can be "resolved, lessened or contained through the use of 'medical diplomacy' or health-oriented superordinate goals" (MacQueen and Santa Barbara 2000, p. 294). Second, health may contribute to peace because of the solidarity of health workers to people and groups that are themselves involved in peace-building. Next, the delivery of healthcare can contribute to transcending social differences, thus rebuilding or strengthening the social fabric. The fourth way in which health can contribute to peace is by dissent—that is, by encouraging views that depart from the prevailing ones. Health knowledge and provision can provide the expertise or legitimacy with which people express their disagreement or seek to redefine a situation. As MacQueen and Santa Barbara (2000, p. 295) put it,

> [b]y redefining the situation, parties attempt to gain control over issues that have been defined by those with formal political power as "none of their business" or "outside their field of expertise". Healthcare workers have at times been successful in redefining war as a public health prob-lem rather than a strictly political problem, thereby creating a space for the exercise of their knowledge and opinion.

For these two authors, the final contribution of health to peace is the possibil-ity of reducing the destructiveness of war: here, the expertise and legitimacy of health workers can contribute to the restriction or abolition of policies or weapons that are particularly destructive.

Another way in which the peace-building efforts of health workers have been analyzed is by distinguishing different levels: (1) primary prevention, or "direct action to identify and combat the root causes of violence"; (2) second-ary prevention—that is, to "directly curb violence and address any consequent health effects on the affected population"; and (3) tertiary intervention, which "seeks longer-term rehabilitation for individuals and societies suffering from exposure to violent warfare" (D'Errico, Wake, and Wake, 2010).

It should be recognized that health can only have a transformative political effect when conjoined with other political initiatives. Simon Rushton (2005, pp. 451–52) notes that health initiatives need to be seen as "part of a broader agenda encompassing democracy, good governance, the availability of the nec-essary financial resources . . . and the infrastructure to deliver improvements in services on the ground." The potential that health interventions hold for long-term change thus resides in their ability to strengthen the social contract and to interact with other developments in the social and economic sphere. Along the same lines, Natalie J. Grove and Anthony B. Zwi (2008) have argued that in order to have a sustained peace-building effect health initiatives should not be perceived simply as technical projects. For these authors, it is important to go beyond an exclusive focus on infrastructure, human resources, or equipment and recognize that health can work in less tangible ways by helping to promote social cohesion, social justice, and good governance.

HBP can serve as a powerful inspiration of how health work can be geared toward political change even in non-conflict settings. Once we go beyond the strict definition of peace as absence of military conflict and conceive it more broadly as the alleviation of multiple forms of vulnerability and harm—that is, effectively, as security—one can begin to see how health interventions can also be a bridge to security. The example of HBP suggests that there is scope for MSF to adopt a more explicit political role. It also shows that the MSF workers are in a privileged position to contribute to political transformation. This is because the transformative potential of health workers does not reside simply on what they can do, but also on what they know and who they are. Neil Arya (2004, p. 247) has argued that health workers have the capacity to act for peace because they are "generally perceived to possess character traits such as altruism, impartiality, trustworthiness, intelligence and analytic skills." In addition to this, they have expert knowledge that is widely considered to transcend political and social divisions.

By relying on their unique combination of character, knowledge, and activity, MSF workers can assume a political role that seeks not merely the immediate alleviation of suffering but also the redressing of longstanding vulnerabilities. This in no way questions the crucial humanitarian work focused on containing outbreaks or responding to crises. However, there needs to be a more explicit recognition that any work of a humanitarian kind is intrinsically political insofar as it relies upon an assumption of how the political order should be organized so as to avoid the reproduction of environments where humanitarian crises emerge. It is in this context that MSF has an opportunity to emphasize and reinvigorate its position. Collaborating more intensely with other actors, it can articulate more systematically its humanitarian work with proactive and sustained efforts toward advancing an agenda of health promotion and crisis prevention.

Conclusion: Doctors Against Borders

A politics of fear now pervades the global health agenda. This politics manifests itself in the tendency to securitize health issues—framing them as existential threats demanding exceptional measures—or to perceive them as uncertain risks needing to be contained. The politics of fear has led to a short-termist agenda focused on crisis management and disease containment.

The politics of fear can be countered with a politics of solidarity based on a global responsibility toward the health of others—that is, toward the alleviation of harm and vulnerability. Alleviating harm and vulnerability amounts to advancing a health security agenda that is focused on the promotion of individual autonomy—the capacity of individuals and groups to make decisions and act in matters pertaining to their own lives. Ultimately, such an understanding of health security calls for broader political change—the transformation of the conditions that enable health problems to emerge and perpetuate themselves.

This politics of solidarity is aligned with the ethical commitments of MSF. This chapter argued that overcoming the tension between humanitarian work and political intervention via the notion of health security can be the first step for MSF to fully embrace this agenda. Nonetheless, the politics of solidarity should continue to be navigated in a careful and self-reflective manner. This is because MSF also has as one of its mainstays the notion of borderlessness (DeChaine 2002). If left unexamined, this idea runs the risk of being detrimental to solidarity. As Brauman notes, for MSF the idea of borderlessness was from the outset connected with "the 'right' that humanitarian doctors gave themselves to cross borders clandestinely in order to reach certain war zones to which access was prohibited" (Brauman 2012, p. 1526). More recently, the idea of borderlessness has become popular in global health in connection with the idea that "diseases know no borders" or that we are all "united by contagion" (Zacher and Keefe 2008). Both of these conceptions have important limitations. According to the former, borderlessness refers mainly to the activity of doctors, who have the right to disregard borders when responding to emergencies. The latter makes an assumption of unity in global health that is highly problematic. Both suffer from elitism, overlooking the persistence of the multiple inequalities and exclusionary practices that shape global health. On the one hand, not everyone has the capacity to cross (territorial) borders at will. On the other, the experience of health and disease is everything but homogeneous. Rather, it is traversed by the systematic production of vulnerabilities—"borders" that go well beyond territorial ones.

Unquestioned claims of unity have been at the heart of appeals to solidarity. As Didier Fassin (2012, p. 183) has noted, humanitarianism has been built upon the mobilization of emotions and "the production of an illusory equality of conditions" in the aftermath of disasters. Grounding solidarity upon such illusory equality serves to reinforce the tragic (in the sense of unavoidable) nature of events like the Ebola outbreak. Assuming that we are all equally exposed to disease in a "globalized world" erases agency from the picture, eliding the fact that outbreaks are not simply natural but also political disasters—the result of actions and inactions that affect people differently according to their socioeconomic status. Indeed, as Fassin (2012, p. 182) recognizes, however well intentioned they may be, these calls to unity have a fleeting effect, as "the reality of inequality and conflict quickly reasserts itself."

A more activist conception of borderlessness is required, one that recognizes the persistence of borders pertaining not simply to geography but also to the reinscription of harm and vulnerability based on differences of gender, race, class, or sexual orientation. The politics of solidarity should not start from the supposed fact of borderlessness and unity. Rather, solidarity will be all the more powerful if it unpacks and questions the very idea of borderlessness. More than an emotional appeal that arises from a situation of supposed convergence or unity, solidarity should be seen as a "political relation that shapes different ways of challenging oppression and inequalities" (Featherstone 2012, p. 8). It is a "world-making process" that enables the invention of "new ways of relating and being in the world" (Featherstone 2012, pp. 245, 254).

MSF is in a privileged position to spearhead such a politics of solidarity, but it needs to revisit its conception of borders. This chapter has suggested some ways in which it can continue its self-reflection along these lines. Borders are everywhere for the majority of the world's population, and particularly for the poorest and most vulnerable. They have an impact upon vulnerability to disease and injury, and upon the ability to deal with harm when it occurs. Borders still separate, exclude, disable, wound, and kill. MSF has the responsibility to help bring down the walls of global health.

Acknowledgments

The author would like to thank Sokhieng Au and Michiel Hofman for their useful comments on an earlier version of this chapter.

References

Abeysinghe, Sudeepa. 2016. "Ebola at the borders: Newspaper representations and the politics of border control." *Third World Quarterly* 37: 452–67.

Alcabes, Philip. 2009. *Dread: How fear and fantasy have fueled epidemics from the black death to avian flu.* New York: Public Affairs.

Aradau, Claudia, and Rens Van Munster. 2007. "Governing terrorism through risk: Taking precautions, (un)knowing the future." *European Journal of International Relations* 13: 89–115.

Arya, Neil. 2004. "Peace through health I: Development and use of a working model." *Medicine, Conflict and Survival* 20: 242–57.

Beck, Ulrich. 1992. *Risk society: Towards a new modernity.* London: SAGE.

Beigbeder, Yves. 1998. "The World Health Organization and peacekeeping." *International Peacekeeping* 5: 31–48.

Bigo, Didier. 2002. "Security and immigration: Towards a critique of the governmentality of unease." *Alternatives* 27: 63–92.

Booth, Ken. 2007. *Theory of world security.* Cambridge, UK: Cambridge University Press.

Brauman, Rony. 2012. "Médecins Sans Frontières and the ICRC: Matters of principle." *International Review of the Red Cross* 94: 1523–35.

Buzan Barry. 1991. *People, states and fear: An agenda for international security studies in the post-Cold War era.* Boulder, CO, and London: Lynne Rienner Publishers.

Buzan, Barry, and Lene Hansen. 2009. *The evolution of international security studies.* Cambridge, UK: Cambridge University Press.

Buzan, Barry, Ole Wæver, and Jaap de Wilde. 1998. *Security: A new framework for analysis.* Boulder, CO, and London: Lynne Rienner Publishers.

Curley, Melissa G., and Jonathan Herington. 2011. "The securitisation of avian influenza: International discourses and domestic politics in Asia." *Review of International Studies* 37: 141–66.

D'Errico, Nichole C., Christopher M. Wake, and Rachel M. Wake. 2010. "Healing Africa? Reflections on the peace-building role of a health-based nongovernmental organization operating in Eastern Democratic Republic of Congo." *Medicine, Conflict and Survival* 26: 145–59.

DeChaine, D. Robert. 2002. "Humanitarian space and the social imaginary: Médecins Sans Frontières/Doctors Without Borders and the rhetoric of global community." *Journal of Communication Inquiry* 26: 354–69.

Elbe, Stefan. 2006. "Should HIV/AIDS be securitized? The ethical dilemmas of linking HIV/AIDS and security." *International Studies Quarterly* 50: 119–44.

Elbe, Stefan. 2008. "Risking lives: AIDS, security and three concepts of risk." *Security Dialogue* 39: 177–98.

Fassin, Didier. 2012. *Humanitarian reason: A moral history of the present.* Berkeley: University of California Press.

Featherstone, David. 2012. *Solidarity: Hidden histories and geographies of internationalism.* London: Zed Books.

Fourie, Pieter, and Martin Schönteich. 2001. "Africa's new security threat: HIV/AIDS and human security in Southern Africa." *African Security Review* 10: 29–42.

Garber, Randi. 2002. "Health as a bridge for peace: Theory, practice and prognosis—Reflections of a practitioner." *Journal of Peacebuilding and Development* 1: 69–84.

Garrett, Laurie. 1995. *The coming plague: Newly emerging diseases in a world out of balance.* London: Penguin Books.

Givoni, Michal. 2011a. "Beyond the humanitarian/political divide: Witnessing and the making of humanitarian ethics." *Journal of Human Rights* 10: 55–75.

Givoni, Michal. 2011b. "Humanitarian governance and ethical cultivation: Médecins sans Frontières and the advent of the expert witness." *Millennium: Journal of International Studies* 40: 43–63.

Goodin, Robert E. 1985. *Protecting the vulnerable: A reanalysis of our social responsibilities.* Chicago and London: University of Chicago Press.

Grove, Nathalie J., and Anthony B. Zwi. 2008. "Beyond the log frame: A new tool for examining health and peacebuilding initiatives." *Development in Practice* 18: 66–81.

Hansen, Lene. 2000. "The Little Mermaid's silent security dilemma and the absence of gender in the Copenhagen School." *Millennium: Journal of International Studies* 29: 285–306.

Hayden, Erika C. 2015. "MSF takes bigger global-health role." *Nature* 522: 18–19.

Hayden, Patrick. 2012. "The human right to health and the struggle for recognition." *Review of International Studies* 38: 569–88.

Horton, Richard. 2009. "The occupied Palestinian territory: Peace, justice, and health." *The Lancet* 373: 784–88.

Huysmans, Jef, and Alessandra Buonfino. 2008. "Politics of exception and unease: Immigration, asylum and terrorism in parliamentary debates in the U.K." *Political Studies* 56: 766–88.

Kaldor, Mary. 1999. *New and old wars: Organized violence in a global era.* Stanford, CA: Stanford University Press.

Kaplan, Robert D. 2002. *The coming anarchy: Shattering the dreams of the Post-Cold War.* New York: Vintage.

Krause, Keith, and Michael C. Williams. 1997. "From strategy to security: Foundations of critical security studies," in *Critical security studies: Concepts and cases,* edited by Keith Krause and Michael C. Williams. London: UCL Press.

Leach, Melissa. 2015. "The Ebola crisis and post-2015 development." *Journal of International Development* 27: 816–34.

Leebaw, Bronwyn. 2007. "The politics of impartial activism: Humanitarianism and human rights." *Perspectives on Politics* 5: 223–39.

Linklater, Andrew. 2011. *The problem of harm in world politics: Theoretical investigations.* Cambridge, UK: Cambridge University Press.

Long, William J. 2011. *Pandemics and peace: Public health cooperation in zones of conflict.* Washington, DC: United States Institute of Peace.

MacQueen, Graeme, and Joanna Santa Barbara. 2000. "Peace building through health initiatives." *British Medical Journal* 321: 293–96.

Markel, Howard, and Alexandra M. Stern. 2002. "The foreignness of germs: The persistent association of immigrants and disease in American society." *The Milbank Quarterly* 80: 757–88.

McInnes, Colin. 2006. "HIV/AIDS and security." *International Affairs* 82: 315–26.

McInnes, Colin. 2016. "Crisis! What crisis? Global health and the 2014-15 West African Ebola outbreak." *Third World Quarterly* 37: 380–400.

Médecins Sans Frontières. 2007. *Dialogue 4: Protection,* accessed May 6, 2016. http://www.msf.org.uk/sites/uk/files/Protection_printable_version_200902034541.pdf

Médecins Sans Frontières. 2009. *Dialogue 8: Responsibility to Protect,* accessed May 6, 2016. http://www.msf.org.uk/sites/uk/files/MSF_Dialogue_No8___R2P_200904012144.pdf

Médecins Sans Frontières. 2010. *International justice—pragmatism or principle?,* accessed May 6, 2016. http://www.msf.org.uk/sites/uk/files/MSF_Dialogue_No9___International_Justice_201007270041.pdf.

Médecins Sans Frontières. 2012. *Fighting neglect: Finding ways to manage and control visceral leishmaniasis, human African trypanosomiasis and Chagas disease,* accessed May 11, 2016. http://www.msf.org.uk/sites/uk/files/Fighting_Neglect_May2012_201206081400.pdf.

Médecins Sans Frontières. 2014a. *MSF International President: United Nations special briefing on Ebola,* accessed May 6, 2016. http://www.msf.org.uk/node/26146.

Médecins Sans Frontières. 2014b. *International activity report 2014,* accessed May 10, 2016. http://cdn.msf.org/sites/msf.org/files/msf_international_activity_report_2014_en.pdf.

Médecins Sans Frontières. 2014c. *It's not just about drinking tea: Dialogue between MSF, its patients and their communities,* accessed May 11, 2016. http://www.msf.org.uk/sites/uk/files/a5_not_just_tea_corrected_may_6_2014_msf.pdf.

Médecins Sans Frontières. 2015a. *Pushed to the limit and beyond: A year into the largest ever Ebola outbreak,* accessed May 6, 2016. http://www.msf.org.uk/sites/uk/files/ebola_-_pushed_to_the_limit_and_beyond.pdf

Médecins Sans Frontières. 2015b. *An unprecedented year: Médecins Sans Frontières' response to the largest ever Ebola outbreak,* accessed May 10, 2016. http://www.msf.org/sites/msf.org/files/ebola_accountability_report_final_july_low_res.pdf.

Médecins Sans Frontières. 2016. "MSF to pull out of World Humanitarian Summit," accessed May 10, 2016. http://www.msf.org.uk/article/msf-to-pull-out-of-world-humanitarian-summit.

Nettleton, Sarah. 1997. "Governing the risky self: How to become healthy, wealthy and wise," in *Foucault, health and medicine,* edited by Alan Petersen and Robin Bunton. London and New York: Routledge.

Norwegian Nobel Committee. 1999. *The Nobel Peace Prize 1999—Award ceremony speech,* accessed May 12, 2016. http://www.nobelprize.org/nobel_prizes/peace/laureates/1999/presentation-speech.html.

Nunes, João. 2014. "Questioning health security: Insecurity and domination in world politics." *Review of International Studies* 40: 939–60.

Rushton, Simon. 2005. "Health and peacebuilding: Resuscitating the failed state in Sierra Leone." *International Relations* 19: 441–56.

Skinner, Harvey A., and Abi Sriharan. 2007. "Building cooperation through health initiatives: An Arab and Israeli case study." *Conflict and Health* 1: 1–9.

Taylor, Charles. 2004. *Modern Social Imaginaries.* Durham, NC: Duke University Press.

Weir, Lorna, and Eric Mykhalovskiy. 2010. *Global public health vigilance: Creating a world on alert.* Abingdon, UK: Routledge.

Wolff, Jonathan. 2009. "Disadvantage, risk and the social determinants of health." *Public Health Ethics* 2: 214–23.

World Health Organization. 2014. *Statement on the 1st meeting of the IHR Emergency Committee on the 2014 Ebola outbreak in West Africa,* accessed May 6, 2016. http://www.who.int/media-centre/news/statements/2014/ebola-20140808/en/.

Zacher, Mark W., and Tania J. Keefe. 2008. *The politics of global health governance: United by contagion.* Houndmills, UK: Palgrave Macmillan.

2

Whose Security?

Militarization and Securitization During West Africa's Ebola Outbreak

ADIA BENTON

In September 2014, more than six months into what would become the largest Ebola outbreak on record, Médecins Sans Frontières (MSF) urged governments of rich nations to send military medical and biohazard personnel and assets to respond to the Ebola crisis (Hussain 2014; Médecins Sans Frontières [MSF] International 2014). The recommendation by MSF was controversial, given the organization's typically cautious approach to military involvement in humanitarian emergency response. It also posed a conundrum, in that it clearly outlined the terms for military involvement to exclude quarantine, crowd control, and containment and to include clinical care and improved logistics for the diagnosis and management of patients. MSF's strict guidelines for military involvement implied that it was possible to deliver military medicine without military might. Indeed, as I have written elsewhere, by the time MSF had issued its call for military assistance, the question was not whether the military would or should be involved in responding to the Ebola crisis, but which model of intervention—one of benevolent, efficiently deployed assistance or one of containment, isolation, and force—would prevail (Benton 2014a). Neither model alone is sufficient to describe what happened during the two-year outbreak.

As the crisis escalated in mid-2014, the presidents of the countries most affected by the West African outbreak, Guinea, Liberia, and Sierra Leone, had already mobilized their security forces to contribute to Ebola control efforts. Military and police action in all three countries included maintaining checkpoints, patrolling country and locality borders, enforcing village-level and district-wide quarantines, and taking punitive measures against individuals found in violation of government mandates for burials, case reporting, and caregiving (Gbandia 2014; Harmon 2014; Human Rights Watch 2014; McNeil Jr. 2014). These efforts provoked a range of responses by the communities hardest hit by the disease—from acceptance or reluctant acquiescence to outright resistance. Domestic security forces performed much-needed public health functions, but they were also implicated in egregious abuses of power that only intensified mistrust of state actors and policies related to Ebola prevention and treatment.[1] International troops, in contrast, took on a low-risk approach to Ebola by focusing their efforts on construction, logistics and protection of their citizens (DuBois et al. 2015, p. 38).

This essay is an attempt to contextualize community and regional concerns about the use of security forces during a peacetime public health emergency, while addressing the question of whether military might and military medicine—military logics and military logistical apparatus—can ever be productively uncoupled. It is an urgent and important question as security paradigms regain prominence for preventing and responding to future outbreaks, and as we take stock of actual security measures put in place to support the Ebola response (Heymann et al. 2015; Kickbusch et al. 2015). In this essay, I address this question by focusing on *whose security* mattered during this outbreak, and security *from what*. Differing perspectives on this issue, I argue, shaped Ebola control interventions and their reception.

My analytic approach is anthropological, in that it centers on social and cultural forms of humanitarian response. It also highlights various communities' responses to military interventions and securitized approaches to health.[2] Thus, the essay is based upon knowledge developed from intensive, continued engagement and study in the region in 2003 to 2007, training in outbreak investigations and complex humanitarian emergencies, and triangulation of textual and visual data collected from a range of sources: the MSF archives, government testimony and communications, local and international news print and multimedia sources, social media, scholarly and gray literature, and informal conversations with frontline responders who were health workers, social scientists, and epidemiologists in the three countries.

The argument unfolds along two paths. First, I describe the deep ambivalence about military intervention in humanitarian crises among aid agencies and affected communities, and of the broader use of security paradigms for addressing public health crises. I argue that pro-military and pro-security stances attempt to shore up uncertainty and ambivalence by de-emphasizing militarization, securitization, and attendant problems with these frameworks. I also provide an account of how public health and humanitarian assistance are "always already" securitized, despite attempts to balance concerns about health and aid worker security with care and empathy for communities under duress.

In part, the difficulty of decoupling security and aid is related the "defensiveness" embedded in the aid landscape and everyday aid practices.

Second, during this outbreak, the postconflict security apparatus has operated in ways that mirror and perpetuate existing inequalities. Too often—and this was certainly the case with Ebola—the domestic military and police are mobilized against certain segments of the population in defense of elites and special interests, while foreign militaries were perceived to operate benevolently (but still in the interests of foreign elites). To understand and draw conclusions about the perceived differences between domestic and foreign military intervention during the West African Ebola outbreak, I suggest that it may be productive to recast the tension between security and empathy in terms of another dualism: (1) a politics of flight and rescue and (2) the logics of coercion and criminalization.

In a politics of flight and rescue, the commitment to care for Ebola-affected communities is often at odds with the safety and security of international aid workers and local health authorities. Foreign militaries were most closely associated with a politics of flight and rescue. In this epidemic, a politics of flight was expressed in terms of who is eligible to be shuttled away for care through institutional and citizenship-based evacuation procedures and policies (Ivers 2012). The military's capacity to rescue sick foreigners and evacuate them but *not* to be capable of extending even the most basic forms of care in country to country nationals is crucial for a politics of flight. It is therefore important to ask whether the rescue logics of natural disasters, for which the military appear to be fairly well equipped, can be applied to epidemics like Ebola, where the duty to provide care and treatment is more important than evacuation plans, armed protection for personnel and property, and immediate disaster relief.[3]

The logics of coercion and criminalization of "recalcitrant" or "rebellious" populations were strongly associated with the efforts of domestic militaries, with some buy-in and support from foreign forces. Unlike foreign militaries' responsibility to provide logistical support to health authorities and protect and rescue foreign nationals, domestic militaries were deployed for discipline and coercion—to ensure compliance with public health measures and government dictates (whether those dictates are supported by sound public health science or not). Coercion and criminalization were default logics for this group because it is what they are trained to do, and professionalization within the military's ranks has been focused on these dimensions in the three countries—even if measures to deescalate tensions or withhold force were unsuccessful. Thus, soldiers' capacity to aid in humanitarian missions was also uneven. Some domestic military personnel have clinical and laboratory training, but few were prepared to rapidly build out infrastructure to assist with diagnostics, care, and treatment (Woods 2015).[4]

"The Military Is All We've Got": Critiques of Military and Security Paradigms

The Ebola crisis was framed not only as a humanitarian crisis and a public health emergency, but also as a threat to regional stability and security (UN Security Council 2014). This framing, along with MSF's call for military biohazard assets, profoundly shaped international intervention in the final months of 2014 and early 2015. In response to MSF's call for medical reinforcements, U.S. President Barack Obama announced his plan to deploy 3,000 troops to combat Ebola in Liberia, giving rise to a range of critiques. Some of the more compelling critiques were presented in visual form. Brazilian political cartoonist Latuff, for example, penned a cartoon captioned "Obama to send 3,000 troops to fight Ebola in Liberia . . ." In the cartoon, Liberia is a man sick in bed with Ebola. U.S. soldiers in combat gear, guns raised, kick open his bedroom door as they shout, "Humanitarian aid!" (Fig. 2-1).

James David (JD), a young Monrovia-based artist, reimagined Latuff's cartoon. In JD's version, bedridden Liberia and American soldiers remain as key figures but the U.S. "invasion" is not central; rather, it is nested between stacks

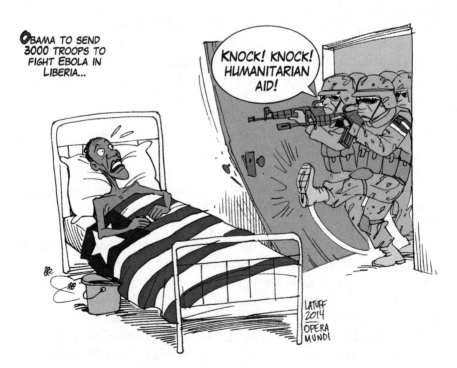

Figure 2-1 "Knock! Knock! Humanitarian aid!" Reprinted with permission of Latuff.

of U.S. dollars and the words, "my contributions," in a thought bubble above the head of President Obama.

A third cartoon, by American cartoonist Ted Rall, extends these critiques (Fig. 2-2). In the drawing's foreground, an American soldier wears a cargo vest whose pockets are filled with hand grenades. The soldier points his gun at a clinician wearing scrubs, who remarks, "We were kind of hoping for doctors." The soldier replies, "We're the United States. The military is all we've got!" In the background, which features a few makeshift buildings and a military helicopter, a soldier shoots a rocket launcher and exclaims "Ebola!" Another soldier comments, "Send in the drones . . . just because."

Like many critics of military intervention in humanitarian and health emergencies, Latuff, JD, and Rall questioned whether the military should play a prominent role in responding to crises like Ebola. The artists differ in how they depict motivations and justifications for military interventions, however. For JD, the U.S. motivation for sending troops to Liberia is "self"-centered and rooted in anxieties about national security and aid transactions. Critics like Latuff and Rall suggest that for the United States, Ebola operates not only as a viral disease harbored in bodies but also as a hostile, occupying actor to invade, dominate, and conquer. Ebola is weaponized.

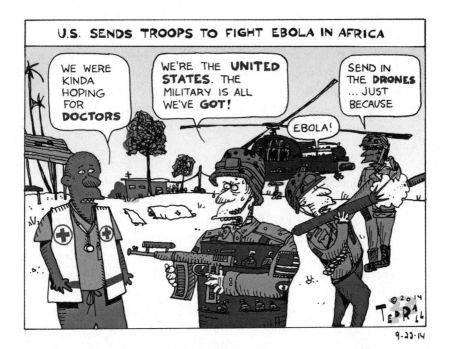

Figure 2-2 "We were kinda hoping for doctors." Reprinted with permission of Ted Rall.

The tendency to use the military to contain Ebola reflects the extensive investment in defense when compared to other forms of humanitarian aid delivery mechanisms (McGovern 2014). JD centers and places Obama and his cash contributions in the same frame with military assistance, explicitly linking deployments of foreign troops to Liberia, Sierra Leone, and Guinea to colonial ties of patronage and trusteeship. All three cartoons implicitly acknowledge that too few efficient and effective mechanisms exist to deliver medical assistance during an epidemic of this scale and scope. The cartoons depict the ambivalence characterizing militarized approaches to the Ebola outbreak. Foreign troops in humanitarian situations operate in a zone of indistinction between care and security, assistance and coercion.[5] Domestic troops, rendered invisible in these cartoons, operate in similar kinds of zones of indistinction but must also contend with their rootedness in local and national political conflicts.

Military Norms, Military Values: Critiques of Militarization

Foreign military responses were generally rolled out along national lines, linked to historical legacies of colonialism and current economic arrangements, as JD noted in his cartoon. These were varied, depending on the military capacity to assist in outbreaks and the expressed motivations and objectives of the national governments providing military personnel. Collaboration among international security forces was, in large part, coordinated under national government agencies organized to address the Ebola epidemics. Countries sending military personnel included China, the United Kingdom, the United States, Canada, Germany, and France. The African Union also sent military personnel with outbreak experience. Of the countries sending military assistance, China was exceptional in providing mostly medical personnel from the People's Liberation Army, providing an opportunity for China to flex its humanitarian "muscle."[6]

Critics of militarization are not simply decrying the use of military assets to address humanitarian crises; they are also pointing to how values and norms of militarization pervade humanitarian missions. "Belief in hierarchy, obedience, and the use of force," as Cynthia Enloe reminds us, are chief among these norms and values. Militarized perspectives presume that these beliefs associated with militarization work for a range of problems, and that these solutions are uniquely suited to the problems to which they are applied. Militarization is also a process that "involves an intensification of the labor and resources allocated to military purposes, including the shaping of other institutions in synchrony with military goals" (Lutz 2002, p. 723).

For anthropologist Catherine Lutz, the militarization of social life reflects a "shift in general societal beliefs and values in ways necessary to legitimate the use of force, the organization of large standing armies and their leaders, and the higher taxes or tribute used to pay for them" (2002, p. 723). Or to recall cartoonist Rall's assertion about the skewed priorities of the United States: "the military is all we've got!" As official responses to the Ebola crisis show, even when a military solution may not yield optimal results, it becomes *the solution* most readily available to bridge gaps in medical, public health, and humanitarian capacity. Militarization, when coupled with humanitarian practices, helps to define the conditions under which life is protected, rescued, and saved in the name of humanity. More specifically, the conscious coupling of military and humanitarian approaches demands that we ask whose lives are amenable for protection and rescue through the threat of force, which people may demand obedience from Ebola-affected communities, and on whose terms these demands can be made. Ultimately, this helps us to understand whose security is prioritized and from what dangers or threats they are being protected.

Security Before Humanity: Critiques of Securitization

Security approaches to public health share similar problems with military approaches to humanitarian assistance. Public health measures during any outbreak tend to be coercive because they often require that people prioritize community protection in relation to public health messages over conflicting community priorities and individual concerns. During the Ebola crisis, official health security approaches emanating from the West emphasized containing Ebola to mitigate the threats it posed to privileged others elsewhere. Domestic security concerns may not have emphasized privileged others residing elsewhere, but they were applied unevenly, and often along lines of social status (e.g., skin color, class, ethnicity, geography).[7] Both types of security measures, according to critics, place uneven emphasis on containment and isolation of the disease and its hosts, often to the detriment of care and empathy toward individuals suffering from Ebola and their families. Such measures are premised on "an approach which puts physicians and public health personnel in the position of border guards" and undermines the kind of "solidarity and mutual support" required to bring an epidemic under control (Farmer 2001).

MSF workers openly expressed ambivalence about security paradigms. Commenting on the West African Ebola outbreak, Peter Redfield pointed out that this ambivalence among MSF employees was not recent. In fact, it was a topic of serious discussion when the organization convened to reflect upon its response to a 2005 Marburg virus outbreak in Angola:

A member of the audience described that we were reduced to "health police," while another expressed regret concerning the remote, paranoiac attitude of the majority of caregivers, increasing the gap that already exists between doctor and patient. Most ultimately agreed that the brutality of the operation was regrettable. (Redfield 2015)

In such cases, health security (protection from threats to health) is all too often collapsed into national security (protection from threats to sovereign power and representatives of the state).[8] In some communities, state institutions like public hospitals and the police, nongovernmental organizations (NGOs), and the Ebola virus all posed a significant threat to survival. These countries' leaders—all of whom declared Ebola a national emergency within the first six months of the outbreak—had similar concerns about Ebola's threat to national security. Among the threats to national security were the Ebola virus and the health systems that failed to contain the virus's spread. Unlike marginal communities, however, government leadership also perceived "resistant" (or reticent, in official Guinean parlance) communities to be a threat to national security. Initial messages urged people to stop eating bushmeat; to transfer sick family members to treatment centers, where they were very likely to die; and to bury the dead in ways that defied social norms. In addition to displacing concern for humanity, these pronouncements were backed by the threat of (legitimate) force (Frankfurter 2014; Redfield 2015). Such measures, therefore, were certain to face some resistance, as first-line responders and members of affected communities balanced on a tightrope between security and care, coercion and negotiation, suspicion and trust.

Circumventing Critiques? The Politics of Rescue and Flight

Groups favoring military involvement in the Ebola outbreak are well aware of these critiques and of the potential for militarized interventions to spark conflict. They divert these critiques by focusing on the presumed capacity of the armed forces to quickly deploy humanitarian and medical assets to the most affected communities (Abramowitz, Rodriguez, and Arendt 2014). Rightly so. The height of the epidemic coincided with the height of the rainy season and the scaling back of international flights in and out of the Ebola-affected region; it also coincided with the departure of personnel from development-oriented NGOs and private-sector actors. An "air bridge" that could facilitate the movement of clinically trained staff, equipment, supplies, and patients was sorely needed. Well-defined protocols for evacuating the foreign sick, as aided by military personnel, purportedly encouraged the participation of international volunteers. Thus, the physical, geographical, technical, and infrastructure conditions under which Ebola flourished in the region required allotting resources to address these gaps.

The disorganization of the international response, it has been argued, required the order, discipline, structure, and *inflexible flexibility* that the military represents.[9] In other words, military blueprints for disaster relief operations could be modified slightly to address the specific challenges of the West African rainy season and massively depleted infrastructures and health systems. Rapid construction of health infrastructure and hierarchical but sufficiently flexible command structures could impose order on an otherwise chaotic process. Yet it appears that whatever postconflict international assistance Western governments provided to "professionalize" police and military in the three countries had not adequately equipped them to carry out the tasks that foreign militaries were expected to perform during a humanitarian emergency: build and staff Ebola treatment units (ETUs), transport samples, and facilitate the movement of supplies provided by aid agencies. Instead, they learned many of these tasks on the job (Beaubien 2014; Pellerin 2014).

If we are to take their official communication seriously, foreign militaries had no intention of providing the scale of support for clinical care MSF requested (Benkimoun et al. 2015; Castner 2015). Once they arrived on the scene, they were largely preoccupied with protecting themselves. In an interview with journalist Sophie Arie, MSF International President Joanne Liu remarked, "Countries are approaching this with the mindset of going to war. Zero risk. Zero casualties." She equated early military efforts with "airstrikes without boots on the ground" and argued that they needed to balance efforts to build ETUs and move supplies with a greater number of clinicians (2014).[10] Later assessments of the U.S. military response would show that the construction of ETUs in Liberia came too late and resulted in a large number of empty, unused facilities (Onishi 2015). The United Kingdom, which organized its military efforts under the auspices of the Department for International Development, also embedded with the Republic of Sierra Leone Armed Forces, which meant greater support of the military. MSF later reported that less effort should have been spent on building ETUs and more on recruiting and placing clinicians to provide care at the height of the epidemic (House of Commons 2016).

Comments like Liu's stood in stark contrast with those that lauded foreign military efforts in Sierra Leone and Liberia. Apparently, if they had just "shown up" and done nothing else, their work would have been deemed a success (Kamradt-Scott et al. 2015, p. 12). But military presence was more than political theater, and was perhaps perceived to be as coercive as any domestic security actions. As World Vision officially noted in its testimony to the British House of Commons:

> The use of the military to support the command and control centers had its advantages. They were particularly useful for enforcing the emergency regulations and providing security. From our experience in providing support to set up and run the Command and Control centers in each district, World Vision noted that using the British military has worked well. This is in terms of putting in place efficient processes and systems. They enforced some rigor in the management of alerts of sick or dead people and encouraged adherence to standard operating procedures.

Managing Military Visibility and Everyday Security

MSF and others decided that because the Ebola-affected countries were not in the midst of active conflict, a foreign military presence would not pose a threat to efforts to curb the spread of Ebola.[11] Yet they were preoccupied with maintaining a strict separation between their activities and those of visible military actors. Although military informants noted that they collaborated well with MSF, other international NGOs did not receive such generous assessments. In a report on civilian–military cooperation authored by Kamradt-Scott and colleagues, one officer remarked that he "would have preferred if the NGOs did more to support us by 'getting behind the mission', but they instead appeared to be preoccupied with 'their reputation'" (Kamradt-Scott et al. 2015, p. 8).

These international NGOs were not alone in their concerns about their reputations, or about how communities perceived their relationship to the military. Internal memos from the MSF archives included talking points and guidelines for managing the organization's visual and semantic proximity to armed forces and their most powerful symbols. For example, they emphasized that military personnel could not act as personal security for staff or patients and could not be posted near MSF-run health facilities. MSF also offered pointers to employees about how to discuss the role of the military in the overall response. Staff members were told that any discussion of the military must be in close proximity to a statement about their "medical assets." In discussions with media, they were to exercise vigilance about any discussion of security and to direct their responses accordingly.[12]

Cultural Logics of Securitization

Even as organizations carefully managed their interactions with the military, securitization in the field is so common that it escaped comment by people accustomed to living its reality. International staff of humanitarian and development NGOs in the Ebola-affected countries live in "compounds" tucked behind guarded gates and high walls, adorned with barbed wire and broken glass. These enclosures ensure a sharp demarcation between foreign and local elites and everyone else. The mobility of workers within countries—yet another marker of status and prestige—is usually facilitated by access to sport utility vehicles (SUVs), built to move effortlessly through difficult terrain, as they also move comfortably above the rabble (Smirl 2008).

Security briefings and protocols are developed and presented to incoming workers, providing a detailed cognitive map of all possible dangers present in the workplace and its surroundings. These accounts by employers, as presented to their staff, provide a road map and set of prescriptions and proscriptions for risk avoidance. The safety and security of expatriate workers, moreover, is explicitly codified in their contracts, with provisions for medical evacuation as a prerequisite condition for service. Medical evacuations, as Duncan McLean's chapter in this volume (Chapter 10) shows, was a topic of significant negotiation during the outbreak and occurred along lines of citizenship and nationality. For some observers evacuation decisions made solely on the basis of citizenship and nationality were also interpreted in terms of racial difference and globalized racial hierarchies (Benton 2014b). Rotation of international staff in and out of the affected areas was characterized in terms that prioritized an efficient, effective and psychologically hale mobile international workforce.

Writing of the general conditions of emergencies, Didier Fassin and Mariella Pandolfi argue that

> beyond the differences between humanitarian actors and the military that the aid organizations insistently highlight, the two sides come together on the same scene, in a reciprocal and asymmetrical dependency—the military increasingly calling on the humanitarians to legitimize their interventions and the latter needing the former to ensure their safety. (Fassin and Pandolfi 2010, p. 15)

Kamradt-Scott and colleagues demonstrate just that: personnel evacuated by international NGOs in the initial months of the outbreak soon felt comfortable returning once Western leaders had committed troops to be deployed to the region (Kamradt-Scott et al. 2015, pp. 8–9). Although each of these militaries was tasked with performing non-security duties—and considered themselves to be subordinate to NGO and Intergovernmental organization (IGO) coordination mechanisms—the security of workers arriving from wealthier nations providing aid appeared to be of primary concern. The military's relationships to international NGOs, moreover, helped to legitimate their humanitarian work: in the case of the United Kingdom, for example, the defense medical services were the only British organization equipped to roll out a rapid medical response for this type of emergency (Bricknell et al. 2015).

This is not to say that security measures, as enforced by military or police, or as carried out in NGO security policies and protocol, are not developed in response to actual threats. Ebola's etiology and modes of transmission require both vigilance and some degree of separation for at least two reasons. First, encouraging workers to help with the response requires some assurances that considerable effort will be taken to ensure that they will not become infected and, therefore, will be available to participate in the treatment and management of patients and other Ebola mitigation projects. Second, some forms of segregation are necessary for providing care to sick patients. Personal protective equipment, when used correctly, protects against viral transmission between patients and health workers; separate lanes for entry and exit from the treatment wards allow for sanitary and safe passage for individuals who are performing care and treatment duties, as well as those being discharged "Ebola-free." But the "viral" spread of security measures themselves also builds barriers that foster community resentment of those providing health care. They shape the subjectivities of aid and health workers.

Secure Spaces and the Psychic Brutality of the Barracks

Security paradigms erect and enforce physical and social segregation. They also organize capital, labor, and the interior lives of people engaging with securitized spaces. African militaries—Sierra Leone, Liberia, and Guinea among them—are increasingly involved in commercial enterprises. Security is privatized (De Waal 2002).[13] Guards hired to protect U.S. government–sponsored Ebola treatment facilities during the Ebola outbreak were subcontractors with Intercon, a private military and security corporation known for its expertise in providing security for the U.S. embassy during Liberia's civil war and safeguarding the personnel and property of mining companies (Mathieu and Dearden 2007, p. 746; Associated Press 2013). As Denielle Elliott (2015) poignantly illustrates in a photo essay about the U.S. military's Liberia mission, security protocols for civilian workers in the U.S. government treatment facilities strictly enforced segregation. They were not allowed to leave the worksite unaccompanied; their movements were limited to U.S. embassy–approved locations. The design of spaces for use by these workers was developed toward similar security aims.

On empty fields, barracks-style accommodations were built for epidemiologists, lab technicians, and clinicians. Barbed wire fences enclosed these spaces. "Communication with patients," Elliott adds, "whether infected or only suspected, occurs through a fence, or with medical personnel in full protective gear . . . Security guards are local Liberian men, stationed approximately every thirty meters within the walls, who police who may enter and exit" (2015). Elliott also notes how sequestered U.S. civilian workers were frustrated by the limits placed on their mobility. Like those MSF Marburg responders in 2005, the U.S. government health workers posted in Liberia were experiencing the "brutality" of barracks living, even if they did not express their feelings of frustration in these visceral terms. Such sharp divisions and segregations, designed with security in mind, also shape how communities respond to interventions.

In Guinea, security designs more modest than those described by Elliott had profound effects on how NGO efforts were received. Anthropologist Sylvain Faye, deployed to Guinea between July and September 2014, described how fear motivated the Red Cross to modify how it approached communities. These modifications had a negative impact on how they interacted with communities and how communities perceived the organization. By February 2015, the Guinean Red Cross reported that their mobile teams had experienced at least 10 attacks per month throughout the country (Hussain and Farge 2015). Faye writes:

> Because of the painful experiences of volunteers, the Red Cross recommended that [when they enter villages for outreach], their vehicles be placed in starting positions, so that they could escape physical violence. They also asked that team members wear clothes that would make traveling easier (in anticipation of violence in the field). Protective aprons [for example] used at funerals were made detachable, in order to escape potential captors. Even if these recommendations were useful, they hardly seemed conducive to peaceful and positive interactions with the population, or to achieving dignified burials. For example, every time members of the communities expressed their discontent or wanted answers to certain questions, volunteers would interpret them as signs of "reticence," justifying their withdrawal from the community. Thus, they forgot that they had found communities there, suffering. (Faye 2015, my translation)

Faye's observations echo those of critical geographer Lisa Smirl, who remarked that security design practices—even ad hoc measures like the ones described by Faye—influence how people internalize, behave, and respond to securitized initiatives (Smirl 2008; Duffield 2012). Security mobilized against communities experiencing profound distress, rather than in acknowledgment of their fears, desires, and preferences, may inspire acts of resistance. A heightened awareness of *insecurity* among aid workers may compel them to interpret overt challenges to their authority as a threat to their security; it may inspire further acts of defensiveness.

Checkpoints, Roadblocks, and "Invisible" War

Checkpoints staffed by the military and police stoked suspicion among people working and living near those sites. A typical checkpoint is set up to "mitigate risk"—in the case of Ebola, the risk is the spread of the virus. Individuals wanting to pass through the checkpoints erected at various points along roads in the region had to wash their hands at a chlorine station at the entry point of the monitoring area, move through a narrow tarpaulin-covered passage, and take a seat on a bench so that they could have their temperature taken by a digital thermometer pointed at the temple, described by many as resembling a gun (CNN 2014). Effectively stemming the spread of the virus means regulating the scale, tempo, and rhythm of people's movements. Checkpoints do this work, officially, though it is clear that there are many strategies that people use to avoid these regulations—for example, taking footpaths through the forests and using fever reducers to avoid being detained. Sometimes workers shirk their responsibilities (Maxmen 2015; Searcey 2015). There are also people for whom these regulations do not stringently apply. Under the conditions of the blockade announced by the Sierra Leonean government on August 6, 2014, aid workers and businesses carrying certain supplies into communities had unrestricted access to the eastern provinces, while the movements of others were heavily regulated. This practice extended to include people who were marked as foreigners either by their traveling in NGO vehicles or their white skin (Bah 2014; Shepler 2015).[14]

Writing from Freetown in mid-July 2014, citizen-journalist Bankolay Turay noted that the "war" against Ebola was a fight against an invisible enemy. Turay, like many others, compared the "invisible war" waged against Ebola to the country's civil war. He notes, "The neighborhood watch rekindles memories of the war, with the Community Defense Unit (CDU) set up to aid the warring factions then, and now enforcing the Public Health Emergency declared by the President" (Turay 2015; Gbandia 2014). While Ebola is indeed invisible, physical structures like checkpoints mark the landscape, making it difficult to ignore memories of the war. Traces of the war—alongside previous iterations of warfare and resistance—are embodied in individual and collective memories of place and comportment (Shaw 2002). They also produced local responses that included mobilizing traditional and ad hoc policing and protection mechanisms for affected communities.

Domestic Militaries and the Logics of Criminalization and Coercion

The responses by national governments appear to be fairly uniform in the sense that they were deployed to maintain order, enforce borders, and control flows of people between and within countries (Fofana and MacDougall 2014; Harmon 2014; Human Rights Watch 2014). How communities understood and responded to the use of military and police force, of course, varied across communities (and within communities) on the basis of their histories and experiences with security forces and public services sectors more broadly. Historians of the region have documented cases in which punitive, coercive, and violent public health measures were actively resisted in the past (Rashid 2011; Cole 2015; Lachenal 2015). As the armed extension of state power, the military could therefore be perceived as an extension of political grievances and machinations, backed by the threat of force.

This does not mean that community responses and resistance to military interventions were universally predictable, however (Fairhead 2014). In some cases, domestic military forces were praised for maintaining order and assisting health workers to safely complete their duties; indeed, the Republic of Sierra Leone Armed Forces had successfully participated in a 2012 response to an outbreak of cholera (Gbandia 2014). Foreign militaries were a welcomed and highly anticipated dimension in a coordinated response (Muchler 2014; Castner 2015; Kamradt-Scott et al. 2015, p. 17). Any assistance with building health facilities, staffing them, and making general improvements in the clinical care and public health practices represented a step in the right direction. Yet acts of violence and suppression occurred with some frequency among vulnerable and marginal communities, suggesting that military and police action taken in the name of protecting the public's health often came at the expense of the most marginal.

In the following subsections, I briefly describe three such diagnostic events, using them to analyze broader trends associated with the role of security forces in public health emergencies (S. F. Moore 1987). Events like these reflected, and to some extent shaped, how members of these communities reacted to perceived transgressions to their autonomy and humanity. While physical violence against health workers was not the most frequent or even common mode of resistance, these incidents reveal how even the *threat* of force and awareness of past transgressions may have affected interactions between Ebola response teams and affected communities.

Justice for Shaki: West Point, August 2014

In early August 2014, international media outlets covered a violent clash between Liberian security forces and residents of the Monrovia neighborhood, West Point, when the government's Ebola task force decided to put it under quarantine and place an Ebola containment center in a local school building. Area residents say they were not consulted, and they suspected that the government was bringing nonresidents into the holding center, thereby bringing infection into the community. The evacuation of the West Point area commissioner, writes Luke Mogelson, "tipped the outrage into violence" (2015). The clash became a prime example of a militarized response gone wrong when police and military opened fire and used tear gas against area residents. One teen resident, Shaki Kamara, died of gunshot wounds to his leg; several others were injured.[15]

The incident represents more than the disproportionate use of force by security forces, a measure of the effectiveness or practicality of quarantines, or even an indicator of enmity toward and distrust of government efforts. Understanding the motivations behind and the repercussions of this event also requires, at the very least, a basic assessment of how West Point figures into the local cartographies and explanations of security. It also requires understanding how the area's residents interpret and respond to these explanatory models. Before the incident, the neighborhood was described in news media and the "gray literature" as an urban slum characterized by high levels of violence and crime, a refuge for veterans of Liberia's civil war. West Point residents also believe the community has been deliberately marginalized in discussions about how social services and development efforts are conducted and distributed—even as they have become an target of such efforts. Cameron Zohoori interviewed and photographed several hip-co music artists from the neighborhood in 2011. One artist, Takun-J, summarized West Point's reputation:

> If you come from West Point, people might not take you to be a good person, criminals come from there, rogues, thieves. But a lot of good people live there, a lot of families. They feel like they are outcasts, like nobody pays attention to them. (Zohoori 2011)

Development projects in West Point have focused on housing security, environmental degradation brought about by its precarious location on the coast, waterborne illnesses, waste management, and other infrastructure problems associated with "urban slums." The neighborhood has also served as a venue for testing and evaluating community policing efforts in the postconflict reconstruction era, and for developing community-based development projects that mobilize youth and women (Patton 1988; Stephens 1991; Mensah 2006; Kaufmann 2011; MacDougall 2016). Alongside these efforts, neighborhood residents have been involved in collective organizing for justice reform, women's empowerment, and broader community development issues.

West Point residents' treatment by security forces during the outbreak, however, seemed to focus on the criminal elements rather than on the potential strengths of and dialogue with community institutions. Anger at the authorities was rooted in lack of advance notice of the quarantine and the transfer of nonresidents into the neighborhood holding center, where no care or treatment for visibly sick people was provided. Although anger was directed toward these issues, the turning point, according to some residents, was when the military came to evacuate the neighborhood commissioner and her family—again raising questions about how security is imagined and reinforced, against what and whom (J. Moore 2014a, 2014b; Mogelson 2015).

Voice of America journalist James Butty spoke with area residents after the government lifted the 10-day quarantine. Residents noted that the quarantine made them feel "dehumanized" and "as if they were in a high-security prison." The quarantine, and indeed the press coverage of protests and the military police crackdown on area residents, had stigmatized their neighborhood, according to resident and youth leader, James Weah: "We have been called all sorts of names. People point fingers at us labeling us to be Ebola patients. We want the government to tell the public that the people from West Point are indeed Ebola-free" (Butty 2014).

The Crackdown at Womey: September 2014

Similarly, the relationship between national authorities and residents in Guinea's Forest Region, where the outbreak began, was characterized by decades of perceived discrimination and social claims remaining ignored by successive regimes (Wilkinson and Leach 2014, p. 143). As anthropologist Julienne Anoko noted in her account of a "listening exercise" in 26 villages in the region, "The outbreak of EVD has become, for these rebellious communities, an arena in which to be heard and to hope to obtain solutions for unemployment and poverty, access to education and health, new schools, bridges and roads, among other things" (2014).

Local and international media reports about acts of resistance to Ebola highlighted recent histories of mistrust between government authorities and citizens—most often by focusing on acts of violence against health workers. Reporters have been less attentive to the histories of mistreatment and malfeasance, both government and intracommunity, that persisted in collective memory and in everyday interactions.

In September 2014, residents of Womey, a town in the region, murdered eight people, Guinean journalists and health workers who had traveled there to conduct Ebola education and outreach. The murders attracted international media coverage. In the international press, the tragic events were often presented as an example of villagers' ignorance and recalcitrance rather than an incursion rooted in long-term mistrust. If deep-seated mistrust was mentioned at all, it was solely located in the Forest Region, which had a reputation for being notoriously "reticent," despite the fact that resistance to government and NGO interventions was documented elsewhere in the country (Assessment Capacities Project [ACAPS] 2015).

Womey was in the news again after the Guinean military invaded and looted the town shortly after the killings, sending thousands fleeing their homes and seeking refuge in the bush for several weeks (Brittain 2015). As many tried to make sense of both the murders of health workers and the military's retaliation against the town's residents, varied accounts surfaced about the conditions shaping and leading up to these events.

Abdoul Goudoussi Diallo, a Guinean geographer, suggested that violence against health workers might have been related to their arrival during a secret initiation ceremony. He writes:

> It was difficult to verify if the people were murdered at Womey because they interfered with an initiation ceremony in the sacred forest. . . . However, we are entitled to question the underlying reasons why the Guinean authorities cracked down so hard on the inhabitants of Womey, who were forced to flee and hide in the bush for about one month while the area was militarized and subject to all kinds of looting their homes and their property. Why have defense and security forces prevented the representatives of the NGO Lawyers without Borders from conducting their investigations in the field? (Diallo 2015, p. 29, my translation)

A firsthand account from an Ebola response team member who survived the attack, Guinean sociologist Marie Ouendeno, further complicates this narrative by suggesting that other regional political grievances—which by extension included an appointed official as a member of the team—increased hostility toward the team and its message. Ouendeno sensed this tension during the meeting, but when she suggested that they abandon the site, other team members assured her that she was overreacting (Ouendeno 2014; Oosterhoff and Wilkinson 2015). Whatever precipitated the violence in Womey, it is important to understand how interventions, no matter how benign in their intentions, may also be rooted in a longer local history of how such interventions have been interpreted. In other words, attempts to align community priorities with public health ones should be attentive to and demonstrate willingness to address exist-ing asymmetries lest they reproduce the conditions of structural and physical violence that beget resistance, recalcitrance, and more violence.

State of Emergency: Koidu, October 2014

On October 21, 2014, two residents were left dead and the community was placed under curfew in the mining town of Koidu after Ebola contact tracers attempted to take the blood of a 90-year-old woman against the wishes of her family. They insisted that she had been chronically ill and was convalescing at home for some time and had not been exposed to Ebola. The family sought assis-tance from neighbors to remove the officials from the area, and a clash between the community residents and security forces ensued (Calain and Poncin 2015). As in the incidents reported in Womey and West Point, international reports depicted the youths as "machete-wielding" "hordes" resistant to public health efforts, not taking into account local interpretations of the extractive quality of various encounters—especially where youths are concerned (Perez 2014; Ruble 2014).

Around the time of this incident in Koidu, President Ernest Bai Koroma trans-ferred Ebola leadership from the Ministry of Health and Sanitation (MOHS) to the Ministry of Defense (MOD), citing the military's enhanced capacity for coordinating logistics and other activities related to the Ebola response road map. For some political commentators in Sierra Leone, the shift of operations from MOHS to MOD was a political statement in which the president conferred greater legitimacy for handling national crises—public health or otherwise—to the military. The decision had some wondering if the newly minted Ebola czar, Major Palo Conteh, wasn't also being groomed to take over the presidency upon President Koroma's departure (Thomas 2014). After taking up his new respon-sibility, Conteh explained what he felt would be the best approach to seemingly indifferent and recalcitrant populations. People who refused to obey the official Ebola mandates laid out by the government were criminals, their refusals overtly criminalized:

> I am now using the "carrot and stick approach," I have been giving out
> the carrot since I took over but our people still do the wrong things.
> When I start using the stick, I will see all kinds of headlines in papers
> and radio programs but will not be deterred by them. (*Awoko* editorial
> staff 2014)[16]

By November 2014, District Ebola Response Centers were set up with military officers taking the lead. MSF appeared to be troubled by this shift and the potential risks to security that it imposed:

> They are taking a very military approach and advising that the Sierra Leone government deploy more police and military to ENFORCE the quarantine measures at the household level . . . we have the opportunity to negotiate with them to have responsible operational model in these to help the effort without getting anyone killed. THIS MUST BE DONE in a forthcoming and diplomatic manner or we risk to clash and people will die if we don't sort this out.[17]

Despite efforts to "humanize" the official Ebola response by international and local actors, Conteh's perspective had changed little in those eight months of coordinating the response to the Ebola crisis. Food and supply shortages during a countrywide lockdown in late March 2015 set off another set of clashes between security forces and communities in Freetown (Olu-Mammah and Fofana 2015). During a press conference in June 2015, Palo Conteh remarked that "lawlessness keeps the virus alive: people still wash dead bodies and bury them secretly; the sick still visit herbal healers instead of going immediately to treatment centers. And they still flee quarantine and infect others" (Gbandia 2015). While it is possible to read Conteh's pronouncements as merely performative and as a spectacle without the "teeth" of enforcement—and some of my interlocutors working in the region have argued this—it is important to note that threats of violence may be sufficient to force compliance *and* foster resistance.

Conclusions

Can military logics be productively uncoupled from military logistical apparatus? Not really. The military have long been involved in public health, often focusing on minimizing threats to the nations they are employed to protect, as they have also sought self-protection in their overseas military campaigns. Similarly, responses to epidemics have long been securitized, in the sense that they have often focused on coercion; enforcement of public health measures may be supported by criminalization of protocol violators and punitive measures. However, any outbreak response effort must be attentive not only to these realities, but also to the fact that some communities have long been suspicious and fearful of domestic police and military forces. These suspicions and fears usually reflect histories in which they have been disproportionately subject to structural and physical violence at the hands of these actors. Moreover, securitized public health efforts—those primarily preoccupied with containment, coercion, and criminalization—may fail if they are not accompanied by attempts to provide care and comfort. This includes how foreign forces choose to align themselves with national security forces. An effort to demilitarize and downplay the coercive effects of public health requires dialogue and deep understanding of local political and social conflicts.

Notes

1. Although feelings were mixed about military intervention in all three countries, domestic militaries were too often perceived to be acting in their own interests or in the interests of political elites and their associates. Liberian human rights attorney Samuel Kofi Woods openly expressed concerns about how the Armed Forces of Liberia (AFL) had long been used to commit acts of state violence against its citizens. During a speech for Armed Forces Commemoration Day in February 2015, Woods outlined a history in which the AFL was a "vehicle of the political establishment using brute force and naked power." He forcefully argued that distrust lingered in communities where the military had acted with impunity through the civil wars and in their aftermath (Woods 2015). In Sierra Leone, rumors circulated that the All People's Congress party had sent troops to spread Ebola in the majority Sierra Leone People's Party eastern region. In Guinea, similar concerns were raised, even as marginalized people saw the emergence of Ebola in the region as a way to bring attention to ongoing struggles with social, political, and economic marginalization. Additional details are provided in a detailed mission report by an anthropologist working in the area (Anoko 2014).
2. In this essay, "communities" refers to diverse groups, from international humanitarian agencies and nongovernmental organizations to towns and villages affected by Ebola and "international publics" who shaped and responded to international media reports, ongoing intellectual debates about the disease, and so forth.
3. Flight and rescue might also be considered in relation to country nationals, with flight from quarantine figuring in opposition to the impossibility of "being rescued." Similarly, international forces, when embedded with national security forces, were sometimes deemed complicit in criminalization and coercion.
4. While military laboratory and clinical personnel from the Sierra Leone Armed Forces helped to provide care, the care was as limited as in other places due to the sheer number of cases presenting at hospitals and the number of staff available to provide care and diagnostics capacity.
5. Compare to zones of indistinction outlined, via Agamben, by Constantinou and Opondo 2015, p. 4.
6. China was in a precarious position in this regard; they were at first criticized for doing too little, given their much-debated economic investment in the region. For additional information about China's involvement, see Tiezzi, "China's Military Wages War on Ebola"; Larson, "China Ramps up Efforts to Combat Ebola"; Goldstein, "White-Coat Warriors: China's Heroic Fight against Ebola." When China offered funding, supplies and medical personnel numbering in the hundreds, their contributions were underplayed, if not ridiculed, by representatives of Western governments, suggesting that these developments were as much political maneuvering as they were rooted in a sense of empathy and care. For examples of this official response from the United States, see Leins, "China's Evolving Ebola Response: Recognizing the Cost of Inaction." Also note response in late October 2014 by White House Secretary Josh Earnest to criticism that the United States had not done enough to help Ebola efforts: "When we have a situation like this on the global scene, people aren't wondering what the Chinese are doing to respond to it. People aren't picking up the phone and wondering if Vladimir Putin is going to commit Russian resources to this effort . . . People want to know what the United States of

America is doing about it." This was quoted in Rajagopalan, "China to Send Elite Army Unit to Help Fight Ebola in Liberia."

7. Notable exceptions include remarks made by Presidents Sirleaf (Liberia) and Koroma (Sierra Leone), which focused on protecting Americans and other foreigners from the disease. See also Benton 2016.

8. While there have been many attempts to resuscitate health security frameworks to be more equitable and to eliminate the us/them dichotomy that it often presumes (human security frameworks are an example of this), these are largely abandoned in actual health security practices. See Deloffre 2015.

9. In fact, one of the questions posed directly by the House of Commons in their inquiry regarding the British response in Sierra Leone was "Was using the military more efficient than using NGOs?" This suggests that they assumed there was a testable relationship of militarization to capacity to achieve desired results in a timely, relatively inexpensive manner, in comparison to those efforts by NGOs. See House of Commons 2016.

10. According to Vickie Hawkins, MSF's executive director in the United Kingdom, MSF may have also overestimated the biohazard capacity that more than a decade of biosecurity funding and research should have produced (Blunt 2015).

11. "On the use of military assets in response to Ebola outbreak: Basic elements of reflexion and positioning," October 7, 2014, internal MSF memo.

12. MSF's UN Security Council Ebola talking points, updated September 18, 2014, read: "We continue to call for states with biohazard disaster response capacity (civilian or military) to act now. When mentioning military, make sure you always use it in the same sentence as medical assets (or synonym). We cannot afford any confusion about MSF calling for military intervention."

13. Weapons procurement for the Sierra Leone police force in 2010, for example, was the subject of public scrutiny, with the UN officially expressing its concerns and the opposition political party, SLPP, making it into a marquee issue during the 2012 election season.

14. Anthropologist Susan Shepler describes the checkpoints erected and staffed by community members in urban Freetown neighborhoods. Volunteers staffing the checkpoints also faced some resistance to their demands. But while these operated under a rubric of suspicion, they also became more accepted modes of surveillance than those mediated through the military or police.

15. Many more were likely affected by the release of tear gas into the neighborhood, resulting in a kind of "atmospheric violence" as has been argued in other contexts, like Istanbul, Turkey, and Ferguson, Missouri (Lippmann 2015; Aciksoz 2016).

16. This speech was delivered on November 20, 2014, within just a few weeks of his becoming head of the national Ebola response.

17. Andre Heller, Report, Field Support Visit-Magburaka-Tonkolili District, November 26–28, 2014.

References

Abramowitz, Sharon, Olga Rodriguez, and Greig Arendt. 2014. "The effectiveness of U.S. military intervention on Ebola depends on the government's will and vision to direct vast military resources towards a public health response." *LSE American Politics and Policy*. Released April 24, 2015.

Assessment Capacities Project (ACAPS). 2015. "Ebola in West Africa. Guinea: Resistance to the Ebola response." Thematic Note. http://www.acaps.org/special-report/ebola-west-africa-guinea-resistance-ebola-response.

Aciksoz, Salih Can. 2016. "Medical humanitarianism under atmospheric violence: Health professionals in the 2013 Gezi protests in Turkey." *Culture, Medicine and Psychiatry* 40(2): 198–222.

Anoko, Julienne. 2014. "Communication with rebellious communities during an outbreak of Ebola virus disease in Guinea: An anthropological approach." Geneva. http://www.

ebola-anthropology.net/wp-content/uploads/2014/12/Communicationduring-an-outbreak-of-Ebola-Virus-Disease-with-rebellious-communities-in-Guinea.pdf.

Arie, Sophie. 2014. "Only the military can get the Ebola epidemic under control: MSF head." *BMJ (Clinical Research Ed.)* 349 (oct10_5): g6151. doi:10.1136/bmj.g6151. http://www.bmj.com/content/349/bmj.g6151.

Associated Press. 2013. "Embassy guard bears witness to years of Liberia's grisly wars." *New York Times*, October 30. http://www.nytimes.com/2003/10/30/international/africa/30LIBE.html.

Awoko editorial staff. 2014. "We will use force if . . . NERC boss." *Awoko (Freetown)*. http://awoko.org/2014/11/20/sierra-leone-news-we-will-use-force-if-nerc-boss/.

Bah, Saidu. 2014. "Flaws uncovered at Ebola check points." *Awoko (Freetown)*. http://awoko.org/2014/11/26/sierra-leone-newsflaws-uncovered-at-ebola-check-points/.

Beaubien, Jason. 2014. "U.S. military response to Ebola gains momentum in Liberia." *Goats and Soda, National Public Radio.* http://www.npr.org/sections/goatsandsoda/2014/11/05/361796044/u-s-military-response-to-ebola-gains-momentum-in-liberia.

Benkimoun, Paul, Gilbert Potier, Michel Janssens, Frédéric Le Marcis, and Antoine Petibon. 2015. "Ebola: chronique d'une catastrophe annoncée." *Humanitaire*, no. 40 (May). Médecins du monde: 12–31. http://humanitaire.revues.org/3130.

Benton, Adia. 2014a. "The epidemic will be militarized: Watching outbreak as the West African Ebola epidemic unfolds." *Hot Spots, Cultural Anthropology Website.* http://www.culanth.org/fieldsights/599-the-epidemic-will-be-militarized-watching-outbreak-as-the-west-african-ebola-epidemic-unfolds.

Benton, Adia. 2014b. "Race and the immuno-logics of Ebola response in West Africa." *Somatosphere.* http://somatosphere.net/2014/09/race-and-the-immuno-logics-of-ebola-response-in-west-africa.html.

Benton, Adia. 2016. "What's the matter boss, we sick? A meditation on Ebola's origin stories." In *Ebola's Message: Public Health and Medicine in the 21st Century*, edited by Nicholas G. Evans, Tara C. Smith, and Maimuna S. Majumder. Cambridge, MA: MIT Press.

Blunt, Elizabeth. 2015. "A marriage of convenience: The UK military and NGOs." *IRIN.* http://www.irinnews.org/timeline/2015/03/03.

Bricknell, Martin, T. Hodgetts, K. Beaton, and A. McCourt. 2016. "Operation GRITROCK: The Defence Medical Services' story and emerging lessons from supporting the UK response to the Ebola crisis." *Journal of the Royal Army Medical Corps*, June; 162(3): 169–175.

Brittain, Amy. 2015. "The fear of Ebola led to slayings—and a whole village was punished." *Washington Post*, February 28. https://www.washingtonpost.com/world/africa/the-fear-of-ebola-led-to-murder--and-a-whole-village-was-punished/2015/02/28/a2509b88-a80f-11e4-a162-121d06ca77f1_story.html.

Butty, James. 2014. "Liberia's West Point: Life after Ebola quarantine." *Voice of America.* http://www.voanews.com/content/liberias-west-point-ebola-quarantine-lifted/2434374.html.

Castner, Brian. 2015. "Hearts, minds, and Ebola: The US Army drops in on Liberia." *Vice News.* https://news.vice.com/article/hearts-minds-and-ebola-the-us-army-drops-in-on-liberia.

CNN. 2014. "Go through an Ebola checkpoint: Ebola checkpoints in Sierra Leone aim to stem the virus' spread. CNN's David McKenzie takes you through one." http://www.cnn.com/videos/health/2014/08/06/erin-dnt-mckenzie-ebola-checkpoint-sierra-leone.cnn/video/playlists/gupta-ebola-virus/.

Cole, Festus. 2015. "Sanitation, disease and public health in Sierra Leone." *Journal of Imperial and Commonwealth History* 43 (2): 238–66.

Constantinou, C. M., and S. O. Opondo. 2016. "Engaging the 'ungoverned': The merging of diplomacy, defence and development." *Cooperation and Conflict*, September 51(3): 307–324.

De Waal, Alex. 2002. *Demilitarizing the mind: African agendas for peace and security.* Lawrenceville, NJ: Africa World Press.

Deloffre, Maryam Zarnegar. 2015. "Human security in the age of Ebola: Towards people-centered global governance." *Global Policy Journal.* http://www.globalpolicyjournal.com/blog/21/01/2015/human-security-age-ebola-towards-people-centered-global-governance.

Diallo, Abdoul Goudoussi. 2015. *Et vint le virus Ebola: Rumeurs, stupeurs et réalités en Guinée.* Paris: L'Harmattan.

DuBois, Marc, Caitlin Wake, Scarlett Sturridge, and Christina Bennett. 2015. "The Ebola response in West Africa." HPG Working Paper, London.

Duffield, Mark. 2012. "Risk management and the bunkering of the aid industry." *Development Dialogue* 58: 21–37.

Elliott, Denielle. 2015. "Other images: Ebola and medical humanitarianism in Monrovia." *MAT: Medicine Anthropology Theory* 2(2): 102–24.

Fairhead, James. 2014. "The significance of death, gunerals and the after-life in Ebola-hit Sierra Leone, Guinea and Liberia: Anthropological insights into infection and social resistance." October. http://opendocs.ids.ac.uk/opendocs/handle/123456789/4727.

Farmer, Paul. 2001. "Russia's tuberculosis catastrophe." *Project Syndicate.* https://www.project-syndicate.org/commentary/russia-s-tuberculosis-catastrophe.

Fassin, Didier, and Mariella Pandolfi. 2010. "Introduction: Military and humanitarian government in the age of intervention." In *Contemporary States of Emergency: The Politics of Military and Humanitarian Interventions,* edited by Didier Fassin and Mariella Pandolfi, p. 403. New York: Zone Books.

Faye, Sylvain Landry. 2015. "L'« exceptionnalité » d'Ebola et les « réticences » populaires en Guinée-Conakry. Réflexions à partir d'une approche d'anthropologie symétrique." *Anthropologie et Santé,* no. 11 (November). Association Amades. doi:10.4000/anthropologiesante.1796. http://anthropologiesante.revues.org/1796.

Fofana, Umaru, and Claire MacDougall. 2014. "Sierra Leone, Liberia deploy troops as Ebola toll hits 887." *Reuters Africa.* http://www.reuters.com/article/us-healh-ebola-africa-idUSKBN0G41CK20140804.

Frankfurter, Raphael. 2014. "The danger in losing sight of Ebola victims' humanity." *The Atlantic,* August. http://www.theatlantic.com/health/archive/2014/08/the-danger-in-losing-sight-of-ebola-victims-humanity/378945/.

Gbandia, Silas. 2014. "Soldiers manning Ebola checkpoints bring back war memories." *Bloomberg.* http://www.bloomberg.com/news/articles/2014-08-20/soldiers-manning-ebola-checkpoints-bring-back-memories-of-war.

Gbandia, Silas. 2015. "Sierra Leone's deadly virus—Corruption cost lives in Ebola outbreak." *Le Monde Diplomatique.* http://infoweb.newsbank.com/resources/doc/nb/news/156FC3B147C92230?p=WORLDNEWS.

Goldstein, Lyle J. 2015. "White-Coat Warriors: China's Heroic Fight against Ebola." *The National Interest.* Washington, D.C. http://nationalinterest.org/feature/white-coat-warriors-chinas-heroic-fight-against-ebola-13135.

Harmon, William Q. 2014. "Sirleaf mandates AFL, LNP to enforce Anti-Ebola compliance." *The Liberian Observer,* July 23. http://www.liberianobserver.com/news/sirleaf-mandates-afl-lnp-enforce-anti-ebola-compliance.

Heymann, David L., Lincoln Chen, Keizo Takemi, David P. Fidler, Jordan W. Tappero, Mathew J. Thomas, Thomas A. Kenyon, et al. 2015. "Global health security: The wider lessons from the West African Ebola virus disease epidemic." *The Lancet* 385(9980): 1884–901.

House of Commons, International Development Committee. 2016. "Ebola: Responses to a public health emergency." London. http://www.publications.parliament.uk/pa/cm201516/cmselect/cmintdev/338/338.pdf.

Human Rights Watch. 2014. "West Africa: Respect rights in Ebola response." https://www.hrw.org/news/2014/09/15/west-africa-respect-rights-ebola-response.

Hussain, Misha. 2014. "MSF calls for military medics to help tackle West Africa Ebola." *Reuters Africa.* http://af.reuters.com/article/topNews/idAFKBN0GX1QP20140902?pageNumber=2&virtualBrandChannel=0.

Hussain, Misha, and Emma Farge. 2015. "Red Cross Ebola teams in Guinea attacked 10 times a month." *Reuters.*http://www.reuters.com/article/us-health-ebola-guinea-idUSKBN0LG1GO20150212.

Ivers, Louise. 2012. "Humanitarian aid, impartiality, dirty boots." In *Haiti After the Earthquake*, edited by Paul Farmer, pp. 308–18. New York: Public Affairs.

Kamradt-Scott, Adam, Sophie Harman, Clare Wenham, and Frank III Smith. 2015. "Saving lives: The civil-military response to the 2014 Ebola outbreak in West Africa." Sydney.

Kaufmann, Andrea. 2011. "Mobilizing for improvement : An empirical study of a women's organizaton in West Point, Liberia." *Social Movements in Africa*. http://edoc.unibas.ch/33064/4/Stichproben20_Kaufmann.pdf.

Kickbusch, Ilona, James Orbinski, Theodor Winkler, and Albrecht Schnabel. 2015. "We need a sustainable development Goal 18 on global health security." *Lancet* 385(9973): 1069.

Lachenal, Guillaume. 2015. "Outbreak of unknown origin in the Tripoint Zone." *Limn* 1(5). http://limn.it/outbreak-of-unknown-origin-in-the-tripoint-zone/.

Larson, Christina. 2014. "China Ramps up Efforts to Combat Ebola." *Science*. http://www.sciencemag.org/news/2014/11/china-ramps-efforts-combat-ebola.

Leins, Chris. 2014. "China's Evolving Ebola Response: Recognizing the Cost of Inaction." *Atlantic Council*. http://www.atlanticcouncil.org/blogs/new-atlanticist/china-s-evolving-ebola-response-recognizing-the-cost-of-inaction.

Lippmann, Rachel. 2015. "Settlement reached: Police must warn before use of tear gas or other chemical agents." *St. Louis Public Radio*. http://news.stlpublicradio.org/post/settlement-reached-police-must-warn-use-tear-gas-or-other-chemical-agents.

Lutz, Catherine. 2002. "Making war at home in the United States: Militarization and the current crisis." *American Anthropologist* 104(3): 723–35. doi:10.1525/aa.2002.104.3.723.

MacDougall, Claire. 2016. "Fearing the tide in West Point, a slum already swamped with worry." *New York Times*, March 16. http://www.nytimes.com/2016/03/16/world/africa/fearing-the-tide-in-west-point-a-slum-already-swamped-with-worry.html?_r=0.

Mathieu, Fabien, and Nick Dearden. 2007. "Corporate mercenaries: The threat of private military & security companies." *Review of African Political Economy* 34(114): 744–55.

Maxmen, Amy. 2015. "In Sierra Leone's chaotic capital, Ebola found fertile ground." *National Geographic*. http://news.nationalgeographic.com/news/2015/01/150127-ebola-virus-outbreak-epidemic-sierra-leone-freetown-photos-pictures/.

McGovern, Mike. 2014. "Bushmeat and the politics of disgust." *Hot Spots: Cultural Anthropology Website*. http://www.culanth.org/fieldsights/588-bushmeat-and-the-politics-of-disgust.

McNeil Jr., Donald G. 2014. "Using a tactic unseen in a century, countries cordon off Ebola-racked areas." *New York Times*, August 12. http://www.nytimes.com/2014/08/13/science/using-a-tactic-unseen-in-a-century-countries-cordon-off-ebola-racked-areas.html.

Médecins Sans Frontières (MSF) International. 2014. "MSF international president United Nations special briefing on Ebola." http://www.msf.org/article/msf-international-president-united-nations-special-briefing-ebola.

Mensah, Anthony. 2006. "People and their waste in an emergency context: The case of Monrovia, Liberia." *Habitat International* 30(4): 754–68.

Mogelson, Luke. 2015. "When the fever breaks." *The New Yorker*, January. http://www.newyorker.com/magazine/2015/01/19/when-fever-breaks.

Moore, Jina. 2014a. "Mob destroys Ebola center in Liberia two days after it opens." *Buzzfeed*. http://www.buzzfeed.com/jinamoore/two-days-after-it-opens-mob-destroys-ebola-center-in-liberia#.bkdRzOzReQ.

Moore, Jina. 2014b. "Mistrust and confusion swirl around Ebola reports in one Liberian neighborhood." *Buzzfeed*. http://www.buzzfeed.com/jinamoore/in-a-liberian-neighborhood-mistrust-and-confusion-swirl-arou#.ugER1m1Rqa.

Moore, Sally Falk. 1987. "Explaining the present: Theoretical dilemmas in processual ethnography." *American Ethnologist* 14(4): 727–36.

Muchler, Benno. 2014. "Hope sparks in Liberia as US soldiers arrive to help fight Ebola." *Voice of America*. http://www.voanews.com/content/hope-sparks-in-liberia-as-us-soldiers-arrive-to-help-fight-ebola/2459616.html.

Olu-Mammah, Josephus, and Umaru Fofana. 2015. "Police fire tear gas on crowd during Sierra Leone Ebola lockdown." *Reuters*. http://www.reuters.com/article/us-health-ebola-leone-idUSKBN0MO0RQ20150329.

Onishi, Norimutsu. 2015. "Empty Ebola clinics in Liberia are seen as misstep in U.S. relief effort." *New York Times*, April 11. http://www.nytimes.com/2015/04/12/world/africa/idle-ebola-clinics-in-liberia-are-seen-as-misstep-in-us-relief-effort.html.

Oosterhoff, P., and A. Wilkinson. 2015. "Local engagement in Ebola outbreaks and beyond in Sierra Leone." IDS. http://opendocs.ids.ac.uk/opendocs/handle/123456789/5857.

Ouendeno, Marie. 2014. "Report of the Mission in the Sub-Prefecture of Womey, Prefecture N'zerekore of September 16, 2014." Unpublished field report.

Patton, Carl V. 1988. *Spontaneous shelter: International perspectives and prospects.* Philadelphia: Temple University Press. https://books.google.com/books?hl=en&lr=&id=8d6nJVcd5NAC&pgis=1.

Pellerin, Cheryl. 2014. "DoD threat reduction agency builds anti-Ebola capacity." *DoD News, Defense Media Activity.* http://www.defense.gov/News-Article-View/Article/603780.

Perez, Chris. 2014. "Machete-wielding mob kills 2 over Ebola testing." *New York Post.* http://nypost.com/2014/10/22/machete-wielding-mob-kills-2-over-ebola-testing/.

Rajagopalan, Megha. 2014. "China to Send Elite Army Unit to Help Fight Ebola in Liberia." *Reuters.* http://www.reuters.com/article/us-health-ebola-china-idUSKBN0IK0N020141031.

Rashid, Ismail. 2011. "Epidemics and resistance in colonial Sierra Leone during the First World War." *Canadian Journal of African Studies/La Revue Canadienne Des Études Africaines* 45(3): 415–39. http://www.tandfonline.com/doi/abs/10.1080/00083968.2011.10541064#.Vw6AMxMrLOY.

Redfield, Peter. 2015. "Medical vulnerability, or where there is no kit." *Limn* 1(5). http://limn.it/medical-vulnerability-or-where-there-is-no-kit/

Ruble, Kayla. 2014. "Ebola riots in Sierra Leone highlight marginalized youth population." *Vice News.* https://news.vice.com/article/ebola-riots-in-sierra-leone-highlight-marginalized-youth-population.

Searcey, Dionne. 2015. "The last place on Earth with Ebola: Getting Guinea to zero." *New York Times*, November 6. http://www.nytimes.com/2015/11/07/world/africa/the-last-place-on-earth-with-ebola-guineas-fight-to-get-to-zero.html.

Shaw, Rosalind. 2002. *Memories of the slave trade: Ritual and the historical imagination in Sierra Leone.* Chicago: University of Chicago Press.

Shepler, Susan. 2015. "Community organized checkpoints." *Sierra Leone's Invisible War (Blog).* http://slinvisiblewar.blogspot.com/2015/01/community-organized-checkpoints.html.

Smirl, Lisa. 2008. "Building the other, constructing ourselves: Spatial dimensions of international humanitarian response." *International Political Sociology* 2(3): 236–53.

Stephens, Carolyn. 1991. "Back to basics: A community-based environmental health project in West Point, Monrovia, Liberia." *Environment and Urbanization* 3(1): 140–46.

Thomas, Abdul. 2014. "Army Major Palo Conteh to soon become head of state." *Sierra Leone Telegraph*, October 26. http://www.thesierraleonetelegraph.com/?p=7852.

Tiezzi, Shannon. 2014. "China's Military Wages War on Ebola." *The Diplomat.* http://thediplomat.com/2014/10/chinas-military-wages-war-on-ebola/.

Turay, Bankolay. 2015. "An invisible war." *On Our Radar.* http://www.onourradar.org/ebola/2015/01/29/bankolay-turay-an-invisble-war/.

UN Security Council. 2014. Resolution 2177.

Wilkinson, A., and M. Leach. 2014. "Briefing: Ebola—Myths, realities, and structural violence." *African Affairs* 114(454): 136–48.

Woods, Samuel Kofi. 2015. "AFL Day keynote address." *The Inquirer (Monrovia)*, February 11. http://allafrica.com/stories/201502121692.html.

Zohoori, Cameron. 2011. "In pictures: Liberian Hip-Co." *Al Jazeera.* http://www.aljazeera.com/indepth/inpictures/2011/08/201188114721700943.html

A Few Days in July

LINDIS HURUM

July 26, 2014—Monrovia, Liberia

The dial tone sounds repeatedly.[1] Reminiscent of church bells, my heartbeat seems to be as long as every dial tone. As usual, it is raining— it rains every damned day—and I am soaked to the skin. I am standing outside, because I do not want anyone to listen to my conversation.

Finally, Marie-Christine, head of the MSF Emergency Pool in distant Belgium, answers. It is Saturday evening and I can hear from her voice that she is expecting bad news, like every time I call. Every day since I arrived four weeks ago has contained bad news. This time, however, the news is worse than ever. "Marie-Christine, Dr. Kent has tested positive for Ebola." "Oh no." Not much more needed to be said to express the despair this information provoked; we both knew instantly this would have a huge impact on our operations here. In her usual comforting and calm way, she urged me to investigate how this could have happened and if any in our team could have been exposed to the virus as well. She ended the call by affirming we are ready to do everything we can to help evacuate him home

I have just returned from the office of Samaritan's Purse, where Kendell, the head of its operations in Liberia, let me know that Kent has contracted Ebola. Kendell must be well over six feet tall. His hair and his well-groomed beard are both gray, and he speaks with the kind of serene baritone voice I'm thinking you often hear in people who are very strong in their belief in Jesus. His demeanor was calm when we spoke, but the knuckles on his folded hands were white and I could see that he had been crying.

Lance, the project manager of Samaritan's Purse who flew in from Texas when we decided to work together to build and run a new and bigger Ebola center, keeps taking his black baseball cap off and putting it on again, as if he's struggling to make it fit properly on his head. He is rubbing his hands—his eyes are red too—before he finally sits down, his head hanging heavy from his shoulders as if it were a lead ball on a pendulum. I want to give them a hug, but I cannot. Touching one another on an Ebola mission is forbidden.

Our collaboration with Samaritan's Purse is a rather peculiar one. It is an American organization with a strong religious foundation and politically conservative; MSF is religiously neutral and fiercely politically independent. We find ourselves on the opposite ends of the spectrum of aid organizations, but we have found common ground in our shared commitment to stop Ebola. We share both humanitarian principles and a self-proclaimed mandate to help individuals in need. It is also an improbable collaboration, in the sense that MSF normally doesn't collaborate this closely with anyone; we stubbornly prefer to do everything ourselves, as this is usually faster and we can operate exactly the way we want. Other organizations, sometimes justly, perceive us as a rather arrogant organization. Samaritan's Purse shared this opinion until we issued a desperate call for help in June, as we had no more resources ourselves to fight the virus. The people at Samaritan's Purse were the only ones to resolutely raise their hand and declare their willingness to help. "We have never worked with Ebola, but we are willing to help if you hold our hands and guide us through it." It was a courageous offer we could not refuse, and since then we have tried to work hand in hand, albeit with protective gloves, in the fight against Ebola.

Samaritan's Purse has been working in Liberia for over 15 years. Among other projects, it has been a faithful supporter of the private missionary hospital "Eternal Love Winning Africa," or ELWA (as it is more commonly referred to). We have no more doctors to send, but they do. We train their staff and draw the blueprints for a new Ebola treatment center according to our standards; they send more people, they provide additional funds and together we start construction. Different forces drive us, but that doesn't matter because our motivations are strong enough to compel both of our organizations to go far beyond our comfort zones. They are pleasantly surprised by how agreeable we can be in person, and we are equally surprised by how many dirty jokes they find funny. We make fun of each other while we build a small team bridging the gap between godliness and secularism, bound together in our work to save the people of Monrovia from Ebola. Dr. Kent bravely ran a small Ebola clinic in the chapel belonging to Samaritan's Purse when we arrived in June after having received training from a small MSF team in April. He followed the rules to the letter and knew the guidelines by heart. We have recently moved the patients to a bigger building that was supposed to become a new kitchen and laundry room for the hospital, but which now has been turned into a reception center for Ebola patients instead. Dr. Kent is one of the key people in the running of what we call ELWA 2: an Ebola treatment center run in collaboration between the Ministry of Health, Samaritan's Purse, and MSF. Alone, none of us has the resources to operate an Ebola center, but together we are able to make it work.

Dr. Kent is the kind of blond-haired and bearded guy you can easily imagine trekking for miles in the mountains without tiring. He is just lanky enough to give me the urge to serve him doughnuts and hot chocolate every time I see him. He is a part of our team now, and he spends every day working with our Dr. Sarah from Belgium, who arrived here recently as a much-needed reinforcement.

Now he is locked away in his small house, with only the fever and a bolted door to keep him company. Ebola.

A few hours later, Kendell calls again to tell me that Nancy has contracted Ebola too. Nancy is an older woman who helps out at ELWA 2, mainly with sterilizing the equipment we reuse, such as boots and protective goggles. For the first time in history, two Americans have been infected with Ebola. I know this will change everything.

July 27, 2014

The atmosphere in the room was thick as porridge during this morning's meeting in the Ministry of Health. The news about Kent and Nancy was received with bewildered uneasiness. For a while, no one spoke. The silence was heavy, as if empty cartoon speech bubbles were floating around the room, and I tried to fill them with the cold facts of the case: we were not able to evacuate them from the country because no insurance companies would take on the task. In a neutral voice, I inform those present that Kent and Nancy's conditions have worsened during the course of the night, Samaritan's Purse has pulled all its staff from ELWA 2 until we can ascertain whether anyone else has been infected, and the center is now severely understaffed, as we still only have one doctor and two sanitation experts from MSF. I rub my aching neck with my hand—the same hand with which I had promised to hold Kent's—and I add that nothing like this has ever happened in our organization, despite having worked with Ebola for over 20 years.

The Minister of Health asks us whether the equipment we use is truly safe. He questions whether our "golden guidelines" are actually good enough. My gaze wanders and finds the ice-blue eyes of Kevin from CDC [the U.S. Centers for Disease Control and Prevention]. He saves me by asserting that if it were so, we would have a lot more cases on our hands. "A human error has probably occurred." I certainly feel like a human error.

Before we have time to dwell on what has happened, I receive a phone call from the staff of our Ebola center in the north, close to the Guinean border, which we also run in collaboration with Samaritan's Purse. They call to inform us that they are in the process of evacuating across the river to our project in neighboring Guinea. One of their teams has been attacked not far from their clinic. They were on their way to pick up an Ebola patient when an angry mob set fire to the ambulance and assaulted the driver with a hammer. They are now surrounded by the mob, who refuses to allow them to pass. The mob believes that we, the white people, have brought Ebola to their country. There appears to be no limit to how much bad news a single day can bring.

July 28, 2014

"In 48 hours there will be no place left for Liberia to send their Ebola patients," I inform Dr. Nestor from WHO [the World Health Organization]. He is only there because, after some effort, I managed to persuade him to attend an emergency meeting with Kevin, Kendell, and myself. We are almost alone in the cafeteria of the Health Ministry. We drink bitter coffee, and Nestor has helped himself to a piece of cake with an overly sweet pink glazing. He looks at me and nods. Not one muscle in his face stirs. I lean in, as close as I can get without actually touching him, and repeat: "Do you understand what I'm telling you? In 48 hours, there will be no isolation center for Ebola in the entire country. Not a single one. Zero." He pulls out a notepad and writes "48 hrs. SP leaving." He thanks us for the information. For a split second, I imagine my hands encircling his thick neck and squeezing. Instead, I ask him what he is planning to do about it.

Kevin makes an effort to explain, expressing himself in a different way in order to make him comprehend the gravity of the situation. "After the last couple of day's tragic occurrences, Samaritan's Purse has decided to evacuate its entire staff, completely withdrawing from the country. MSF still does not have the capacity to run an Ebola center all by itself, and without support from SP, it is far too dangerous to be at ELWA 2, which is drowning in patients. In the morgue, the body bags are piling up in stacks." I add that if none of us is there to ensure safe patient care and sufficient supplies of protective equipment, it is likely that many of the public health workers will not dare to show up for work. Far too risky. From Wednesday, the patients may therefore be left to fend for themselves. Kevin and I request that Dr. Nestor take responsibility and tell his superiors in Geneva that I am right when I say that things are already out of control, that the time for WHO to sound the alarm is far overdue. This is not something Liberia can handle by itself. WHO needs to take the lead now. His response is a shrug of his shoulders as he rises and leaves the cafeteria. If I were to sum up WHO's involvement in this crisis so far, this would be it: a shrug.

Kendell tells me he is filled with guilt, but headquarters has ordered them home. His fingers hammer at the table. I look at the freckles on his hand, the hand I promised to hold.

This was but a few hours ago, and now I have just met with my little team consisting of two doctors and two water and sanitation experts, plus the two new arrivals of today—one administrator to help with salaries and recruitment and an anthropologist who will be in charge of health promotion, working on how to change attitudes in the local population.

Even before sitting down, Dr. Sarah declared that this is by far the worst scenario she has ever seen—and this is her third Ebola project. She likens ELWA 2 to the gates of hell; there are dying patients lying side by side with the deceased that no one has taken care of. There is no room for more people, living or dead. Outside, people are lying under the trees, waiting to be admitted. Other patients let them in when the guards are not looking. There is a desperate lack of experienced health personnel now that Samaritan's Purse has left. Sara doesn't feel safe. We are struggling to respect our own rules, as we are overworked and short on staff.

I listen to Cokie, the experienced British water and sanitation expert, describing the horrific scenario, telling us that it is pure hell. She is normally witty and fun, but now she looks gray and pale, completely exhausted. I am forced to make their day even worse; I have to tell them that Kent has started bleeding and has become weaker, that the chances of evacuating the two are slim. No countries will permit them to transit or even let them into their airspace. Irrational, global panic. Kent and Nancy have both accepted that they will die here. Sara and Cokie are crying. I gaze at our small team and think how insignificant we are in comparison with the slow, viral tsunami descending upon us. We might have managed to run a small clinic, but a center with 120 beds, like the one we are building now, is impossible. It is too dangerous. We always have to weigh our safety against the actual possibility of making a real difference, of saving lives. I ask my team what they want to do: Should we remain, capable only of advising the authorities, or should we too leave, believing the danger to our lives is greater than our ability to make a difference?

It feels like the virus is everywhere, surrounding us, an invisible enemy threatening us no matter where we are. It is an impossible choice, but we agree to leave. Could we perhaps mobilize more personnel so that we can return soon? Maybe our cries for help will be better heard from Brussels? Marie-Christine says what I knew she would say—that it is my choice and that she supports me no matter what. "Always the right to leave, never the obligation to stay" is our carved-in-stone, most fundamental safety principle.

July 29, 2014

The Minister of Health is a former surgeon in his 70s. When he was appointed, he probably had his mind set on a quiet and comfortable end to his career, filled with public receptions and a decent salary. I bet he feels cheated now that the laurels have been replaced with the responsibility of stopping a raging, deadly virus. His demeanor toward me has been pleasant ever since he received me in the leather sofa in his large office on my first day here, July 1. In this first meeting a few weeks ago, he informed me that he placed his trust in me, in MSF. He spoke with great warmth about everything we did during the years of war and conflict: that we were the only ones who did not go back home, and that once again, we are their saviors.

Now he is punching the table, repeatedly, standing up and yelling at me with such force that pearls of spit fall on the polished table between us. "If you have decided to leave, do so at once. Get out, we don't need you anyway!" He is right. I'm useless. I feel my neck burning, a deep red patch of shame.

A few hours later, the car drops me off right outside the entrance of the Department of Internal Affairs. I wash my hands in chlorine and send my handbag through the security; my temperature is measured with a temperature gun held against my temple. I think the people who invented this instrument should have created a design that does not evoke associations of being shot. But even a plastic gun pointed to my head has become routine now. Over the last weeks, everything has become routine. I am operating on autopilot. I have never washed my hands this often or this thoroughly. It is like a fixation, paired with an obsession to avoid all bodily contact. For a month I have not given nor received a single hug, shaken a single hand, or held a single person in my arms. The speed with which that rule became an internalized reflex perplexes me. It is odd how it is possible to get used to avoiding the touch of fellow human beings. Fearing other people's skin. Frightened of a hug.

The great, marbled-floored hall is nearly empty. I am late. A guard pulls aside the massive, moss green curtains covering the doors to the conference room. Behind them, a layer of red velvet drapes the room, where a large assembly is seated. There must be several hundred in attendance; they are tightly packed around the tables arranged in a horseshoe pattern. I recognize the American ambassador, the head of the UN forces, heads of departments, and other people with position and power within the country. They are all recently appointed members of the president's new Ebola task force. This is their first meeting, and any illusions I harbored that this was to be a smaller, more efficient working group are immediately shattered. This is as official and inefficient as it gets.

I feel slightly out of place, wearing my large MSF vest over a, fortunately, clean shirt, but my trousers are covered in chlorine spots and my hair is frizzy with sweat and rain. I scan the room, find Kendell and Lance, and hurry across the room to them. I see my name on a chair, take my seat quickly and feel my hands tingle from stress, heat, and raging thoughts. I try smiling at Lance; he looks down at the floor. Kendell gives a silent nod. His eyes are red, his hands folded. Lance is holding his iPhone, manically turning it on and off, making the screen image of his wife and children continually disappear and reappear. Again and again.

Ellen Johnson Sirleaf, president of Liberia—or President Ellen as we know her— speaks into the microphone, hands it over to someone else, takes it back. Their voices are somber—I register words like *serious, deaths, help, need, funerals.* However, I am unable to follow the discussion, as my mind is firmly fixed on what I am about to stand up and proclaim—that we are leaving, that MSF lacks the staff and Ebola experts to remain here, that we cannot help them. My hands are sweaty; I rub them against my trousers, where the imprint of my hand remains clearly visible for a few seconds before disappearing into the orange linen.

Suddenly, Kendell rises. This large white man who has been living here in Liberia for the last 14 years gets up and speaks into a microphone someone hands him: "Monrovia is my home. You are my people. My family belongs here. Nevertheless, we have to leave." His voice is cracking, he emits a sobbing sound and he draws his coarse hand across his eyes, but I can still see his tears. I shut my eyes to stop my own. Kendell, in an unsteady voice, explains that two of his colleagues are gravely ill from Ebola. He tells the story of his other colleagues in the north, who were attacked by angry villagers believing Samaritan's Purse to be the cause of the virus. He says that they are in far over their heads. That they are in shock and grief. That the headquarters has requested that they go home to recover, to head home in order to return stronger. It does not sound particularly convincing.

But his thanks, his words of pain and sorrow and how much it breaks his heart to have to leave are beyond doubt. President Ellen thanks him, tells him she understands, and expresses sympathy for his colleagues who have fallen ill. She says all the right words, but her face is drawn. She looks weighed down, older. She falls heavily back into her chair, her hand fleetingly touching her forehead. The room is completely quiet. It is strange how so many people can make so little noise.

I get up quickly and as I stand there, with hundreds of eyes upon me, I experience a change of heart and I hear myself saying, "I am very sorry that we haven't been able to help you more; that we don't have more doctors or experts. I know we have far too little to offer as of now, but I promise that we will stay nonetheless. MSF stayed for the whole duration of the war; we will stay in this war too." A shared, inaudible sigh comes from the assembly. It feels like a window has been opened and the air has become a bit lighter.

It is impossible to leave. I understood that if we leave, they will lose hope. Our mere presence—that our logo is seen on a few cars or on my chest during meetings—gives some sort of hope. Nevertheless, it also feels like a betrayal, as I know that we are not doing enough. The responsibility that comes with our logo, especially in this country, is enormous. I feel that I am letting them down with each passing day. But I have to stay. It is possible that the others in this room are relieved by what I have said, but I feel the weight of tremendous responsibility pressing me back into the chair.

Afterwards, many approach me to express their sincere gratitude. The president thanks me and tells me she trusts me. It is absurd— they are standing in the middle of an escalating catastrophe and are thanking me for being here, even though my contribution can do nothing to stop the imminent wave of Ebola that threatens to engulf the country, to drown us all. Do they not understand that at this very moment, the virus is looking for new, unsuspecting bodies in which it can live and thrive, while the body dies? And while the victims are dying, the virus spreads to the next of kin who love the bleeding and dying victims so deeply that they cannot resist holding and hugging them. Ebola is the mass murderer that kills through love.

I feel deceitful, and I am barely able to receive all the gratitude, repeating that I hope that we can do more soon. If I were the president, I would have reproached me, not thanked me.

Back in our house I have to tell the team that yesterday's decision no longer stands, that it is impossible for MSF to abandon the Liberians now. I tell them that everyone is free to leave, even the ones who are not at the end of their mission.

No one leaves.

Note

1. This essay has been translated from Norwegian from Lindis Hurum's book "Det finnes ingen de andre, det er bare oss," ("There are no 'the others', there is only us") the chapter entitled "Monrovia." It is being translated and republished with the kind permission of the Cappelen Damm publishing house.

THE SYSTEM

3

The "Humanitarian" Response to the Ebola Epidemic in Guinea

Between Routines and Exceptions

JEAN-FRANCOIS CAREMEL, SYLVAIN LANDRY B. FAYE,
AND RAMATOU OUEDRAOGO

"Exception" was probably one of the words most commonly used to describe the Ebola epidemic that hit West Africa between 2013 and 2016. The term denotes a number of truths:

- The unprecedented number of cases and deaths associated with the virus
- The size of the areas affected
- The fear it caused in the region and beyond its borders
- The initial delay in responding, followed by the *en masse* international response
- The methods used in this response, with the resulting "resistance"[1] by the people
- The disease's visibility in political arenas and the international press

But "exception" is not simply a description of the situation. The term also provides an essential framework of interpretation.[2] The discourse that results is both normative and performative at the same time: *exception* is useful for describing a situation but also organizing an regime of action. In this chapter, we will examine this "exceptionality" and focus on it as a central theme to explore, from the ground, the international response processes around the epidemic. In doing so we propose going beyond the presentation of the response as a formulaic "blockbuster"[3] event incorporating epidemic, international engagement, emergency response, protective/quarantine measures, local and international actors, and so on. Instead we seek to explore, "from the ground up," what lay behind the *economics of technical and scientific promise*[4] that created (or prevented) the capacity to link (or not) humanitarian aid, industry, public and nonprofit research, emergency rationales and local perceptions, geopolitical challenges, states, and nongovernmental organizations (NGOs).

Using "exception" in discourses on epidemics is a form of engagement and a common, or even permanent, form of narrative of both "humanitarian ethics" (Fassin 2010) and global health (Lakoff 2010). Exception is evoked in HIV, the 2005 food crisis in Niger (Crombé and Jezequel 2007), the tsunami in Southeast Asia, the landslides in South America (Revet 2009), the issue of asylum seekers, victims of sexual violence (Fassin 2010), and so on. Looking at the extensive use of this semantic in the management of the Ebola response enables us to explore the underlying aid processes and to ask, in this particular case, what was (or was not) exceptional about them. The anthropological materials we will use in this article come from interviews and observations made in Conakry, Foyah, and Forécariah, Guinea, during the summer of 2015. This fieldwork concerned the stories created by different social groups around the epidemic, enabling us to compile the experiences of a variety of people involved in the epidemic and its management (e.g., members of the national coordination team, NGOs, international institutions, survivors, affected or unaffected families, community leaders). Using these data, we will examine an interlinked and apparently contradictory phenomenon: the "exceptional" nature of the epidemic resulted in major mistrust by international players regarding local "state" capacity and led to rationales and to structure the response with routines and aid bureaucratization, that were not remotely exceptional. Exceptionality also led to mistrust among international players in how to manage an "evil" (Ebola) whose etiology and causality were disputed. In other words, by reviewing the narratives and response measures, we will look beyond the media image to what was actually "exceptional", or not, in the epidemic response.

We will look at these issues in three stages. In the section that follows, we will review the methods of risk construction. We will explore the humanitarian and biosafety construction of Ebola and the way in which the resulting interpretations are based on failings in state functions in the countries where the aid community was operating. This premise for action would appear to contradict the many local/popular explanations for the epidemic, which are based on distinct relations/perception of the state and its powers. This discrepancy between popular and biomedical perceptions of the epidemic and its responses will help us in the second part to explore how the legitimacy of a humanitarian response program is constructed and to explain the central role that standardized models and routines play in it. These are complex systems and "travelling model" that, when applied to local and often misrepresented contexts, construct partial chronicles of success foretold (Olivier de Sardan, in press). To conclude, we will demonstrate that, barring a few exceptions, the "exceptional" dimension of the Ebola epidemic response seems to refer more to a traditional type of "government of exceptions" rather than "government by exceptions" (Nguyen 2009).

Forms of Risk Construction and Epidemic Response Methods, or How Biomedicine Was Overwhelmed by Popular Perceptions

Although scientific research has, since the 1970s, constructed the "natural" biological existence of the Ebola virus,[5] the specifics of the epidemic that hit West Africa from 2013 to 2016 posed challenges that were as much social and political as they were technical and medical. That is why a socio-technical analysis (Akrich 1991) of the material expressions of the response is essential. In Guinea and the other West African countries, the epidemic systematically impelled a range of technical and medical measures (e.g., images and posters, awareness messages, handwashing systems and lotions, Ebola treatment centers, protective suits, ambulances, body bags) that, by their associations with the disease, in many ways came to symbolize it, (re)shape its contours, and modify its realities/perceptions.

The analysis of the sociotechnical frameworks (e.g., technologies, treatment centers, coordination meetings, projects and logical framework, quarantine areas, vaccine trials) permits an exploration of the many interpretations given to the measures of the response Apparatus (*Dispositif*).[6] If we are to give them a voice, and also take what they have to say seriously, the narratives of the actors about their experiences of the epidemic and responses to it provide a door to their rationalizations that shed light on the discrepancies between biomedical and popular perceptions. It then becomes possible to go beyond interpretations of locals based on "resistance;" although these are very convenient in justifying the limitations of the response, they sterilize the analysis and limit advances in practices (Faye 2015; Bradol 2016).[7]

The Interpretation by the Aid Community: Ebola Between Biosafety and Humanitarian Issues

The international response to the epidemic was based on forms of risk construction that refer to two standard rationales for global health interventions: biosafety and humanitarian objectives (Lakoff 2010). These rationales and resulting responses by the aid community sometimes (if not often) present two contradictions: the difficult link between these two justifications and the discrepancy they often represent with local perceptions, which we will explore in the next section. Humanitarian and biosafety rationales clashed in the field and were highly controversial, sometimes within the humanitarian teams and particularly within the medical teams. It is these negotiations that one can follow, for example in the change from the name "quarantine zones" to "surveillance zones" in the vaccination trial, or in the heated discussions within MSF in 14 letters published on the MSF Intranet in response to the open internal letter "Ebola: A challenge to our humanitarian identity" (Balasegaram et al., 2014) examining MSF's response to the epidemic. The same tension is seen in practice, be it in the Ebola treatment centers, during health education campaigns, or through the definition of national and international policies; the priority given to humanitarian versus safety rationales involved a complex balancing act.[8]

On the one hand, the virus and the epidemic are essentially seen as a threat to global biosafety.[9] This argument linked the virus to failings in health monitoring services, poor hygiene measures, severe overcrowding, individual travel, and the "cultural resistance" of the people. It framed the response as a fight against a wide-scale contamination representing a major threat in the epicenter, and a risk for countries in the subregion. This approach led to measures focused on surveillance and local and international quarantine to contain a proven threat.

On the other hand, the response to the epidemic as a humanitarian issue creates different imperatives. Because the virus exposes people to direct risks (contamination, death) and indirect risks (rising food insecurity, increased mortality from other diseases with the dysfunction of health systems), it involves humanitarian emergency responses. These responses articulate a need for compassion and at the same time impel reduction in the risks taken by those involved in the response. This engagement, unlike the first, reflects a form of transnational civic response to general dysfunction in the global system that should be regulated through direct action (in this case treatment), sounding the alerts, and witness accounts.[10]

In the field, the domination of one interpretation over the other changed, depending on the space available in the treatment facilities, the deployment level of the responders, their objectives and resources, their respective influence and their alliances, the number of countries affected by the epidemic, the developments in scientific knowledge, the possibilities of diagnosis and treatment, and (the lack of) communications.

But while there are undeniable differences between the biosafety and humanitarian rationales,[11] it should be noted that they both resulted in the following phenomena being considered as problems during the response to the epidemic:

- Travel, whether regular, local travel (e.g., visiting family) or forced or migratory travel
- Certain traditional practices (e.g., funeral rites) or routine practices (eating habits, individual hygiene) not meeting biomedical hygiene requirements
- Limited access to basic services

This method of risk construction encouraged an interpretation essentially focused on the incapacity or "failure" of the state that was "incapable of keeping its population in one place," of "changing traditions and promoting good hygiene practices," and of "guaranteeing the operation of the health systems." This interpretation legitimized the rationales behind the provision of the aid provided by international players. During the Ebola epidemic, as in many other cases, the supposed failure of the state[12] largely ignores its actual modes of its local expressions (Biershenck and Olivier de Sardan 1993) and the operation of the state "under an aid regime" as an underlying cause of their fragility. This rationale removes, fairly systematically, the role of international policies as one of the causes of the problem (Chabrol 2014), making it possible to confine exclusively aid as a solution in an emergency situation.[13]

The Six Major Popular Categories of Explanation for the Disease and the Reactions to the Aid Measures

The bases of health and biomedical response were simple yet difficult to reconcile with the many local interpretations of the disease and the epidemic that prevailed, for example, in Conakry and in the coastal region of Guinea. As already highlighted in other works, the perceptions of the disease and the interpretation of the response apparatus measures deployed by the aid community and the Guinean State were out of sync with popular perceptions and expectations.[14] Contrary to the interpretation by the responders, the "beneficiaries" were nearly always the first to react[15] to the epidemic, well before any international measures were deployed. This initial reaction involved the use of protective and isolation rationales, far from the wait-and-see attitude and passiveness ascribed in awareness and health education messages,[16] the majority of the time, to the populations, as well as treatment response strategies. Ignorance and, even more so, misunderstanding of these local strategies explain some of the "hostility" to which the Apparatus (*Dispositif*) and the apparatus measures became "victim" (Anoko 2014; Faye 2015). In seeking to understand the rationales behind the popular reactions, we were able to empirically identify six major recurring patterns for explaining the disease and the reactions to measures against it. Although several of these explanations may be used successively by a single interviewee during an interview and, perhaps also because they were open and complementary, these categories of interpretation of the international response can help shed new light on the rationales behind the local mistrust in Guinea toward the medical and prevention measures and their implementers.

Witch Doctor State

One of the prevailing explanations for the epidemic is that it is a manifestation of a witch doctor state, an occult power. The history of Guinea is largely interpreted by local populations from two angles, (1) that of the manipulation and mismanagement of successive governments and (2) that of the predatory extraction strategies by major powers. The recurring "magical-religious" explanations during interviews underscore the beliefs and mentalities in which the *conspiracy economy* figures prominently. Ebola is part of these occult interpretations and reinforces them.

The explanation of the epidemic's emergence in Guinea is based on a central argument: a postcolonial "white" conspiracy, a local origin of the disease introduced to the country by the government to retain control.[17] From this angle, Ebola (and the Apparatus) is interpreted as a means used by the president to win the local elections and legitimize the use of armed forces. These explanations are consistent with the interpretation of Guinea's history as a "victim" of the terms of its independence, the desire for its mining resources, and the aspirations of its politicians.

This interpretation is supported by the popular explanation of the spatial dynamics of Ebola. Its appearance in the forest and expansion to coastal Guinea and the fact that it spared Kankan, the region of origin of the president, is interpreted as a sign of historical revenge for Conté's (Sousou) repression of Diara's (Malinké) 1985 coup attempt.[18]

The geography of this "evil" is bolstered by highly local explanations for the disease. Some youth demonstrations are partly explained by the observation that it was women who were dying in the Ebola treatment centers, which reinforced the idea of an international conspiracy whereby the disease was a method by foreign powers to wipe out the Guinean people and attain its rich mining resources.

The focus on witch doctor/occult rationales partly explains the fear of the Ebola treatment centers. Those providing medical care and the response measures are considered to be linked with death, not just because of the absence of treatment available for the disease but also due to widespread rumors that Ebola was transmitted by the medications and injections that are given at Ebola treatment centers, so that the body can be used for harvesting organs (e.g., genitals, hands, eyes) that are sold on as part of the preparations to ensure financial success, political success, and so forth.

The same goes for the strategies aimed at reducing contamination from dead bodies. For example, the suspension of traditional, ritual funeral practices and the requirement to use body bags in "safe and dignified burials"[19] is interpreted as a strategy by the government to prevent the deceased's spirit from leaving the body, exposing Guineans to vengeance/'*fossi*' from beyond the grave. Likewise, by prohibiting pilgrimages to Mecca, the epidemic prevented one of the pillars of Islam, interpreted by some of our interviewees as a personal/family threat, often interpreted from an ethnic angle.[20]

Sovereign State/Police State

At the same time, the response to the epidemic is interpreted as a reassertion of the sovereign state through the manifestation of the monopoly on "legitimate" violence seen in the authoritarian nature of the Apparatus and its measures. This reassertion of the state's power over its people is particularly evident in the declaration of a state of emergency, the obligation to carry out safe and digni-fied burials for the victims of Ebola, the systematic application of this treatment for all dead bodies (including stillborn babies and drownings), the develop-ment of travel control procedures, and the monitoring of "foreigners"[21] or through the "reacquisition" of the national space by the state's central authority against local powers, with the use of armed forces to support prefects in "open-ing up" reluctant villages to allow the actors in the response "free access" to the quarantine zones.

International aid provides the resources to enable the operation of many sovereign functions of the state and the improvement of public services (armed forces, police, civil protection, epidemiological surveillance). This action strengthened the administrative network of the national territory particularly by bringing back prefectoral committees, the development of coordination plat-forms, and the engagement of mayors and community networks that are more associated with state-appointed local than with traditional local powers.

Biomedical State and Healthcare Bureaucracy

These examples illustrate the close link frequently made between aid, a police state, healthcare bureaucracy, and biopower.[22] Nevertheless, the biomedical state does have certain specific features.

Contrary to the police state, the healthcare state in the Ebola epidemic response apparatus largely concerned outsiders. It involved infiltrating the area via the omnipresence of chlorinated water buckets and sprays for disinfecting in front of all public buildings, most of the time bearing the logos of the donors, and the visual and auditory presence of ambulances (from health facilities, MSF), and funeral vehicles (Red Cross 4x4s), the intrusive free movement of the response apparatus community (screening, treatment, contact follow-up, body management, information, village and neighborhood surveillance). All these apparatuses are associated with the epidemic and act as a reminder, if not of its reality, then at the least of the methods used, which were in contrast with those available to the health system before the epidemic.

This infiltration of the territory by the "Apparatus" measures led to the construction of administrative categories for individuals (e.g., "foreigner"/resident, survivor/case/contact) and zones (e.g., risk zone, quarantine zone/surveillance zone), contributing to the rezoning and reconfiguration of the social space by the biomedical government.

The biomedical government also asserts itself as a biopolitic through its capacity to produce numbers and data that are the key focus of coordination meetings, produced by each of the services involved in the response apparatus (e.g., communications, safe and dignified burials, call centers). These are in many ways the drivers of the response apparatus, around which it organizes itself and through which it assesses itself and is assessed. These data concerning cases and contacts are, along with the funds made available to the state, the key pieces of information in the media (e.g., TV, radio). The visibility of such data contributes to the construction of one form of reality of the epidemic. The healthcare state becomes the sponsor of a biomedical police state and a form of a providence state through the money raised and distributed.

Providence State and Organizer of the "Ebola Business"

Now we come to another popular category frequently used to interpret the epidemic response, that of the "Ebola business." Even though a significant number of the people interviewed called into question the existence of Ebola, there was wide consensus that saw the epidemic response apparatus as a new avatar of the income economy of aid, income of which everyone wanted a part.

If we analyze the content of "popular" discourses, the notion of "Ebola business" systematically refers to the actors in the response who "eat Ebola money," first in line being the state, followed by all the individual "Apparatus" workers.

In local interpretations, the ability of those involved in the response apparatus, particularly the state, to harness the Ebola income is not necessarily negative; it is, so to speak, just part of the game. The state is then perceived as a providence state that, in its management of the income, plays a redistribution role, even though the majority of this redistribution is to its profit and to that of its staff. This windfall is shared among:

- Financing/salaries of temporary health workers, particularly the switch from unpaid "intern" to "international response agent" employed by international institutions (e.g., World Health Organisation, UNICEF, International Monetary Found, USAID) with high incomes

- The bonuses paid and training given to the various health system executives who are leading the coordination
- The training and/or short contracts for awareness or surveillance actions for taxi unions, imams, and the police, which provide opportunities to pay daily allowances and thereby help improve the end-of-month pay of these categories
- The same goes for community engagement with village surveillance groups, neighborhood surveillance groups, and community workers.

By becoming a form of income, "Ebola money" gradually became less problematic and everyone hoped to "eat it," as is the case with other emergency and development aid project money.

Operator and Predator State

The Ebola response is, in popular perceptions, a source of income. It is redistributed by the state or the response apparatus community. Nevertheless, for a large number of those interviewed affected by the response apparatus measures, particularly the many who doubted the existence of Ebola, there is a major discrepancy between the funds raised in the fight against Ebola, and which were heavily reported on the television and radio, and the funds actually deployed in the field.

Here the discourse shifts from providence state to operator state, or even broker state (Sardan and Biershenk 1993), whose goal is to maintain its predatory power. Many illustrations were collected from the field[23] highlighting that "everyone is eating Ebola money," money that arrived in huge quantities and that fueled an urgently mounted response that remained largely ineffective in the eyes of the players, especially with regard to the resources it was consuming.

Collaborator State / State Under Aid Regime

In the epidemic response apparatus, the forms of police and healthcare state, in other words the biomedical and police powers, found, due to the methods of financing public policies in Guinea, a vast majority of their resources under another form of state: the state under an aid regime, portrayed as a collaborating power.

Indeed, the Ebola response apparatus underscores the financial and technical dependency of the Guinean state in the implementation of responses that aim to preserve the lives of the people it is responsible for. This asymmetry in its response capacity led to coordination methods that made the Guinean state a state "under an aid regime." An examination of the methods of organizing the response apparatus reveals the predominant role of United Nations agencies (e.g., WHO, UNICEF) and international nongovernmental organizations (e.g., MSF, Action Against Hunger, Save the Children). The omnipresence of these organizations is particularly significant in peripheral coordination facilities, where they accounted for two thirds of the participants at meetings and the vast majority of the resources used (Fig. 3-1).

This typology resulting from the interviews makes the complexity and diversity of the local perceptions of the disease more explicit. It also sheds light on the popular view of the "Apparatus" and helps explain the reactions to the prevention and treatment measures deployed, which were quite out of sync with local perceptions.

Varying Reasons for Mistrust Toward the State and the Many Consequences

This difference in interpretations by international players and local players nevertheless shares a common point. Whether they be popular or emanating from the transnational health system, the explanation for and the response to

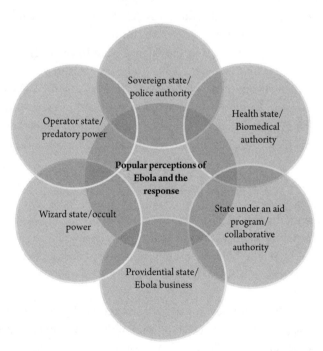

Figure 3-1 Synthesis of different popular perceptions of state power in the response to the epidemic.

the epidemic differ on the role and function of the state. Faced with the emergency, local interpretations essentially speak of the dysfunctional operation[24] of a state power that remains very present. Conversely, the interpretations by international players suggest rather the nonfunction, real or expected, of a sovereign and social state that is seen as (nearly) absent. While these interpretations both reflect mistrust toward the state,[25] they are very different. On the one hand, popular perceptions tend to interpret the epidemic, with its many explanations and apparatuses, as the manifestation of a state power that has always been present and that is acquiring, via the "Apparatus," new resources that are reinforcing its violent and intrusive power. Conversely, the interpretations at the basis of the aid community's response strategies assume a lack of a sovereign and especially socially responsive state, which leads them to position themselves either as an alternative[26] or as a support on the state's return.[27]

Routine in Emergencies and the Urgency for Routines: Ebola, Journey of a Partial Success Foretold

These Ebola risk construction methods and the oft-examined balance between biosafety and humanitarian strategies provided a very strong, implicit foundation on which to structure the organization of the epidemic response apparatus. Indeed, mistrust in the capacity of the state, considered a "failure" by the aid community, is a strong motive for legitimizing its work and offers a structural framework for designing the response strategies. In the emergency, the states affected by the epidemic were often, explicitly or implicitly, considered "incapable." As such, they had to be replaced by humanitarian players or helped by them to make a comeback and reassert themselves.[28] It is here that, in the epidemic response, a form of state within a state, a nongovernmental state (Nguyen 2010), comes into being.

The Nongovernmental State, Reasons and Methods at Local Level

This nongovernmental state is based on an initial double negation, not just of the state, as we have briefly mentioned, but also of the community. This double negation does not lead to a void but to a process of reconstruction-renegotiation of these two entities by the aid community.

The initial negation of the "community" is particularly sensitive and paradoxical. This becomes evident when looking at the aid community's (non) recognition of local strategies initially used against the disease (essentially organized by family members, neighbors, authorities, and local health staff, whether they practiced traditional medicine or biomedicine). These initiatives were at best ignored, or at worst undermined and disparaged in the name of the risk incurred and the primacy of biomedical competence in this field. This initial negation is especially contradictory given that the notion of "community engagement" is at the heart of aid rhetoric in general and was particularly so in the epidemic response. There are many types of participation rhetoric, community "activation" encouraged by the international aid community in the field: community motivators, Comités de Veille Villageois (village surveillance groups), Comités de Veille de Quartier (neighborhood surveillance committees), operational units, and so forth. Initially restricted to the villages and neighborhoods affected by Ebola, they were rapidly extended across the entire territory, becoming an exogenous network and control measure. "Local participation" in the epidemic response apparatus as part of this measure is based on a local destruction-reconstruction process implemented by the aid programs. Be it intentional (which is rarely the case) or otherwise, this discrediting of popular responses is based on contradictory images of the community as both ignorant and needing to be enlightened and empowered, and united, which is embodied by community participation and demonstrated by "voluntary" engagement.[29]

This dominant interpretation[30] of the "community" led to an initial move to negate-reconstruct the other, making it possible to replace its specifics with a generic approach transposable anywhere, a "travelling model." This interpretation of the "community" led to the development of a response apparatus that was not founded on local reality, expectations, or capabilities but on an image that is often illusory, or at least extremely simplified, of popular perceptions of the disease, power struggles, and the mechanisms of solidarity. A substantial part of the work by the aid community therefore consisted in gradually incorporating, with difficulty, local realities into the aid response or gradually modifying it, often by adding additional measures, at the cost of complexity for the "beneficiaries" and a significant waste of energy and resources.

This standardization process should have facilitated rapid deployment of the aid, justified by the risk of wide-scale contamination and later, when therapeutic solutions came into being, by the need for early treatment. This process, which at least initially overlooks popular perceptions and an understanding of local disease management processes, is not singular to the Ebola epidemic; on the contrary, it is fairly typical of aid rationales. In the case of Ebola, food, or nutrition crises, this is based on an attempt to relegate local strategies to the ranks of palliative care or even as a problem for aid deployment. These approaches endorse and maintain the discrepancies between the "aided" and the "aider" and lead to discourse on the need for external aid, which is based partly on a lack of understanding of the complexity of local resilience mechanisms that are often interpreted as the "resistance" of communities.

The urgency of the epidemic, the initial scarce resources, and the demands for the deployment of a rapid response largely explain the thrifty analysis of local processes and the early attempt to replace them by those of the aid community. Yet, although the strategies of these two groups are often the same (e.g., isolation, quarantine, limited contacts, specific hygiene measures), their physical and symbolic realities are not. The first uses local resources and people, whereas the second resorts to new exogenous response measures (e.g., Ebola treatment centers, transit centers, protective clothing, body bags). The quarantine methods used by the aid community as part of the response apparatus (Le Marcis 2015a, 2015b) transformed, became standardized and then systematised during the course of the deployment of the "Apparatus." The people implementing them also rapidly changed. Local/community players were replaced by NGO workers, and other "projects" evolved under a variety of different names (community motivators, village or neighborhood surveillance committees), which covered as many functions (e.g., the Red Cross' Safe and Dignified Burial teams, contact and lost case search teams, flashers, alerters, WHO vaccination teams, mixed security teams) in which traditional players became at best auxiliaries and at worst, as was most often the case, illegitimate. This displacement is part of and reinforces the popular interpretations and explanations of the epidemic: the WHO, Red Cross, and UN agencies were linked together and working for a power state with a complex past.

In fact, the reality of this transfer of responsibility for the cure and care and the implementation of quarantine was partial. The initially scarce resources to cover needs followed by the gradual extension of the "risk" situations, particularly with the controversial systematization of safe and dignified burials, led to the continuation of primary care by the family, which was a kind of public secret (Geissler 2013; Redfield 2013). At the same time, the increase in the number of external players encouraged a second kind of quarantine. While the patients and their contacts where placed in quarantine, enclosed and monitored in centers, in a symmetrical analysis one could talk of a collective and individual self-quarantine by the responders. This resulted in the "no-touch policy" of the response's staff,[31] reinforcing the "them" and "us" rationale and making the sensitive knowledge of the operational settings illusory.

The appearance of the epidemic in Guinea with the late *en masse* international response, the forms of mutual isolation, and the challenges of coordinating the

many players involved led to a sort of extraterritorial state. Such a nongovernmental state is regularly highlighted in the interviews:

> In the beginning, we did as we wanted . . . you talked with two or three
> people [from the Ministry of Health] and you reacted . . . now that
> things are calming down, you have the state and the agencies taking
> control. (Interview in Conakry with an executive from an NGO that
> carried out a number of missions in Guinea during the epidemic, 08/
> 10/2015)

This initial "nongovernment state" phase of the epidemic's management, characterized by the presence of just a few players, is also seen as a time long ago that the
response apparatus workers remember fondly. It contrasts with the "Apparatus"
that symbolizes the "nongovernmental state," fossilized by its routines, politics,
and power struggles, as illustrated in this quote from a health worker:

> In the initial phase of the epidemic in Conakry [at a time when most of
> the humanitarian community were in the forest zone of Guinea] we had
> fewer difficulties, we were paid less, but we worked well . . . Since then,
> there are rules, regulations, but behind all that, where is the national
> sovereignty? I have often said no [to the responders], but I am just a
> technician [and there are other financial and political issues]. (Interview
> with a regional executive responsible for health management and the
> response to the epidemic, Conakry, 08/04/2015)

This initial response was gradually expanded as the epidemic ended in the
forest zone and the teams redeployed on the coast. The residents of Conakry
and the Basse-Côte then saw an increase in the symbols that represented the
response apparatus: the sirens of ministry or MSF ambulances in particular; Red
Cross vehicles loaded with burials; the rented white 4x4s with their many stick-
ers; awareness campaigns and other posters; Ebola treatment centers; door-to-
door teams; the diverse array of T-shirts, jackets, caps, and logos; the presence
of security forces or civil protection forces in/around health facilities; and more.

In this case, the apparatus deployed is similar to the healthcare system.
However, even though it often shares the same spaces (e.g., health centers, hospitals) and the same human resources (e.g., nurses, doctors), it reflects opposing rationales—mobility versus immobility, lack versus abundance of resources
and salaries—which reinforces the temptation for local health workers to find
a place within the "Apparatus."[32] Once again, this endorses the popular perceptions of an "Ebola business," all the bigger and more complex given the number
of responders involved.

The Nongovernmental State: The Strength of Aid Routines and the Conditional Return of the State

The risks inherent to the Ebola response, the complexity of any action involving multiple players demanding independence, and the challenges of rationalizing and coordinating are all reasons that are regularly given for the introduction of information sharing and regulation measures. And so, the response apparatus was soon in a situation in which the prevention measures and the complex and changing treatment measures were superimposed by an administrative system composed of many layers, clusters, focal points, and so forth at different levels, from the local (health posts) to the departmental, regional, national, and ultimately transnational levels. Those involved varied according to these various levels (with the embassies being present only at the top), but not only that. Indeed, the segmentation was not just horizontal but also vertical, with some institutions taking "the lead" over traditional functions, while others competed in their usual area of expertise (as is the case, for example, with the support of the WHO by the U.S. Centers for Disease Control and Prevention [CDC] in collecting and managing data). The approaches were segmented both geographically and thematically: UNICEF in communications, the WHO in surveillance and the management of Ebola data with new support from the CDC, MSF-Alliance for International Medical Action (ALIMA) in treatment, and the Red Cross in the management of dead bodies.

But this "structuring," although aspiring to "good governance," is also a black hole in which a large amount of time and energy were spent, often with only relative success, on key activities like information sharing, approach coordination, and data production. This organization and its output sustained a complex system that seemed to be driven by its own routines and administrative requirements (e.g., situation reports, daily data, activity reports).

The complexity of these measures and the resources they require to be represented,[33] and more importantly to be a full-fledged player, led to significant asymmetries. It is in this highly restricted context that what the fieldworkers referred to as the "return of the state" occurred. This is demonstrated by the appointment of a certain number of influential figures at the head of these measures, with the priority given to strong policy guidelines from top political figures, sometimes out of touch with the realities of the field,[34] and the return of certain administrative obligations (e.g., systematic use of mission orders approved by the administrative authorities), which often tended to add a layer of complexity to the response apparatus. Both expected and feared, this "return of the state" occurred, despite everything, in a complex system that was essentially "designed" and developed by the aid community based on their resources, administrative requirements, and operational objectives, which aimed to respond to the epidemic through interventions, while taking into consideration the contractual obligations imposed by their sponsors. Here we are confronted with the second public secret, that of the asymmetry in the partnership. We arrive, therefore, at the same conclusion concerning Ebola as that made by K. Glenzer (2007, p. 130) on the governance of early warning systems:

> Discourses on good governance thereby accomplished the feat of making governments [. . .] on the African continent responsible and accountable for the development and humanitarian assistance efforts which are, however, planned, conceptualised and standardised by international experts and financed by leaders in developed countries. In this context of "partnership," "cooperation" and "mutual support," it seems absurd for a developing state to be able to take on the system since it is supposed to fully participate in the decision process. [. . .] Ultimately, while increasing their hold over the decisions of these countries, international players gradually absolve themselves of all responsibility and obligation.

Beyond Routines, Perceptions, and Demands for Action: "Ebola Is Version 2.0 of the Emergency Bullshit"

The analysis is harsh but does sum up the consequences and the many overlapping demands for action and management of the administrative and political issues that each of the players had to address. Once again, this configuration is not specific to the epidemic response; it can be seen in many other crisis situations, be it in Niger with the 2005 food crisis or in natural disaster situations such as the earthquake and cholera epidemic in Haiti or the tsunami in Southeast Asia. But, as the people working in these contexts themselves admit, these difficulties took on new proportions with Ebola. As pointed out quite simply by an executive from a major international emergency NGO who had been in Guinea for over a year when we interviewed him about the mechanisms of the coordination, the succession of strategies driven by the UN agencies, and the challenges of reporting to donors: "Ebola is version 2.0 of the emergency bullshit."

Despite its succinct nature, this quote illustrates one of the widely recognized exceptions of the response:

> Ebola has become a profitable emergency because it has generated fear across the developed "North," so lots of money and a lot of players, not always with the capacity to spend it, or at least as one should . . . if you compare the sums injected with the [number of] positive cases, it'll bring tears to your eyes . . . all for the 18th-ranked disease in terms

of the country's mortality rate. (Interview with an executive responsible for the epidemic response from an international NGO, Conakry, August 2015)

The increase in players and donors led to a multitude of administrative procedures and coordination platforms that can be interpreted at the same time as (1) the symptoms of aid management in an increasingly complex system and (2) a consequence of the influx of players and resources. The result of this process was the development of a sizeable, and mostly non-field, administration, which sought to manage both the epidemic and the income associated with it. This further reinforced the popular perceptions of an "Ebola business."

The massive, non-field nature of the response apparatus led to an increase in response strategies and reinforced negation of the "community." This led to the term "resistance" being used to describe what was the majority of the time a discrepancy between the images constructed by the external players (and supported by the local players) of a united "community" requiring information and resources in the epidemic response, and the local realities, which were often far removed from the perceptions of the aid community and had a social complexity that found opportunity in the aid response to reorganize (and sometimes renegotiate) statuses and social positions.

Exception? Did You Say Exception?

When seeing the close link between the studies of the epidemic response and those of the anthropology of development, one can ultimately ask what was exceptional in this case. Of course, the fact that it was an Ebola epidemic of unprecedented scale tends to illustrate that the people and the aid community were dealing with an extraordinary situation. Although the initial reason for action was exceptional, what about the results of the response?

An anthropological examination of the responses that were deployed in Guinea leaves food for thought. In the unfolding response there were typical idiosyncrasies in humanitarian and biosafety responses:

- The rapid construction of an "expert" and "transportable" know-how
- Discrepancies between popular and biomedical perceptions
- A "project-based" response
- Time-consuming and inefficient coordination processes leading to the bureaucratization of the aid
- Perceptions of the community and its "engagement" and "participation" that are closer to illusory constructions and transportable models than an analysis or a rationale of action anchored in reality

In this emergency response, a certain number of factors perceived as new nevertheless came to the fore:

- The reassertion of compassionate medical research
- The collaboration between nonprofit, public, and industrial research
- An unprecedented speed-up in the development of technological and therapeutic solutions[35]
- The raising of private funds and those from philanthropic capitalism alongside public funds
- A new role for social science research in operational responses[36]

These many changes can be interpreted as a *global health* success over traditional transnational medicine, a victory that would leave hope for a promising future in which technology would compensate for the failings in health systems, in which the inefficiency of public financing would be replaced by philanthropic capitalism, and where the intellectual property rights of health products could be made common property.

This idyllic interpretation nevertheless allows us to forget a little too quickly that these changes driven by global health remain within a system of medicine that is still largely "inhospitable," more so now than ever (Jaffré and Olivier de Sardan 2003). Yet it has to be said that this reality and its asymmetries of power cannot unfortunately be solved by technological innovation or performance-based payment. There is good reason to suppose that the commitments to reinforcing the health systems of the countries affected by the epidemic provide only partial solutions by continuing to ignore the previously neglected problems of the health systems.

The revolutions expected from a crisis presented as exceptional therefore do not appear to have happened. The changes that did occur mostly took place outside of the traditional aid mechanisms, as part of fertile interindividual or inter-institutional relations. In other words, using a concept developed as part of the changes resulting from the HIV epidemic, although "the government of exceptions" was necessary in the Ebola epidemic, it seems to us that it was still far from "governement by exceptions" (Nguyen 2009), so inseparable are routines from emergency response systems.

Acknowledgments

The research for this article has been funded by the Horizon 2020 program of the European Union as part of the REACTION! project, coordinated by Hervé Raoul (US003- P4 Laboratory, Jean Mérieux-Inserm).

Notes

1. "Réticence" in French.
2. Here, *essential* should be taken in its various meanings—in other words, referring to the philosophical essence, to the common dimension of what is constitutive and intrinsic as well as to the essential medical definition of the disease whose cause remains unknown.
3. Drawing movie parallels was widely used by the press, but social science researchers also often diffused this presentation and analysis (Lachenal 2014).
4. We are borrowing the concept that Pierre Benoit Joly applies to the analysis of biotechnological innovations and applying it to humanitarian aid innovations (Caremel 2016).
5. It is interesting to note the presence of the virus in images to battle Ebola, an iconic engagement, as if it should demonstrate the existence of the virus.
6. We use the word response Apparatus (*Dispositif*), with a capital letter and in the singular, which is the very Foucauldian name that the response workers in Guinea were given to distinguish them from the response measures (*dipositifs*), without a capital letter and in the plural.
7. Here we should note that this notion of "resistance" used by the aid community to explain the limitations of their response is far from confined to Ebola. It has been used to explain the failure to use treated mosquito nets, the delay in seeking treatment, and the notion of "bad mother"/"social negligence" in the case of malnutrition.
8. The controversy around the suspension of flights to countries affected by the epidemic is a good illustration of the tension between biosafety and humanitarian issues.
9. Recognition of the impossibility of controlling the travel flows of individuals between affected countries and other countries heightened the feeling of vulnerability everywhere, making the epidemic in West Africa a transnational epidemic capable of destabilizing states nationally and internationally. This situation was confirmed by reported cases imported into Europe and America.
10. During our fieldwork in Guinea, we studied, through an anthropology of the awareness-raising messages, the difficult link between individual, local (protect your family and village), and national (protect the nation) citizenship. As this transnational citizenship was taking shape, it sought support from national citizenship.
11. It must be noted that the response to the epidemic mostly mitigated these differences, as the humanitarian aid community focused on biosafety objectives in the first phase of the epidemic, which subsequently made explanations for the shift in strategies, a shift sought by many and implemented by some, fairly complicated if not impossible.
12. For a review of the failure of the state, see Olivier de Sardan 2004.
13. In this case, the distinction between emergency and development is more a rhetorical argument than a real change.
14. These discrepancies are not limited to the Ebola epidemic: the same analyses are at the heart of anthropological works on disease.
15. It should be noted that such phenomena are regularly documented and highlighted during "natural" "humanitarian" disasters, particularly by MSF, be it for example in the tsunami in Southeast Asia or during the earthquake in Haiti. The social narratives we put together acknowledge the spontaneous response of the communities to seek medical treatment, support the response, and demand recognition. However, it seems that as part of an epidemiological risk such as Ebola, for which the biomedical and technical response was designated as the only effective response, these methods of local response, if not widely ignored, are often delegitimized by the aid community.
16. The awareness/health education messages were based on local perceptions and strategies only in exceptional cases; they often began from a clean slate and aimed, without explaining why, to substitute these.
17. This explanation is bolstered by the surname of Alpha Condé as opposed to *khirawouya*, which means "the man with several paths."
18. The Ebola epidemic is thereby interpreted by some interviewees as Comdé's *n'fatarah* ("I did well") in response to Conté's discourse supporting the repression and his famous *wo fatarah* ("you did well").

19. What some of our Guinean interviewees called the ForéSac campaign, from the name given to the black plastic bags that were used at markets and that were the same color as the body bags initially used.

20. As underscored by one interviewee from Conakry: "There hasn't been a pilgrimage to Mecca in two years . . . which affects the Peuhls more than the Sousous or the Malinkés."

21. Which in many respects is similar to the dark periods of colonial and revolutionary/socialist Guinea.

22. We recognize that we are fairly far off from Foucault, who held that the principle behind biopower is internalization and self-control. Biopower is here understood as the form of medical coercion organized by the healthcare system to get people to adopt certain habits based on a health rationale/ethic.

23. A few examples of the operator and predator power state:

   - Fieldworkers mention during coordination meetings that they cannot work because they do not have any telephone credit or money to pay for petrol for the motorbikes; outside the meeting they point out, as an aside, the discrepancy between their needs and the salaries of the consultants.

   - Supplies intended for people in the quarantine zones are diverted by the local/prefectoral/ religious authorities for resale on the market.

   - Motorbikes and telephones given to community leaders by the response apparatus are misused.

   - Rumors circulated about the bonuses paid by the WHO to its agents and the strategies it used to minimize their exposure to the risk and transfer it to community players.

24. There is a difference between nonfunction and dysfunction. The prefix "non-" suggests a failure to operate, whereas "dys-" describes a problematic/incorrect operation.

25. Although this mistrust may seem legitimate in many ways, we aim to give here a description/ analysis that is as factual as possible.

26. Which was somewhat schematically the position of the emergency NGOs at the start of the epidemic.

27. Which was, again, forcing the link somewhat between the position of the development agencies and the UN agencies.

28. Which then forgets, due to the exclusive tropism concerning the management of the epidemic, that the government continues to (mal)function and that reassertion is down to an individual or a facility and cannot be done by another.

29. We will not go into the rationale behind this strategy in greater depth here, nor the practical implementation (e.g., selection, motivation), which have already been widely described and analyzed by aid anthropology and which barely differ in the response to the epidemic.

30. "Dominant" should be understood here in the various commonly accepted meanings of the word: physical dominance/overlook, genetic / prevailing, extensive, legal/ that which places in servitude.

31. It is interesting that the people involved in the response use the term "dispositif" (apparatus, device, response organization) to describe it and refer to themselves as the "apparatus staff or personnel."

32. The opinion held by health workers of doctors and social workers who found a place in the response apparatus is explicit: "These doctors who think they come more under the WHO than the Ministry of Health . . . their reintegration will be a complicated, political process, there will need to be positions and resources" (interview with an executive from the Ministry of Health, Conakry, 7/08/15).

33. This is a common strategy to involve subordinate staff to represent them and collect information at the many meetings so that decision makers need to be represented only at certain strategic meetings. This strategy nevertheless had an immediate crowding-out effect, self-fulfilling expectations, as meetings became by themselves less interesting and only worth the opportunity they offered to informally develop peripheral networks.

34. This is perfectly illustrated by the "zero Ebola in 60 days" commitment from January to March 2015.

35. Conakry had, at the end of November 2015, a workshop focused on speeding up the availability of vaccines that brought together many players (e.g., the firms, the NIH, CDC, INSERM, WHO, UNICEF, embassies, NGOs).
36. Even if this can and should be largely criticized (e.g., Faye 2015, Le Marcis 2015a, 2015b).

References

Akrich, M. 1991. "L'analyse socio-technique." In *La gestion de la recherche*, edited by D. Vinck. Bruxelles: De Boeck, pp. 339–53.

Balasegaram, M. 2014. *Ebola: A challenge to our humanitarian identity, MSF internal open letter, MSF internal website:* http://asso.ocp.msf.org.

Bradol, J.-H. 2016. "La réponse à l'épidémie d'Ebola: négligence, improvisation et autoritarisme." *Alternatives Humanitaires* 1.

Caremel, Jean-Francois. 2016. "Le renouveau «humanitaire» des politiques de la faim au Sahel, (ou) comment la malnutrition est entrée dans la santé globale." *Face a Face* 13.

Chabrol, F. 2014. "Ebola et la faillite de la santé publique en Afrique." *Revue internationale et stratégique* 18–27.

Fassin, D. 2010. *La Raison humanitaire*. Paris: Gallimard.

Faye, Sylvain Landry B. 2015. "L'«exceptionnalité» d'Ebola et les «réticences» populaires en Guinée-Conakry. Réflexions à partir d'une approche d'anthropologie symétrique." *Anthropologie & Santé. Revue internationale francophone d'anthropologie de la santé*, n°11, online https://anthropologiesante.revues.org/1884.

Geissler, P. W. 2013. "Public secrets in public health: Knowing not to know while making scientific knowledge." *American Ethnologist* 40: 13–34. doi:10.1111/amet.12002

Glenzer, K. 2007. "We aren't the world." In *Niger 2005. Une catastrophe si naturelle*, edited by X. Crombé and J-H. Jezequel, p. 117.

Jaffré, Y., and J. P. Olivier de Sardan. 2003. *Une médecine inhospitalière*. KARTHALA Editions.

Jézéquel, J.-H., and X. Crombé, eds. 2007. *Niger 2005. Une catastrophe si naturelle*. Karthala.

Lachenal, G. 2014. "Chronique d'un film catastrophe bien préparé." http://www.liberation.fr.

Lakoff, A. 2010. "Two regimes of global health." *Humanity: An International Journal of Human Rights, Humanitarianism, and Development* 1: 59–79.

Le Marcis, F. 2015a. *La mise en camp de la Guinée*. Presented at the EboDakar, Dakar, Sénégal.

Le Marcis, F. 2015b. "«Traiter les corps comme des fagots» Production sociale de l'indifférence en contexte Ebola (Guinée)." *Anthropologie & Santé. Revue internationale francophone d'anthropologie de la santé*, n°11, online https://anthropologiesante.revues.org/1884.

Nguyen, V. K. 2009. "Government-by-exception: Enrolment and experimentality in mass HIV treatment programmes in Africa." *Social Theory & Health* 7: 196–217. doi:10.1057/sth.2009.12

Nguyen, V. K. 2010. *The Republic of Therapy*. Durham: Duke University Press.

Olivier de Sardan, J.-P., and T. Bierschenk. 1993. "Les courtiers locaux du développement." *Bulletin de l'APAD*, n°5, online https://apad.revues.org/3233.

Olivier de Sardan, J.- P., in press, "Miracle Mechanisms, Travelling Models and the Revenge of the Contexts. Cash Transfer Programmes: a Textbook case" in Cash transfers: an anthropological approach. The revenge of contexts, edited by J-P Olivier de Sardan and E. Piccoli, New York: Berghahn Books.

Redfield, P. 2013. "Commentary: Eyes wide shut in transnational science and aid." *American Ethnologist* 40: 35–37. doi:10.1111/amet.12003

Revet, S. 2009. *Les organisations internationales et la gestion des risques et des catastrophes naturels*. Centre d'études et de recherches internationales.

4

The Initial International Aid Response in Sierra Leone

A Viewpoint from the Field

THOMAS KRATZ

I am a physician and currently working as a research associate in Berlin, Germany. On May 30, 2014, I received an email from my MSF pool manager with the subject heading "Three French speaking medical doctors for asap in Guinea for this Ebola outbreak." This would mark the beginning of my entry into a humanitarian emergency that would be one part drama, one part absurdity, and the largest and most unfortunate part tragedy. Although I had prior experience with one other Ebola outbreak, the early stages of the 2014-15 West African Ebola outbreak unfurled in a manner that neither I nor others experienced in managing such epidemics would have anticipated. While the story that follows was shaped by geography, happenstance, and the bioepidemiology of the disease, the most important part of the story is that it was also shaped by politics, misinformation, and avoidable human error.

How Things Started

When I first viewed that email in my inbox, it took me a moment to understand what was going on. Among my contacts at MSF, there had been some discussion about the spectra of an Ebola flare-up in this region earlier in May 2014, but since then the issue had quieted down. An MSF colleague, Anja Wolz, had just returned from Guinea and held a generally optimistic presentation on the Ebola outbreak in the region at the MSF Germany General Assembly. Only a passing remark from another colleague, Armand Sprecher, one week later in London suggested that the issue was not entirely resolved. While little information was available on the context, a request for three Ebola doctors simultaneously indicated a very serious situation. Thus, I contacted MSF.

The two MSF operational centers (Brussels and Barcelona) mostly dealing with Ebola virus disease (EVD) at the time had a pool of not many more than 100 expatriates experienced in dealing with this disease. All relevant positions, medical and nonmedical, were to be covered by this small emergency pool. Missions are short, and most expatriates are employed on a temporary basis, which means that they have to request time off from their workplace (e.g., in a hospital). Clinicians can confirm that in a busy working environment such as a hospital it is not easy to arrange leave from work at short notice. I know several "Ebola-experienced" colleagues who wanted to be deployed when the situation in West Africa visibly deteriorated but who couldn't, mostly due to their work responsibilities back home.

After negotiations with MSF and my employer at the time, I found myself in the Brussels headquarters of MSF Belgium in early June. There, briefed on the situation, my concern only grew. Information from the field indicated increasing numbers of suspect and confirmed Ebola cases, rumors of movement restrictions, and other patchy and disturbing information. "*Ça part dans tous les sens*" (it's all over the place) was the most conclusive message the MSF emergency unit provided. As the epidemic had started in a remote region of Guinea and moved to the capital, Conakry, I had expected that this was where our efforts would be focused. But, surprisingly, the hot spot had then moved to Sierra Leone, where the situation was deteriorating at an alarming rate, although an epidemic had only been declared there by officials on May 26, 2014. Preparations were made to send me, with my future emergency coordinator, Anja Wolz, to Kailahun, Sierra Leone. Alerts about Ebola from Daru, Koindu, and Buedu in Kailahun province verified by an MSF exploratory team had alarmed the MSF Belgium emergency unit. We departed for the field on June 10, 2014.

Arrival in Sierra Leone

Oddly, the main airport of Sierra Leone's capital city of Freetown is separated from the city by a large bay, and to reach Freetown one must take a speedboat from the Lungi airport. The mission began just as other medical missions I had undertaken for MSF. The streets of Freetown seemed normal, Anja was briefed by coordination, and we slept in the MSF guesthouse overnight. The next day, I set off on the eight-hour car ride across the entire width of the country from Freetown, located on the Atlantic Ocean, to Kailahun, an inland district on the far eastern edge of Sierra Leone. A decent tarmac road of about 350 kilometers long goes from Freetown via Bo and Kenema to Daru. From Daru to Kailahun, it is a further 30 kilometers by dirt track road, which becomes a slippery matter during the rainy season. It took more than one hour to get out of Freetown due to dense traffic. Once outside the capital, the remaining ride was quite straightforward. Nevertheless, the entire journey from Freetown to Kailahun took about eight hours. I passed by the town of Bo, where a large MSF maternal and child healthcare project with an isolation unit for Lassa fever suspect cases is situated—another familiar place I knew from the project a year before. I swapped cars there, a usual process within MSF called "car kiss": one car comes from the departure point and another one from the destination point, with both cars meeting at the midpoint of the itinerary. This allows drivers and cars to get back to their origin as soon as possible, as well as transport of staff and/or materiel in both directions. I had my first indications of the fact that this mission would be exceptional when we met up with a visibly overwhelmed logistician who had to deal with demands from Bo and, increasingly, Kailahun at the same time. The frazzled logistician was perhaps not the norm, but one small exception was easy to dismiss, and I still assumed that this mission would be like my previous ones. This myth was dispelled for me at Daru, a two-hour drive from Bo toward Kailahun, where my driver and I were asked to pick up a water and sanitation expert ("watsan" expert) from our team at a health post. In Daru, we were met by our watsan expert, who was clearly upset, having been left with two dead bodies in the health post, which had provisionally been transformed into a pre-referral center for patients suspected of suffering from EVD. The structure was run by the Ministry of Health (MOH) with support from MSF. Due to rapidity of events and understaffing, the provisional change in status and purpose of the health post was not accompanied by sufficient procedural explanations or supporting human resources. I saw a sprayer who decontaminated staff leaving the high-risk zone. He wore only haphazard personal protective equipment (PPE) including goggles and a hood with missing essential elements of PPE such as a scrub suit and overall. Despite these missing elements, the watsan expert was putting a huge effort into attempting to ensure that nevertheless PPE undressing procedures were done as correctly as possible in this context.

The watsan expert and sprayer were essentially alone with these bodies, as neither the community health officer responsible for the health center nor the burial team could be reached by phone. As, we discovered later, the burial team was also serving as the regional ambulance, it was unsurprising that they were unreachable, as they were overwhelmed by their double duties. When the ambulance/burial team finally arrived, dusk was falling, and my watsan colleague and I were not able to supervise handling of the bodies as thoroughly as we would have liked, as we still had to drive to Kailahun that evening for security reasons.

Work in Kailahun

In autumn 2012, two years before my arrival in Kailahun, I had participated in an intervention on a small Ebola epidemic in the Democratic Republic of the Congo, where there had been 19 inpatients in the treatment center. For these 19 patients, high-ranking experts from WHO, the U.S. Centers for Disease Control and Prevention (CDC), and the Public Health Agency of Canada (PHAC) were on the ground. Their presence during this small outbreak was a boon for me, as it gave me the opportunity to learn a great deal from seasoned experts. The contrast in 2014 was striking. Despite the number of confirmed Ebola patients climbing toward 200 in the region, no experts were present. We were working alone.

Kailahun is a small town in picturesque tropical surroundings. We entered a beautiful hotel compound, Luawa resort, and were welcomed by our logistician Kjell. The hall of the hotel was almost empty, with the exception of a few boxes of PPE lying on the ground. "Guys, are you ready for this?" Kjell asked as way of greeting our four-member team, soon to increase.

The presumed index case (the first case from which the epidemic spread) in the region was a deceased traditional healer from the Koindu area who had previously treated patients in neighboring Guinea. Many rumors were then circulating about sick and diseased people, mainly in the areas around Koindu and Daru, both situated in Kailahun district. Task force meetings consisting of, among others, MOH and MSF on a district level were held daily but, in the beginning, accomplished little. No one could agree on delegation of tasks; no clear authority presided over the meetings. Case numbers were contradictory and the lack of resources was evident. For example, as of May 29, 2014, only three body bags were available for the entire Kailahun district (MSF 2014b). By June 23, the number of confirmed cases in Sierra Leone soared to 163, among them 142 in Kailahun.

Reasons for this vacuum of interest and action have been posited after the fact. For example, an investigative article in the *New York Times* on December 30, 2014 (Sack 2015), would exhaustively describe limitations within the WHO at the time, such as financial shortages, an underestimation of the ongoing outbreak, and clunky governance structures. The WHO was organized with an international office at Geneva where key outbreak experts were based and a largely autonomous WHO-Afro regional office in Brazzaville, Republic of Congo, for Africa. This early stage of the outbreak response was largely led by the WHO-Afro regional office. Apparently communication was weak between the WHO-Afro regional office and the WHO office in Geneva, while local political influence was high. For instance, the WHO-Afro director is appointed by the health ministers of the WHO-Afro region. One of the harshest examples of local politics overriding questions of competence was when WHO-Afro blocked the appointment of one of the most renowned and experienced WHO experts on viral hemorrhagic fevers, Pierre Formenty, from working in Guinea in a coordinating position, in favor of an inexperienced colleague (Sack 2015).

The recent history of Sierra Leone and its existing socioeconomic situation also complicated response to the epidemic. The country had undergone a devastating civil war that ended in 2002. It was ranked 183 out of 187 countries in the human development index in 2013; it had a population with low levels in terms of life expectancy, education, and standard of living. Physicians were so scarce that there were only two physicians per 100,000 inhabitants (data from 2010), one of the lowest ratios in the world (UN Development Programme 2014; Central Intelligence Agency 2016). In fact, community health officers, hierarchically situated in between doctors and nurses, were de facto substitutes for the provisioning of medical care. To become a community health officer, one must receive three years of training and undergo six months to one year of internship (Cobb 2015).

Since March 2014, about 140 blood sample tests for EVD had been performed in Sierra Leone, all negative (Yang 2014). The first blood sample confirmed positive for EVD was recorded on May 26, 2014. However, it is possible, if controversial, that the epidemic had been introduced into Sierra Leone much earlier and had simply gone undetected. Until June, all laboratory testing of blood samples was performed by Metabiota Laboratory in Kenema. Investigative articles indicate that this laboratory lacked necessary diagnostic capacities (Freeman 2015; Sack 2015; Satter 2016). By early June 2014, blood sampling in Sierra Leone was done by the MOH and Metabiota teams as home-based testing: Blood was taken from patients in their homes and driven to the laboratory at Kenema for testing. The results were transmitted one or more days later; if the patient's blood test was positive for EVD, he or she was then transferred to the Ebola Treatment Unit (ETU) in Kenema. This practice was less than ideal, as it compromised the biosafety of the ambulance team, who frequently entered potentially contaminated homes without proper protective clothing, and led to patient flight during the waiting period for the results (Schieffelin 2014; MSF 2014b; Satter 2016).

Beginning in June 2014, MSF planned to give logistic support to improve infection prevention and control measures in Daru, maintain the Daru pre-referral center, and build up another pre-referral center in Koindu. These centers would be managed by Sierra Leone's MOH and would function as holding units for patients suspected of suffering from EVD (so-called suspect cases) with an opportunity for blood sampling. Once cases were confirmed, they were to be transferred and treated, as before, in the Kenema Government Hospital (KGH) which, formerly a Lassa Hospital, had been transformed to an ETU. Furthermore, MSF was in the process of constructing an ETU in Kailahun town to receive patients from Kailahun district and relieve some of the pressure from the KGH. Unlike the MOH-run pre-referral centers at Daru and Koindu, the Kailahun ETU was to be entirely managed by MSF, including staff recruitment, trainings, and salaries.

During this first stage, logisticians and the watsan teams were more critical than doctors and nurses, as the construction of an ETU entails preparing the land, shipping large quantities of construction material and medical equipment, hiring workers, coordinating the construction itself, and facilitating water supply and sanitation in a facility that needs a copious amount of water. Trucks with supplies rolled into the hotel courtyard almost every other night. During this first phase, the medical staff was focused on setting up the pharmacy, mapping cases, and holding trainings for new healthcare staffed hired for the ETU. It was critical that these staff were "polyvalent," as they would be required to take on a host of tasks across different operational functions. While trainings were generally successful due to the eagerness and cooperation of the new staff, mapping became a source of contention as the MOH refused to share data with MSF (Freeman 2015).

Koindu: Where Things Started

Koindu, the location of presumed initial cases in Sierra Leone, is situated a challenging two-hour drive from Kailahun. The town is only accessible to vehicles by a dirt road, difficult at the best of times and sometimes barely navigable during the rainy season. The discovery of the epidemic unfortunately coincided with the start of the rainy season, complicating provision of aid. Further, the somewhat isolated population of the area was skeptical about Ebola and sometimes hostile to measures taken to combat it, leading to concern from local authorities about the security of health staff and others fighting the disease (MSF 2014b). Finally, Koindu borders Guinea and is a short distance from Liberia. The Kissi ethnic group inhabits a territory across the borders of the three nation-states and Koindu served as a focal point for cross-border travel for Kissi with close family and social ties in Guinea and Liberia.

The pre-referral center at Koindu was, as mentioned earlier, an MOH project. MSF planned to provide logistical support for a limited number of items such as tents, PPE, chlorine, and essential drugs, leaving human resources management to the MOH. This strategy ultimately did not work, as the MOH lacked supplies of certain items it was responsible for providing and had immense difficulties recruiting medical staff willing to work in the very basic healthcare facility of Koindu, in a remote region affected by this dangerous virus and surrounded by a hostile population. The district medical officer announced twice that nurses were arriving, but they did not show up. The third time they were announced, the district medical officer himself accompanied six nurses to the facility, announcing. "They are all yours." His smile was in stark contrast to the downcast expression of the nurses, who were coming from outside of Kailahun district. In the days that followed, we improvised as best as we could with the resources we had available.

MSF provided drugs to the Koindu center. Both MSF and WHO donated PPE, leading to confusion due to the different procedures and standards in their use. The MOH provided uncovered mattresses, which sometimes consisted of no more than perforated foamed plastic. Stocks of drugs and PPE were piled up on pallets. In these initial days, despite the rumors of sick individuals, few patients presented at the center. Nurses reported to me that vendors at the Koindu market refused to sell to them, insulting them as "Ebola nurses." At two occasions we tried gathering traditional healers in Koindu for an informational meeting, using the assistance of the village elders. The sensitization of traditional healers is extremely important as they are in frequent contact with sick people potentially infected by EVD. Due to how the disease is transmitted, these healers were at high risk of becoming infected and then themselves spreading the infection in their activities in treating others. Unfortunately, these meetings were unsuccessful, as only three or four healers out of an estimated 100 turned up for each meeting. While the hostility and indifference by local populations to efforts by the state and nongovernmental organizations (NGOs) seemed to deny the existence of the epidemic, other events continued to reveal the growing seriousness of the problem.

One day, we came to a sudden halt on the road to Koindu on discovering a dead body lying there. The legs of the body had rope marks, a sign that it may have been dragged there from another location. We negotiated with the nearby villagers before our watsan team donned full PPE to put the dead body in a body bag, and we arranged for an ambulance team to pick up the body later. Such careful negotiations were necessary as we had learned that the population could get irritated or even aggressive if unannounced people in PPE arrived (Roddy 2007). Fortunately the population cooperated well in this instance. However, the absence of grief indicated again that the dead body was not a known local and was likely brought there from elsewhere. On another occasion, just outside the workplace in Koindu, I spotted two young men in shabby clothing; one of them had dreadlocks and wore a radio that dangled on a strap from his shoulder. This young man introduced himself with the words, "Hi, we are the burial team, and we have been told that there is a body in town. Can you tell me where it is?" While they had motorcycles, they had no other equipment on them, neither PPE nor disinfection material. Indeed, these men had no awareness of the disease. Our watsan expert provided them with basic information on the disease and PPE, supervising the burial to ensure safety. These men were not, unfortunately, exceptional. During this period, the MOH was providing burial teams with incomplete burial kits, and with little or no accompanying explanation on how to use them. With the hostility of the local population, the poor information and training provided to these burial teams, and the lack of adequate burial kits, it is likely that unsafe burials were the norm during this period.

A final striking example of the lack of resources, training, and organization in official efforts to fight the disease can be found in the small details of a blood collecting incident. A member of the MOH ambulance team arrived at the Koindu pre-referral center to take a blood sample from one of our suspect cases. He arrived in full gear, apparently driving to the center wearing his PPE, a completely unnecessary precaution. He then ran into the pre-referral center and took the blood sample. At the same time, he placed a gloved hand in his pocket and then adjusted his goggles. Such actions were against safety protocol and extremely dangerous for him due to the risk of virus transmission through fluids onto the mucous membranes in the face. After securing the sample, he went to the decontamination zone, where he tore off his protective overall abruptly and discarded it—before completing the necessary decontamination spraying step. Such behavior was not only very dangerous to him but also posed a risk to those surrounding him, as his actions could have aerosolized macro droplets that could then fall upon bystanders. Due to the risk of exposure, the nurses and I did not approach him but protested verbally from a distance. He dismissed our concerns, declaring, "I am an epidemiologist." When we encountered this same ambulance nurse later on in Kailahun, we came to realize he was totally exhausted and had received only haphazard training. As a member of MOH, he had followed PPE guidelines from WHO, which at the time recommended a lighter version of PPE than MSF, permitting parts of the face to be exposed. Additionally, unlike the almost ritualized steps of PPE undressing ("doffing") procedures under MSF guidelines, which include a thorough decontamination procedure, WHO recommendations followed a much more simplified doffing procedure with glove and hand disinfection only. It was only in autumn 2014 that WHO recommended more stringent PPE guidelines, although it maintained a much shorter doffing procedure than MSF (Sterk 2008; MSF Training Unit 2014; WHO 2015).

While Koindu, the presumed starting point of the epidemic in Sierra Leone, was astonishingly calm, Kenema and Daru areas were increasingly impacted. To understand this, one must know that in the period from the end of May until mid-June 2014, the majority of suspect cases had their blood samples taken on site in their villages by MOH surveillance teams. The blood was then shipped to the Metabiota Laboratory at KGH for consecutive testing. Once results were confirmed, patients were brought, by an ambulance system stretched over capacity, to KGH. Eighty-two percent of 106 cases confirmed between May 16 and June 18, 2014, originated from the chiefdoms of Jaweih and Kissi Teng with their principal towns of Daru and Koindu (Schieffelin 2014). Patients from Koindu were redistributed to KGH or already had crossed the border to seek medical care in neighboring Guinea and Liberia. In June 2014, testing capacities for EVD in Kailahun district did not exist yet. It took up to three days to get results that were largely orally transmitted; there was no systematic sharing of data. By mid-June, MSF knew that Daru and Koindu were the most affected towns, but we could not obtain data on either exact case numbers or exact locations of affected villages. We were forced to depend on unsystematic information shared orally in the task force meetings. Neither Metabiota Laboratory, nor MOH, or WHO-Afro (whose staff had started to be augmented by mid-June, although there were still no high-ranking experts present) would systematically share so-called line listings with MSF. Line listings comprise patient identifiers and other important data, including their provenance and, if applicable, laboratory results. Metabiota's official reason for refusing to share data was that it was "not authorized to share any results in Sierra Leone to parties other than official health authorities" (Freeman 2015). While MSF had over 14 years of experience in clinical care for EVD (Sprecher 2015), this exceptional lack of information sharing in this crisis made providing such care considerably more difficult. Yet, still at this moment, MSF was the principal actor providing medical care for Ebola, even as it had little access to either the epidemiological data or even the laboratory results for some of its patients. Not knowing the exact number and location of cases immensely complicated targeted activities such as case investigations, contact tracing, and health promotion (Freeman 2015).

On June 23, 2014, the MSF Brussels director of operations issued a strong press statement declaring that the epidemic was out of control (MSF-Belgium 2014). Although I felt very comfortable with this statement, as it corresponded with the situation on the ground, I did not observe any visible impact of it in Kailahun. High-ranking experts from WHO and CDC were still not on the ground and human resource capacities, especially for contact tracing and health promotion, remained low. Three days later, MSF opened the ETU in Kailahun town. The nursing staff there was mostly supervised by Sissel, an expatriate nurse, and Salliah from Kailahun district. Infection and prevention control was, thanks to the thorough trainings performed by the two, very well adhered to. Even once the Kailahun ETU was opened, laboratory testing continued to be an issue for a period. Results given to the ETU by the Kenema laboratory were often unclear. For example, sometimes we would get mobile phone communications from the Kenema laboratory stating, "Patients X and Y are positive, the others are negative." Unfortunately, these negatives were not necessarily negative. Because blood sample transit times to the Kenema laboratory frequently exceeded one day, and at times the laboratory was unsuccessful in testing the blood (due to, e.g., corruption, too small of a sample), the status of these other samples was often not clear. Results that were not positive could either have tested negative or not been tested at all. Significant improvements in testing occurred when an on-site laboratory testing at the Kailahun ETU was implemented by PHAC at the end of June. The PHAC has a mobile laboratory that can quickly be deployed to an outbreak hot spot and installed in any preexisting building or tent. These laboratories were able to quickly and accurately run polymerase chain reaction for Ebola virus as well as differential diagnosis for diseases such as malaria and typhoid fever (verbal communication from PHAC). During an Ebola outbreak in 2012 I had been amazed by their competence, flexibility, and open-mindedness in terms of sharing technical knowledge. The arrival of the PHAC laboratory in Kailahun during the 2014 epidemic permitted clear laboratory results together with patient identifiers within four hours of blood sampling.

Kenema Government Hospital: A Threat to Biosafety

In the meantime, the situation in Kenema remained a challenge. Even though the opening of Kailahun ETU relieved KGH in terms of patients, they continued to trickle in as the disease continued its geographic march westward in Sierra Leone. Key staff members at KGH had significant experience in treating Lassa fever. The chief doctor at the time, Sheik Humarr Khan, was appointed in 2005 to this facility, unique in the world for being dedicated for the treatment of Lassa fever patients. The head nurse, Mbalu Fonnie, co-founder of the Lassa fever program in Sierra Leone, had gained working experience since 1981. Both of them would die of EVD during July 2014 (Bausch 2014) (see also Tim O'Dempsey's chapter in this volume, Chapter 7). On the other hand, KGH staff was not accustomed to the Ebola virus, which is far more pathogenic than Lassa virus. Protective measures, including PPE, are more thorough for EVD than for Lassa fever. The hospital was tremendously understaffed and received little external human resources support (MSF 2014a; MSF-Belgium 2014). Professional exchange between the MOH-run KGH and MSF in Kailahun was complicated by a high workload on both sides and imperfect sharing of patient data. MSF experts from Kailahun frequently visited Kenema in order to get a picture of the situation and to provide feedback on infection prevention and control standards. During a visit by MSF epidemiological, medical, and watsan experts after Dr. Khan contracted EVD in mid-July 2014, the dimensions of the crisis came into clear focus. Lack of human resources was evident, as was a poor separation between low- and high-risk zones. These zones, routinely implemented in Ebola treatment facilities, are crucial to protecting the safety of the healthcare workers and preventing the spread of the infection. Patients with suspected or confirmed EVD are placed in the high-risk zone. Staff entering this zone must wear PPE. On the other hand, the low-risk zone is used for stocking medication and other logistical supplies as well as for accommodating staff during rest, for administrative tasks/handovers, and for donning PPE. Following the correct procedures to move between the high- and low-risk zones is crucial to maintaining the effectiveness of the zones and, indeed, the logic in using the cumbersome PPE. A staff member or cured patient moving from the high- to the low-risk zone must undergo a thorough "doffing" and decontamination procedure.

In Kenema, these precautions were poorly respected. Infected patients crossed into the low-risk zone to get food. Blood sampling of suspect cases was done in incorrect PPE, as the person holding the patient was observed to be more or less unprotected. Staff wearing PPE coming from the high-risk zone crossed through the low-risk zone in order to access another high-risk zone. Patients escaped through the unobserved visitors' zone during several occasions (MSF 2014a).

Hereafter, infection prevention and control activities in Kenema were intensified, including on-the-job-trainings and stays of MSF watsan experts in Kenema for technical support. What happened was a tragedy, both the terrible loss of lives of Dr. Khan and more than 10 of the nurses, as well as the nosocomial spread of the disease.

The End of My Mission

On my last day working on the mission in Koindu, in July 2014, an astonishing number of patients (21) were somehow brought crammed in two ambulance cars from Ngolahun village. Some of these patients had attended a funeral; some were feeling sick; others, although healthy, were concerned and wanted to get tested. All entered the clinic walking, creating a surreal tableau. Their clinical histories did not match typical "cliché" symptoms. No one had hemorrhaging— the patients all had very nonspecific symptoms such as weakness, headache, and nausea. Staff were overwhelmed; I refrained from entering the treatment unit but gave logistical support from the low-risk zone since it was the end of my 14-hour work shift that day. Tests confirmed that 13 out of the 21 patients were infected by Ebola virus. It was discovered later that nearby 40 people from Ngolahun were infected (MSF 2014c).

Once back from the mission, I felt happy and sad at the same time: happy because the mission was over, sad because the epidemic was far from over. Some of the colleagues I met in the field, such as Anja, Kjell, and Sissel, stayed there much longer than me and gained outstanding experience.

Epilogue

Less than a year later, in April 2015, I returned to the epidemic, deployed this time through the WHO mechanism Global Outbreak Alert and Response Network (GOARN) to Guinea. In the intervening year, many things had changed. The WHO had declared the epidemic a public health emergency of international concern on August 8, 2014, unleashing a torrent of international response. And yes, there were indeed a significant number of actors on the ground at this later stage: WHO International, Save the Children, MSF, UNICEF, the French Red Cross, and other governmental and nongovernmental organizations were present and making a huge effort to tackle the epidemic. Resources were available at the remotest locations—for example, donated handwashing points could now be found in even the tiniest and most isolated villages. It was a pleasure to see children being able and eager to demonstrate hand hygiene. Further, patient care was greatly improved. Organizations that had never dealt with EVD before had made significant progress in improving quality of care. Pictures of ETUs in Sierra Leone equipped almost like intensive care units in the Western world were impressive to those of us who still remembered the uncovered mattresses of a year earlier. While improvements in standards of clinical care, patient documentation, and research concerning antiviral therapies, vaccines, and efficacy of supportive care had already been discussed exhaustively in the years before this outbreak (Bausch 2006; Bühler 2014; Kratz 2015), they had never been implemented. On my return, this too had changed. Back in 1995, MSF had started to get involved in the management of epidemics caused by filoviruses (Ebola virus and Marburg virus): first in watsan and then, for the last 14 years, in clinical management. Hence, the management of filovirus epidemics in sub-Saharan Africa had been left as a quasi-monopoly to MSF during this time. Neither planned nor intended by the health actors involved in sub-Saharan Africa, it is debatable whether leaving the situation as such was a "mistake" in light of the events that unfolded. Yet, a year after the epidemic, it is also debatable whether the immense inflow of resources was well distributed. Brand-new cars of UN agencies were parked in villages for well-meaning campaigns to tackle the epidemic, while a few hundred meters next to those cars overworked and underpaid (or unpaid) community health care workers toiled for the same goal (2015). Also, while small children were trained in hand hygiene, basic training of professional health staff for key tasks such as contact tracing continued to be highly variable and sometimes poor.

On one occasion, I encountered a community health worker frantically running around with his thermometer trying to take the temperature of as many people as he could. When I asked him what this was for, he answered, "Contact tracing." I explained to him that contact tracing consists of more than swiftly taking individual temperatures, as the contacts of an Ebola patient must be regularly monitored for signs of disease for the entire 21-day incubation period. This includes, apart from taking body temperature, tracking other key symptoms of Ebola. In my conversation with this health worker, though, it became clear that such thoroughness would not be possible with his caseload, as he had an astonishing 171 contacts to follow up twice daily.

International epidemiological experts who were, in my view, overstaffed in some regions were scarce in other areas because logistics lacked coordination and gasoline supplies. Further, while copious resources were thrown at Ebola, other serious health issues fell along the wayside. Many healthcare facilities dealing with diseases other than EVD were in a neglected state; these facilities and their patients were sorely lacking in resources and were effectively bypassed by the international windfall. In Boffa Prefecture, there was a 10-fold decrease in consultations in healthcare centers in February 2015 compared to February 2014— that is, prior to discovery of the epidemic (author's observation). Mathematical modeling suggests that, in 2014, an excess of more than 10,000 people died due of malaria than usual in Guinea, Liberia, and Sierra Leone (Walker 2015). We have no idea of the true magnitude of this "collateral damage" in terms of overall morbidity and mortality in the region (see also Mit Philips' chapter in this volume, Chapter 5).

The epidemic has been declared finished multiple times with recurring flare-ups. Medical and social problems arising from this outbreak and the weaknesses revealed in the response persist. What could work better in future epidemics caused by highly pathogenic microbes such as Ebola virus? Multiple "lessons learned" processes are ongoing within governmental and nongovernmental institutions that have been involved in the West Africa outbreak. My reflections are based on my personal experiences working both on the "governmental" side in the public health sector in one of the richest countries in the world— Germany—and on the NGO side in the center of the spiraling epidemic in resource-poor West Africa. The differences are striking. MSF has a flexibly adaptable response capacity, well-thought-out logistical planning, and relatively rigorous infection prevention and control, especially when it comes to PPE. On the other hand, when I observed the functioning of high-level isolation units in Germany and the efficiency of the German evacuation airplane for highly contagious diseases, I was thoroughly impressed by high clinical standards of care (Robert Koch Institut 2016).

A pragmatic approach between these two standards, maintaining flexibility and adaptability in the field as well as providing good-quality care for patients, is difficult but not squaring a circle. Mobile solutions for intensive care, which are already common for other non-Ebola settings, could be used in an adapted manner. This would require thorough coordination as well as a good amount of supplementary financial and well-qualified human resources. Acquiring those resources can be difficult if the public interest to combat an epidemic is not there—or not there yet. Clinical/epidemiological data collection and sharing among the partners of an outbreak response is essential. Lassa and EVD are examples where, in the past, laboratory research on pathogens was done pro-actively, whereas clinical and epidemiological data were neglected (Wilkinson 2015). In future outbreaks, clinical and epidemiological data should be col-lected immediately and consistently.

After I met WHO colleagues and infectious disease clinicians from different countries, my impression of these actors became more differentiated than my initial impression of "Where the hell were they when things started?" Currently, clinical networks such as the Emerging Diseases Clinical Assessment and Response Network (EDCARN) from WHO are developing in order to provide an early and flexible aid response. These initiatives are driven by the lessons-learned process from the West Africa Outbreak.

We all work in political and organizational infrastructures that shape the framework of our response capacities. Politics and economics as well strongly influence the relationship between intention and results. The early stage of the EVD outbreak in Sierra Leone was a good example that politics can be a nasty business. If, as it seems, the deliberate withholding of information was done for political reasons, it nonetheless had tragic consequences for the local popula-tions (Freeman 2015; MSF 2015). The story of the fight against the Ebola epi-demic, when seen from the perspective of the people on the ground fighting it, is a story of missed opportunities.

Acknowledgments

I would like to say thank you to Anja Wolz and Michel van Herp, colleagues from MSF, for taking the time to answer questions for this chapter. Thank you to the healthcare workers in West Africa who dedicated a tremendous amount of time and effort to tackle this terrible outbreak. My thoughts are with the patients who have survived or succumbed due to the disease, and their families.

References

2014. Oral communication, KGH staff member.
2015. Verbal communications by staff members from several organizations involved in the national/international WHO aid response; made independently from each other.

Bausch, Daniel. 2014. "A tribute to Sheik Humarr Khan and all the healthcare workers in West Africa who have sacrificed in the fight against Ebola virus disease: Mae we hush." *Antiviral Research*. doi:10.1016/j.antiviral.2014.09.001.

Bausch, Daniel, Heinz Feldmann, Thomas Geisbert, and Cathy Roth. 2006. "Outbreaks of filovirus hemorrhagic fever: Time to refocus on the patient." *Journal of Infectious Disease* 196(Supp 2): 136–141.

Bühler, Silja. 2014. "Clinical documentation and data transfer from Ebola and Marburg virus disease wards in outbreak settings: Health care workers' experiences and preferences." *Viruses* 6: 927–37.

Central Intelligence Agency. 2016. *CIA world factbook*. Accessed January 16, 2016. www.cia.gov/library/publications/the-world-factbook/geos/sl.html.

Cobb, Nadia Miniclier. 2015. "Sierra Leone's community health officers." Transformative Education for Health Professionals Accessed April 20, 2016. http://whoeducationguidelines.org/content/sierra-leone%E2%80%99s-community-health-officers.

Freeman, Colin. 2015. "Guinea and Sierra Leone tried to cover up Ebola crisis, says Medecins Sans Frontieres." *Daily Telegraph*. Accessed January 16, 2016. http://www.telegraph.co.uk/news/worldnews/ebola/11488726/Guinea-and-Sierra-Leone-tried-to-cover-up-Ebola-crisis-says-Medecins-Sans-Frontieres.html.

Kratz, Thomas. 2015. "Ebola virus disease outbreak in Isiro, Democratic Republic of the Congo, 2012: Signs and symptoms, management and outcomes." *PLoS One*, doi:10.1371/journal.pone.0129333.

MSF. 2014a. "Infection prevention and control in KEGH—Results of the visit 22/23 July 2014." Internal Report.

MSF. 2014b. Internal reporting.

MSF. 2014c. "Sierra Leone: Race against time to control the Ebola outbreak." Accessed January 16, 2016. http://www.msf.org/article/sierra-leone-race-against-time-control-ebola-outbreak.

MSF. 2015. "Pushed to the limit and beyond: A year into the largest ever Ebola outbreak." Internal report available at http://www.msf.org.uk/article/ebola-pushed-to-the-limit-and-beyond-msf-report.

MSF-Belgium. 2014. "Ebola in West Africa: Epidemic requires massive deployment of resources." Bart Janssens. Accessed January 16, 2016. http://www.msf.org/article/ebola-west-africa-epidemic-requires-massive-deployment-resources.

MSF Training Unit. 2014. "Ebola practical—undressing." Accessed January 16, 2016. https://vimeo.com/108340219.

Robert Koch Institut. 2016. Accessed January 16, 2016. www.stakob.de.

Roddy, Paul. 2007. "The Medecins sans Frontieres intervention in the Marburg hemorrhagic fever epidemic, Uige, Angola, 2005: Lessons learned in the community." *Journal of Infectious Disease* 196(Supp 2): 162–167.

Sack, Kevin. 2015. "How Ebola roared back." *New York Times*. Accessed January 16, 2016. www.mobile.nytimes.com/2014/12/30/health/how-ebola-roared-back.html?referer=&_r=0.

Satter, Raphael. 2016. "American company bungled Ebola response." *AP: The Big Story*. Accessed April 20, 2016. http://bigstory.ap.org/article/46328e561bfb44b99b2e6937835be957/ap-investigation-american-company-bungled-ebola-response.

Schieffelin, John, Jeffrey Shaffer, Augustin Goba, et al. 2014. "Clinical illness and outcomes in patients with Ebola in Sierra Leone." *New England Journal of Medicine* 371: 2092–100.

Sprecher, Armand. 2015. "How does MSF care for patients suffering from Ebola?" Edited by MSF OCB. MSF website.

Sterk, Esther. 2008. "Filovirus haemorrhagic fever guideline." Edited by MSF. Accessed January 16, 2016. www.medbox.org/filvorus-haemorrhagic-fever-guideline/download.pdf.

UN Development Programme. 2014. *Human development index*.

Walker, Patrick. 2015. "Malaria morbidity and mortality in Ebola-affected countries caused by decreased health-care capacity, and the potential effect of mitigation strategies: A modelling analysis." *Lancet Infectious Disease* 15: 825–32.

WHO. 2015. "How to put on and how to remove personal protective equipment—posters."
    Accessed August 8, 2016. http://who.int/csr/resources/publications/ebola/ppe-steps/en/.
Wilkinson, Annie. 2015. *Lassa fever: The politics of an emerging disease and the scope for One Health.*
    Working Paper Series: Political Economy of Knowledge and Policy.
Yang, Jennifer. 2014. "What went wrong in response to the Ebola crisis?" *Toronto Star.* http://
    m.thestar.com/#/article/news/world/2014/10/17/what_went_wrong_in_response_to_
    the_ebola_crisis.html.

5

Dying of the Mundane in the Time of Ebola

The Effect of the Epidemic on Health and Disease in West Africa

MIT PHILIPS

While Ebola sickened and killed, it also increased vulnerabilities for both survivors of the disease and society at large. Ebola victims who were fortunate enough to recover suffered physical and psychological sequelae, economic loss, and stigmatization. They were often also left mourning for family and friends who did succumb to the disease. But the epidemic also created far-ranging effects on those physically untouched by the actual Ebola virus. In West Africa, it had a cascading impact on many other aspects of society: economic, cultural, social, political (UNDG 2015). To take the example of education, the governments of Guinea, Sierra Leone, and Liberia closed all public schools from the summer of 2014 until early 2015 (Guinea reopened schools in January, Liberia in February, and Sierra Leone in April 2015). During school closures, parents had to find other sources of child care. Some children were unattended and left vulnerable to forced labor, abuse, or criminal recruitment (Save the Children 2015). Rates of rape and unplanned pregnancy spiked during the epidemic, partly due to this phenomenon and partly due to loss of health services, quarantine, and other epidemic-related factors (OCHA 2015; UNDP/Irish Aid 2015). These are just some of countless interlinked negative repercussions of the epidemic on the social fabric of the region.

The majority of people who died during the Ebola epidemic died of something other than Ebola. Many of these deaths were indirectly caused by the crisis. This chapter is focused on this phenomenon, namely the impact of the epidemic on the general health of people in Liberia, Sierra Leone, and Guinea. It provides an overview of the epidemic's ramifications on the health of West Africans physically untouched by the virus, reviewing some of the statistics available on morbidity and mortality in the region. Ebola's impacts on specific areas of health will be further highlighted, drawing from our studies and field assessments, as well as the increasing body of literature on the secondary health effects of the Ebola crisis. The dynamics underlying these impacts on population health will be unpacked as we analyze how the epidemic weakened the health system generally but also eroded interpersonal relations between health workers and patients. The chapter, as it summarizes the effect of Ebola on health care in Guinea, Liberia, and Sierra Leone, interrogates the ongoing narrative constructed in the aid community on this (nearly) post-Ebola moment. Specifically, it calls into question how ideas of "resilience" can be effectively incorporated in the current response to urgent, immediate needs of the region.

As the epidemic began to decline, a grim picture started emerging in the scientific literature of the knock-on effect of the epidemic on health systems and general health in the region. Although there were some early warnings of the attention Ebola was drawing away from other critical health programs, they were muted in the general media (Check 2014; Delamou 2014). More attention was drawn to these issues in early 2015, when a little breathing room developed in the fight against Ebola and the end of the crisis was foreseeable, even if not in the immediate months that followed. While the sickness and death from the virus may have reduced average life expectancy in these three countries from one to five years (Helleringer and Noymer 2015), the widespread social disruption accompanying the epidemic had a cascading effect on other health issues. What that effect looked like was at first uncertain. In late 2014 and through the first half of 2015, public health researchers released a range reports on how the epidemic was potentially impacting other health outcomes (Loubet et al. 2015; Parpia et al. 2015; Takahashi et al. 2015; Walker et al. 2015). These effects, taken from data comparing 2014 (and particularly the second half of the year, when the epidemic was at its peak) to pre-Ebola periods, and the predictions arising from modeling were often alarming. Early 2015 was a unique moment in the epidemic, when tremendous resources were finally arrayed in the fight against the epidemic, only to see it subside quixotically, just as many of these resources were finally ready to be deployed. In this period of epidemic decline, it could be argued that some reports produced were continuing on a tradition of stoking fear as a means of generating interest. However, this phenomenon is also linked to the very real and very recent massive upheavals across the region. From early 2015 to early 2016, an increasingly nuanced understanding of secondary health impacts has emerged as better statistical data on morbidity and mortality become available and the long-term effects on West African health systems come into better focus. Even as increasing numbers of studies with more complete data are published, uncertainty will likely remain on the true impact this epidemic has had on other health outcomes. With the number of new Ebola cases nearing zero, the call to prevent the catastrophic wave of secondary deaths has been increasingly replaced by demands to seize the opportunity to (re)build (resilient) health systems. This shift in priorities may mask some of the lingering problems in the region and could be detrimental to improving the health and well-being of the populations in West Africa.

Ebola's effect on the mortality and morbidity of other diseases could be placed in two phases roughly coinciding with the epidemic's chronology. There was a window of heightened first-order impact, particularly in the period of July to December 2014, when many health services were reduced or suspended. People died as Ebola degraded the healthcare landscape. During this time, people with severe malaria in the most affected regions could have difficulty finding a facility open to see them, a healthcare worker willing to prick their finger for a blood test, or the medications necessary to treat the disease. A woman in labor may have hesitated to go to deliver in the hospital, or perhaps she would have been refused admittance on arrival, and would then be left without emergency care.

What could be called second-order effects followed beyond the peak in the epidemic, as people continued to suffer the after-effects of this reduction in health services. For example, some people living with HIV without access to their antiretroviral drugs were no longer virally suppressed and thus could pass the disease on to others (including mothers to newborn children) or become resistant to the first- or second-line drugs (Loubet et al. 2015; MSF 2016a). For instance, the number of HIV-positive mothers coming to health facilities for treatments to prevent mother-to-child transmission of the virus decreased by 25% in Sierra Leone from May to September 2014 (UNICEF 2015). This decrease represents an additional number of children who will become HIV positive in the following years, and who will need to have a lifetime of antiretroviral drugs to survive. Children unimmunized during the height of the epidemic will succumb to vaccine-preventable disease; child anemia will rise due to previously untreated malaria. Interrupted contraceptive use causes unplanned or unwanted pregnancies. Everything from mental health to blood transfusions, or surgery to malnutrition, has been impacted by the epidemic.[1] The epidemic has such impacts through both a systems effect and an interpersonal effect, although the two are closely linked.

Breakdown of Health Systems, Breakdown of Personal Relations

The already poor health systems in West Africa were weakened even further by the Ebola crisis. In 2010, Sierra Leone ranked fifth, Liberia ranked eighth, and Guinea ranked 13th highest in maternal mortality among 187 countries around the world.[2] These countries also rank at the low end in life expectancy. A child born in 2012 in Canada, Japan, or most of Europe would live on average into his or her 80s. A child in Sierra Leone was expected to live on average 30 years less, with a life expectancy of 50 years; similarly, the life expectancy was 58 years in Guinea and 61 in Liberia.[3] In 84% of districts of Guinea people were using health services less than once every three years on average. In combination with political instability, budget limitations and restrictions in fiscal space[4] have hindered the ability to invest in health systems for decades, leading to rundown facilities, inadequate health staff, insufficient medical supplies, and difficult working conditions (Rowden 2014; Kentikelenis et al. 2015).

Even before the health workers' death toll in the current crisis, the health sector in the three countries faced an important shortfall of human resources (Van de Pas and Van Belle 2015). Liberia had just 57 doctors and 978 nurses and midwives in 2008, while in Sierra Leone 136 doctors and 1,017 nurses were reported, far below WHO recommended minimum standard for staff levels (22.8 health workers per 10,000 inhabitants). At 1.4 health workers per 10,000 inhabitants, the official country figures for Guinea are very low, but this figure includes only staff on the official government payroll and does not reflect the real numbers of trained health staff available in the country. As a consequence of years of recruitment freeze, some health staff worked only as volunteers in the public health system while waiting for an official position to become available and, therefore most qualified healthcare workers are concentrated in the capital or large urban areas where patients can pay for (private) services. Also in Sierra Leone, despite recent funding improvements linked to the Free Health Care Initiative (Witter et al. 2016), the available health workforce is still insufficient, with long delays in absorption of graduates in the public system and an important rural/urban maldistribution. Health facilities are chronically understaffed, with unmotivated, ill-equipped, and overworked health workers, and staff payment being delayed or insufficient to attract and retain health workers in rural areas (McPake et al. 2016). In both Sierra Leone and Guinea, many staff working in the health facilities are not on the official payroll; most earn a living by extracting fees from patients.

Material goods, finances, and human resources were drawn from already fragile and undersupplied health services to the Ebola response. Clinical staff moved to Ebola treatment centers, where financial remuneration and infection protection material were available. Management capacity, often drawn into weekly or daily regional- or national-level meetings on the Ebola crisis, was severely depleted. This created further downstream effects, as some health centers closed (although many fewer than seems to be the general view),[5] and undermanaged or unmanaged supply chains meant stock-outs or low stocks—not only of infection prevention and control (IPC) equipment, but also of essential drugs and medical materials. In Monrovia, Liberia, assessments as late as January 2015 showed critical deficiencies in implementation of IPC in the main health facilities (Cooper 2015). A report on primary health care clinics showed similar problems, including in health facilities with an implementing organization assigned to support them. The necessary accompanying measures such as training, standard procedures, reorganization of patient flow, triage and isolation areas existed in varying degrees of implementation and quality (IPC Partners Mapping 2014; Cooper 2015). Moreover, very little attention and support was being provided to ensure sufficient drug stock availability, basic equipment, and furniture[6] needed for resumption of health services.

Some of the strongest negative effects on the health system could be seen in the supply chain, as resources to maintain the supply of medical commodities and materials were drained for the Ebola response on the one hand, and the drop in demand led to a decrease in supply that was slow to recover as demand returned to normal levels (Government of Liberia 2015). Fewer staff were present not only to provide clinical care, but also to prescribe drugs or monitor adherence. Preventive services were reduced, as supplies of contraceptive drugs became hard to find or healthcare workers were afraid to organize vaccinations.

While the system was hard hit in terms of logistics, human resources, and management capacity, healthcare was also affected by the interpersonal relationships between the healthcare authorities, healthcare workers, and the general population. Reductions in healthcare coverage were caused by trends on both the "supply side" and "demand side" that operated on a systemic but also an individual or interpersonal level. An analysis of various health problems that increased during the epidemic reveals the multilayered processes that drove reduced health service coverage.

Health Facilities Closed or Empty

In November 2015, an MSF team performed an assessment of the health services in the Guinea Forestière region, infamous as the area where the index case (first known victim) of this epidemic died. Examining data collected from 58 health structures (ranging from hospitals to health posts) in Nzerekore, Kissidougou, and Kerouane, the team compared the health services from data for the year 2013 (before the epidemic) through the height of the epidemic (July 2014–December 2014) to October 2015 (when the epidemic was in steady decline). While steep drops in consultations, hospitalizations, and in-hospital births were seen during the summer and fall of 2014, coinciding with the height of the epidemic in that region, hospital service utilization quickly resumed normal levels into 2015 (Telaro and Séverac 2015). Others observed also considerably reduced utilization rates across Guinea in this period: in some places hospital visits dropped by 54%, antenatal care by 59%, and vaccination rates by 30% (Leuenberger et al. 2015; Van de Pas and Van Belle 2015). Such a steep drop in facility usage for the second half of 2014 is also seen for Liberia and Sierra Leone (Government of Liberia 2015; VSO 2015). The data from Telaro and Séverac showed no change in proportional morbidity in Guinea, and one of the surprising results of this assessment was that the health facilities' functioning showed little quantitative difference when comparing the period before the epidemic with the period of epidemic decline (Telaro and Séverac 2015). Similarly, in Sierra Leone, only 4% of peripheral health centers closed at the height of the epidemic (UNICEF 2014).

The continued functioning of health facilities strongly depended on the location and the type of services. An MSF survey found that 60% of health facilities in hard-hit Monrovia, Liberia, remained open in August 2014 (Epicentre Survey 2014). In particular, private facilities remained open or reopened quickly after infective incidents, dependent on revenues from patients. However, hospitalization capacity dropped significantly and hospitalization wards were slow to reopen at full capacity. In January 2015 only 23% of the needed hospitalization beds were available; in pre-Ebola Monrovia there was already an important gap in hospitalization capacity, with only 1,036 beds, or 70% of what is generally accepted as minimally needed[7] for a population of 4.5 million. During the Ebola crisis, about two thirds of this already low capacity fell away.

Vaccine-Preventable Diseases

Vaccination coverage was also greatly reduced during the Ebola epidemic, with an estimated 50% overall reduction in the three countries from January 2014 to June 2015 (ACAPS 2015a; GAVI 2015). An analysis of this phenomenon indicates several different reasons for decreased coverage. In part it was because of the resources diverted toward the Ebola response, the risk perceived in allowing crowds to amass during vaccination sessions, the complexity of dealing with post-vaccine fever, and the technical risk involved with needle injection. But it was also influenced by the relationship between the public and healthcare workers, as the population could be increasingly hostile to healthcare workers, assuming they were associated with often unpopular Ebola measures. For these various reasons, large-scale vaccination campaigns were avoided and delayed, even when clusters of measles were reported.[8] Exacerbating the drop in vaccine coverage, fearful mothers stopped bringing their children to the hospitals for routine vaccinations during the epidemic peak (UNICEF 2014). When routine vaccination finally restarted in health facilities at the beginning of February

2015, this coincided with the start of the Ebola vaccine trials, and the ensuing confusion further worried parents.

One of the most studied examples of decreased vaccination coverage is that of measles vaccinations. A modeling study that predicted 100,000 potential additional measles cases and up to 16,000 deaths due to the lapse in immunizations resulting from Ebola received considerable newspaper coverage after its publication in March 2015 (Takahashi et al. 2015). In keeping with the tone of much reporting on Ebola, several news outlets picked up on this study, warning of an impending measles outbreak representing a second and even more devastating epidemic riding on the tail of Ebola (McKenna 2015; McLoughlin 2015; Taylor 2015). Reports of small measles epidemics would appear on occasion but did not receive the major news coverage comparable to this dramatic forecast (ACAPS 2015a), even if underreporting was likely. Seven hundred measles cases with zero deaths (Suk et al. 2016) seemed not to have the numbers or potential drama to merit media amplification, even if it was a confirmation of an underlying phenomenon. From March 2015 onward, intense vaccination catch-up plans along with a rebound in usage of health structures likely mitigated predicted losses.[9]

Malaria

In a similar vein, but for somewhat different reasons, all evidence indicates that malaria impact rates increased significantly during and after this epidemic. Malaria, with fever as its main symptomology, became quickly entangled with Ebola. Only a blood test could exclude the presence of the Ebola virus and could definitively distinguish one from the other in earlier phases of the respective diseases. Many suffering from malarial fever chose to forego official diagnosis and treatment, likely fearing forcible placement in Ebola treatment centers (ACAPS 2015a; Parpia et al. 2015). Failure to ensure an adequate supply of antimalarial drugs and lapses in delivery of insecticide-treated bed nets contributed to further cases. Again, because routine surveillance data are and were not available, estimates of these additional deaths from these disruptions are largely based on models. One study estimated that there were, across these three countries, a number of additional malaria fatalities (10,900) almost equal to the number of Ebola fatalities (11,308) (Walker et al. 2015). Even more alarming, these estimates did not include deaths caused by disruption in insecticide-treated bed net distribution or the increases in morbidity and mortality of pregnant women from untreated malaria (Walker et al. 2015). In Guinea alone, one research study found that the number of malaria deaths were almost certainly "likely to greatly exceed the number of deaths from Ebola virus disease" (Plucinski et al. 2015). Another study presented even more worrisome data: the authors observed that with a 50% reduction in malaria treatment coverage during the height of the epidemic, malaria-attributable mortality likely increased by 50% in these three countries (Parpia et al. 2016).The study estimated that the greatest impact would have been on children under the age of five years, estimating some 6,800 additional deaths indirectly caused by Ebola among children under five alone in these three countries (Parpia et al. 2016). The country least affected in these models was Guinea, while the country most affected was Liberia, ironically because Liberia had the highest pre-Ebola malaria treatment coverage and Guinea the lowest (Parpia et al. 2016). In the case of Guinea, one cannot lose ground that one has not yet gained.

Mother and Child Health

As the data on malaria and vaccination suggest, maternal, obstetrical, and pediatric care across the region was also clearly impacted by the epidemic. While wide regional variation was noted in Sierra Leone, the country on average saw a 28% reduction in hospital deliveries and cesarean sections from May 2013 to May 2015 (Ribacke et al. 2015). Similar trends were seen in parts of Liberia (Hurum 2015; Iyengar et al. 2015; Lori et al. 2015). In Guinea, a 31% decline in use of reproductive, maternal, newborn, and child health care was observed in comparing October–December 2013 to October–December 2014 (Barden-O'Fallon et al. 2015). This study also observed that the epidemic did not seem to have a wide impact on the *availability* of services (Barden-O'Fallon et al. 2015); however, resort to health structures decreased in facilities that remained open. In some cases avoidance of health structures, combined with measures such as quarantine, actually led to de facto closure of health facilities due to lack of patients (UNICEF 2014). One study found that maternal and newborn care was not strongly affected in terms of human resources, facilities, or equipment availability in Sierra Leone; rather, almost all reductions in service were due to patient avoidance (VSO 2015). A UNICEF study examining the period of May 2014 to September 2014 in selected districts of Sierra Leone made similar observations, noting a drastic reduction in prenatal, maternity, and antenatal care, although most facilities remained functioning with all services offered (UNICEF 2014). Thus, patient choice seemed to be a significant driver in the decrease in reproductive, maternal, newborn, and child health care coverage during the Ebola epidemic. In fact, the decline in mothers bringing children into health facilities represented one of the biggest drops in health facility usage: mothers were afraid to bring their children to the health facilities.

Nonetheless, the loss of available services also had serious detrimental impacts. In Monrovia we documented women who were unable to get timely assistance for safe delivery in August to September 2014, as many maternity units were closed, were functioning at reduced activity level, or were refusing to admit women in labor because of the Ebola virus disease transmission risk.[10] Many women finally had to deliver at home, alone or with the help of a private nurse or midwife (Philips 2015). While there are no reliable figures overall, certain hospitals report during July and August an increased number of dead babies delivered by cesarean section, often interpreted as a sign of delayed care for obstructed labor, with women saying they were unable to get care elsewhere. One study estimated that loss of available healthcare workers alone, irrespective of patient avoidance of services, greatly increased maternal mortality in these three countries and would continue to have a serious negative impact, leading to an increase of maternal deaths of up to 38% in Guinea, 74% in Sierra Leone, and 111% in Liberia (Evans et al., 2015, p. 10).

Interpersonal Interactions and Choices

Here we turn from an examination of specific health issues to highlight how individual choices were negotiated both to maximize healthcare and to minimize risk during the epidemic. Patient and provider decisions were constrained by the existing health systems and resources available but nonetheless also shaped how the system worked. A focus on individual choices and smaller group dynamics reveals that healthcare offering is fungible, and social perceptions deeply impacted how the system was used or if the system functioned at all. The negative impact of Ebola on health went beyond a failure of facilities to remain open or a decrease in service provision. It would seem that the epidemic exacerbated a distrust between healthcare workers and their employer (the state), and between healthcare facilities (perceived) as state enterprises and the individual citizen. This distrust led not just to avoidance but also to a variety of techniques by both providers and patients to cope with risk in an environment of high mutual skepticism and distrust.

The Risks of Being a Health Worker

Those providing healthcare faced the threat of Ebola on a daily basis; their struggle was multifaceted. Healthcare workers were 21 to 32 times more likely than general population to be infected with Ebola (WHO 2015). They died in high numbers, many not well-paid and some not paid at all by their respective governments. They were also ostracized by the general population that was afraid of anyone possibly exposed to Ebola. Understandably, many left their jobs. Tragically, many died (WHO 2015). In some instances healthcare workers protested their poor remuneration and unsafe working environments (BBC 2015;

Telegraph 2015). Clearly, fewer healthcare workers meant less healthcare being offered. The decrease in healthcare offered would increase poor health outcomes in these countries (Evans et al. 2015). However, evidence suggests that a surprisingly large number of health staff continued to soldier on, coming to work during the epidemic and interacting with patients. Those who did remain developed other methods to manage the risk they perceived in their work.

An anthropological study looked at risk perceptions of healthcare workers in Liberia following a case of late diagnosis of an Ebola case in a private clinic in New Kru Town, Monrovia, in January 2015. The misdiagnosed patient had been handled by several healthcare workers using minimal or no IPC. The fear that they expressed after the patient died of Ebola was linked to their insecure environment, variously defined. Beyond fear of infection, they feared losing their jobs or getting blamed because triage did not work; they were uncertain of their knowledge on Ebola and afraid of the stigma that would fall upon them when the case became known. The fear that they felt ultimately derived from management's failure to provide them with basic IPC training and education, and it was also shaped by the lack of effective dialogue between upper management and the workers. These two factors led to a sense of powerlessness and fatalism among the staff, encouraging fear, blaming, and denial (Pellechio 2015).

An assessment by the Liberian Ministry of Health at the end of 2014 found that in many health facilities IPC was still not ensured, despite the known risk and problems of Ebola amplification and spread in healthcare facilities. In our field research, we have found similar effects of the lack of IPC training for staff. A survey by MSF Epicentre of healthcare facilities in Monrovia in August 2014 found that a large proportion of facilities lacked basic infection control material, including 28% reporting a shortage of disinfectant and 25% reporting a shortage of gloves (Epicentre 2014). Considering that IPC training was not provided systematically, and IPC equipment was not always available, healthcare workers found surprising ways to manage their daily fears and triage the risks they perceived in their jobs. Sometimes, workers even found IPC equipment too cumbersome or unfamiliar and opted for other contradictory ways to manage the sources of greatest perceived risks. Such techniques included selective treatment of patients: turning away those perceived as possibly infected with Ebola and refusing to treat patients who were bleeding, vomiting, or otherwise producing possibly infective body fluids. In Monrovia, another tactic was to ask for a negative Ebola test before patients could be admitted. Even if in great distress, patients were left isolated and untouched until test results arrived. Patients had to wait hours to get tested and receive results. Delays were particularly long at night, as testing services were not available 24 hours a day. Sometimes, even in absence of clinical criteria for

Ebola virus disease, patients were sent to Ebola treatment centers solely to get a negative test result.[11]

It is debatable if such measures decreased workers' risk of exposure, or indeed the possibility of cross-contamination of other patients, but it did serve a psychological purpose in giving the healthcare workers a symbolic means to protect themselves in an environment where they felt very little control. Laboratories set up for Ebola virus disease diagnosis did not take into account such "irrational" coping mechanisms relying on negative testing and could not fulfill the expectations of stressed healthcare workers and facilities. Although there are several reports of patients dying during long and complicated referrals, waiting for a hospital to accept them, the lack of systematic monitoring of these incidents means it is hard to gauge the extent of the problem.

Fear of Illness and Fear of Care

Patients also adapted to the essentially hostile healthcare environment created by the Ebola epidemic. Part of this adaptation was simply incorporated through flight and avoidance, as the data on resort to consultations, vaccinations, and hospitalizations across these three countries reveal. As mentioned earlier, patient flight may have been as significant a reason for lower health services utilization as decreased offering of services. For example, an ACAPS study of Sierra Leone comparing 2014 to 2013 data found a serious drop-off in hospital outpatient department attendance at the height of the epidemic, although data toward the end of the study suggested a rebound (ACAPS 2015b). The study observes a specific decrease in consultations for malaria and malaria treatment, suggesting that malaria, with its attendant fevers, may have caused both patient avoidance of health facilities and refusal to treat by healthcare workers (ACAPS 2015b). Further, the spike in stillborn births and maternal deaths seen during the epidemic was likely related to fatal patient postponement to seek medical assistance in difficult cases as much as from lack of appropriate facilities or timely care provision (VSO 2015).

Certainly, fear of hospitals was not completely unfounded, as one report found that hospital infection accounted for 10% of new Ebola cases at the height of the epidemic (UNICEF 2014), certain cases of confirmed nosocomial patient infection have been recorded (Dunn et al. 2016), and the high rate of healthcare worker infection supports at least some workplace infection. Hospitals were seen, not inaccurately, as places of high risk. This particularly impacted child health services in Guinea at least, as mothers stopped bringing in their children for acute respiratory infection, diarrhea, or a variety of other serious ailments (Barden-O'Fallon et al. 2015). A study of perceptions of pregnant and nursing mothers in Kenema, Sierra Leone, in September 2014 (another region with high

Ebola case numbers) found that many such women avoided health facilities for fear of contracting Ebola. This was not simply a fear of nosocomial infection, as many of the women believed that the hospitals were deliberately infecting incoming patients, a belief that lingered long after the epidemic peak (Dynes et al. 2015). What did patients avoiding health facilities do instead? From our field studies, we saw adaptive behavior that included resort to traditional medicine, house calls, and private care including pharmacies. In these three countries, traditional medicine is still an important component of health-seeking behavior and likely continued to serve the health needs of much of the population, even as traditional healers became implicated in the spread of the disease. Private pharmacies provided medicines without the risk of the crowd of the public health facility. Some care providers were also willing to come to the home of the sick patient, given enough incentives.

Distrust, already strong among certain sectors of the population, grew under the pressure of the crisis. Many people blamed the health system for the epidemic itself (Minor Peters 2014; Elston et al. 2015). Healthcare workers, many of whom were already poorly trained and remunerated within the health system, felt further abandoned during the emergency. Populations accustomed to governments that had often failed to fulfill the basic requirements of a social contract (e.g., clean water, education, roads), and a medical system that often seemed predicated on their exploitation—as they were forced to pay for services (even if technically free of charge), for example—readily assigned a nefarious role to official health services in their understandings of the crisis. Already weak systems crumbled further from crises of trust. While distrust of the system continues, recourse to it rebounded as the fear of Ebola subsided. Nonetheless, much remains to be done to improve the health systems and the relations that sustain them.

Six Pillars (Minus Two)

From earlier Ebola epidemics, MSF had developed a "six-pillar" approach to managing and ending Ebola outbreaks (MSF 2016b, 2016c): isolation, contact tracing, community outreach, safe burials, psychosocial support, and general health care provision. During this epidemic in West Africa, the number of sick and nodes of infection spread so widely that some of these pillars were neglected as efforts to simply isolate and care for the sick became challenging. In any Ebola outbreak, the importance of Pillar 6 is recognized: providing access to general healthcare services as part and parcel of the emergency intervention. Besides responding to acute health needs, ensuring functional entry points to care for sick people helps to swiftly identify patients who fit the case definition and to refer them for adequate care and isolation. This last pillar—providing and promoting general health services—also became subsumed to care and isolation for organizations working against the epidemic, including for MSF. During the intensive phase of the epidemic, the overwhelming caseload led to an almost exclusive focus on clinical management and isolation, leaving little space for complementary medico-operational strategies. There were, however, a few notable exceptions, for instance developing and delivering home disinfection kits and distribution of anti-malaria prophylaxis every three months to households in Monrovia and Freetown. Initial attempts to design outpatient consultations that would maintain a safe distance between healthcare workers and patients were rapidly deemed unfeasible and ineffective. Besides these few efforts, MSF did not get involved in non-Ebola care again until late in the epidemic (MSF, 2016b).

While patients and healthcare workers used practical and novel approaches to manage a health landscape changed by the epidemic, the health system generally did not. In large part, nongovernmental organizations also failed to adapt. Besides the distribution of anti-malaria prophylaxis to households every three months, few attempts were made to provide healthcare through alternative channels. Some services could have been moved to peripheral posts or private pharmacies. For example, wide-scale distribution of family planning products could have occurred through such methods. Over-the-counter provision of medicines for malaria or diarrhea has been attempted elsewhere with some success (Roll Back Malaria 2013). Longer refills for patients on antiretroviral or tuberculosis treatment could also have avoided interruption of care. IPC kits could have been distributed more widely; training could have been conducted by non-experts.

In a climate of distrust of health facilities, authorities could have taken measures to provide non–facility-based or decentralized healthcare or at least to ease access barriers to available healthcare. It is well known that in a crisis situation, access to care barriers linked to insecurity, distance, and sociocultural factors are reinforced by financial barriers. Considering this, it is striking that never during this emergency situation WHO's guidance to declare all health services free of charge was applied. For all of the money poured into stopping the crisis (or even the recovery plan), no authority ever suggested waiving or removing patient fees. Even in Liberia, where general essential healthcare was technically already free of charge, private and mixed public–private facilities such as JFK Hospital in Monrovia were charging hefty sums, even requiring financial deposits before patients could be admitted. A January 2015 assessment by MSF in Monrovia showed that among the 355 hospital beds available, 193 required patient payments, with some demanding the equivalent of US$43 to $76[12] before admission was even possible. This meant that only 11% of Monrovia's hospitalization beds came without patient fees. Later, under the services restoration effort, the

Liberian government provided financial support through contracting-out agreements with hospitals run by faith-based organizations, with a 35% reduction of the usual fees, but this still implied very steep fees, representing both an access barrier and an impoverishment risk for patients.

In Sierra Leone, even if the Free Care Initiative greatly improved access to care for children under five and pregnant women, many healthcare workers continued to ask patients for informal fees (Witter et al. 2015). With the economic collapse due to the Ebola crisis, even more people found these payments unaffordable. Measures in this regard might have increased patient access, if not patient trust, in a country such as Guinea, where cost is invariably an important barrier to timely care seeking and potential healthcare workers' revenue can determine choice of treatment. Moreover, with patient fees limiting utilization rates in Guinea to an average of 0.3 contacts per year per inhabitant, one can hardly expect that any health facility–based surveillance system can provide the necessary coverage to detect suspicious cases in a timely manner.

The challenges to provide safe and effective health services for people not suffering from Ebola have become increasingly clear during this outbreak. Only toward the tail end of this epidemic was the sixth pillar of general health services picked up again, mostly under the caption of "post-Ebola" recovery plans. Many of the most ambitious on-paper plans for rehabilitation were programmed for an elusive "post-Ebola" moment. This proved an artificial and fleeting concept, as declaring the end of the epidemic had to be delayed repeatedly due to the continued emergence of new active cases. It has been suggested that flare-ups of case clusters can continue for months or years, or even more troublingly, that Ebola will become an endemic problem in the region. So can we really talk about *post*-Ebola healthcare? If anything, the 2014-15 experience has shown that we need to find a way to provide healthcare while there are Ebola cases present. These "intra-Ebola" times are probably the most dangerous period for transmission as some general health services are just starting up and patients start to seek care again.

Further, the pillar of community outreach, also known to be key in ending an epidemic, did not keep up with the pace of the spreading epidemic; misinformation and distrust spread much faster than education and outreach. In the end, too few actors were on the ground at the height of the epidemic to ensure these services continued. MSF as well failed in this regard, in part due to its burden of care to existing patients (MSF 2016b). This is a great irony, as no epidemic can end without some sort of cooperation by the community. Trust is a necessary component of cooperation, and open communication is a necessary component of trust. This community-based linkage and a functioning health system used by most of the population would also have helped identify early Ebola infections and break transmission chains.

The MSF-run Gondama hospital in Sierra Leone is an atypical example of many of the failures discussed above. At the height of the epidemic, MSF decided to close this hospital preemptively to prevent possible Ebola infections. Remarkably, it is one of the few cases where a secondary care hospital with sufficient staff and funding, and an active patient load, closed. Unlike many of the other facility closures discussed in this chapter, this closure was not based on an actual infection occurring on the premises. Although management had increasing difficulty finding expatriate staff to make up for national staff being funneled into the Ebola response, the hospital was ultimately closed as a precaution against infection. Healthcare was denied to prevent loss of health. This sort of logic is striking but also salutary: fear as a basis for decision making was not only the resort of the uninformed populace or the disempowered healthcare worker.

Fragility of Health Systems: Past, Present and Future

Most health systems in low- and mid-income countries would have struggled with an epidemic of this size in the absence of a timely, effective international response (Philips and Markham 2014; Witter et al. 2016). Even if the Ebola spread benefited from the existing weaknesses in the health systems of West Africa, perhaps it has had its greatest effect by further weakening these systems. Before, during, and after the outbreak, public health officials in Sierra Leone warned of the lack of diagnostic capacities, equipment, human resources, and medicines for basic maternal and child care (UNICEF 2014). In April 2014 (before any confirmed Ebola cases in Sierra Leone), 82% of facilities in Sierra Leone reported having a stock-out of medicines, and although 89% made a request to higher management levels, only 34% received a response (Witter et al. 2016).

Ebola has often been compared to HIV (de Cock and El-Sadr 2015; Drain 2015; Rabkin and El-Sadr 2015), but it should perhaps be more accurately compared to conflict. In conflict, most people do not die of the bullet or the bomb, they die of the mundane: the flu, starvation, a small infection, during child birth —by increased vulnerabilities (Connolly and Heyman 2002). As one study of the Ebola epidemic observed of Sierra Leone, its

> particularly negative effects on vulnerable groups, including women and girls, have been similar to any crisis situation. Women and girls have experienced heightened exposure to the virus due to traditional roles as caregivers and cultural rites, while also being disproportionately affected by the social and economic impacts of the outbreak. (UNDP/Irish Aid, p. 14)

As in conflict, the most vulnerable suffer most: existing vulnerabilities and barriers to effective health care are worsened.

Numerous articles on health and Ebola echo the need to strengthen and improve the health systems, with a major focus on ensuring surveillance and resilience for the next crisis in these countries. But this narrative carries the illusion that healthcare in these countries was mainly the victim of the Ebola epidemic. While aspects of healthcare became direct or indirect victims of the epidemic, good healthcare was clearly lacking before Ebola struck. Why does this matter? Sierra Leone, Liberia, and Guinea were struggling before the epidemic to improve the health of their populations. They were dealing with repetitive outbreaks of measles, cholera, malaria, Lassa fever, and other diseases. Young children died of malaria and women died in childbirth. The most vulnerable had poor access to service. The countries faced, three years ago, many of the exact same issues that they face now that Ebola has come and (largely) gone. To frame their current struggle as only or largely a rehabilitation or recovery effort from the effects of the virus is to miss most of what their health systems are still struggling against: low trust between the state and society, poverty and limited fiscal space for public (health) expenditure, lack of financial and human resources for health, poor infrastructure, inequitable access, vested interests, corruption, and myriad other socioeconomic factors. Ignoring these factors now would mean a repetition of the shortcomings of the past.

Resilience: A Focus on Crises to Come

The current catchphrase of the international health community, the panacea for all future ills, it seems is "resilience," defined as "the capacity of health actors, institutions, and populations to prepare for and effectively respond to crises; maintain core functions when a crisis hits, and, informed by lessons learned during the crisis, reorganize if conditions require it" (Kruk et al. 2015). Thus, for Ebola-affected countries, public health leaders call for a "multisectoral, integrated approach, one that equips countries to absorb unforeseen severe shocks . . . the only way to rebuild the health ecosystem and put these countries back on track for development" (Kieny and Dovlo 2015). Kruk and colleagues identify three elusive "preconditions" and five rather difficult elements or functions that must be achieved for such resilience to be effective. These preconditions— clarity in roles in the global health system, legal and policy foundations for crises response, and a strong and committed health workforce—obviously did not exist in any of these three countries before Ebola. According to the authors the five elements that must be further incorporated in a health system to make it resilient are awareness (good information systems and response), diversity (addressing a broad range of problems), self-regulating, integrated (between different horizontal and vertical programs and actors), and adaptive (able to transform to meet adverse conditions) (Kruk et al. 2015). It is hard to imagine how such elements can come into being with the present policies in place and resources available to West African governments. Indeed, if we consider only one of the so-called preconditions to resilience, a strong and committed health workforce, the path ahead is already quite long. As a World Bank study observed, 43,565 additional doctors, nurses, and midwives would need to be hired in these three countries in order for them to achieve the goal of 80% health coverage of their populations, a number that is completely unachievable in the short run due to their current "fiscal constraints" (Evans et al. 2015). The system will remain under-resourced in the short term.

Ultimately, such systems talk and systems thinking must not mask the concrete problems and health needs of people. The current donor environment has seized upon "resilience" as the solution to wide-ranging humanitarian issues impacting vulnerable populations, while in fact it fosters the elusive ambition to bring a convenient end to the need for humanitarian aid itself (Philips and Derderian 2014; Whittall et al. 2014). Another problem with the concept of resilience, one appropriate to the theme of this book, is that it frames health response on risk rather than need; it is about future strength rather than current vulnerabilities. In line with most of the securitization framework in public health,[13] resilience de-emphasizes the immediate problems faced by a society for a focus on mitigating against future, potential shocks. In doing so, today's problems can be placed in the narrative of the past without actually being dealt with.

Dealing with the Present Before Planning for the Future

It is clear that the people of West Africa are forced to be resilient in the face of systems that are neither sufficiently effective, equitable, nor responsive to people's needs. For these West African nations to recover from the epidemic, individual and community resilience should be capitalized upon and supported in priority. Restoring healthcare systems to pre-Ebola levels will not be enough; it is necessary to improve the access to and quality of healthcare services. The trauma of Ebola left people distrusting health facilities, healthcare workers demoralized and fearful to resume work, and communities bereaved, impoverished, and suspicious. To tackle this present challenge, a thorough revision of pre-Ebola health services is needed, addressing problems and challenges left too long ignored. Longer-term health plans should be adapted to the new situation and should prioritize the population's increased health needs while factoring in the increased precarious conditions of patients and healthcare workers.

Relations between health services offered by the state and the patient must be re-established, or in some cases established for the first time. The deep distrust of sections of the population to state measures taken against Ebola were not irrational considering the nature of the relationship between the state and its population in many of these contexts. Health services were, in the case of Sierra Leone and Liberia, only beginning to show their value in the years leading up to the epidemic. In Guinea, there seemed to be a long and rather static history of poor public health offering before the epidemic began. It is entirely possible that this will continue unless the current dynamic is broken.

While an important opportunity to declare services free of charge for patients was missed during the crisis, the recovery plans also did not include clear measures to improve access to care. Evidence is rife that patient fees deter adequate service use and worsen other access barriers (Leone et al. 2016; Ponsar et al. 2011a, 2011b; Yates 2009); also the quality and efficiency of services are under pressure, as choice of treatment is determined by profits rather than patient needs. However, there has been no clear commitment to ensure that people get the care they need, not only the care they can afford. The issue of free care is closely linked to unpaid or underpaid health staff. When healthcare workers fail to obtain regular and reasonable pay from their employer—the government or the aid agency supporting the structure—they will make their income off their patients, stripping them of their meager resources. Public structures de facto become places of privatized services. In part for this reason, healthcare workers are concentrated in large cities where people are able to pay. Without addressing some of the systemic shortcomings, countries will find it difficult to recruit the needed health workforce.

Further, aspirations to flexibility and adaptability notwithstanding, these regions need "catch-up" plans, some of which have already begun, for services that lapsed during the epidemic. Pentavalent, measles, and other basic vaccinations have recommenced in earnest, and visits to health facilities show signs of being back to pre-Ebola levels, but it is important to remember that these pre-Ebola levels were wretched to begin with. Coverage rates should be higher; the targets should be higher than past achievements. The return of HIV and tuberculosis patients to care needs to be monitored, and we need more data on the continuing needs of people after the epidemic (Mobula et al. 2015; Zachariah et al. 2015; MSF 2016a). These needs do not relate only to post-Ebola syndrome, but also to other vulnerabilities that linger as the disease fades to zero. Instead of abstract notions about a "resilient" tomorrow, ambitions must at the very minimum lead to very practical contingency plans today for response to current and future crises. This would include, for example, several months of antiretroviral drugs supplied for stable HIV patients when access to healthcare becomes an issue, or a backup supply plan for necessary medical supplies should supply chains be cut. Resilience should go beyond an abstract concept of the ability of a health system to merely continue doing what it does (in spite of future shocks). If anything, resilience should be a descriptor of a "healthy health system," able to provide services to those who need it and in particular the most vulnerable.

This crisis presented challenges in keeping health services available and in demand. As many of the examples in this chapter illustrate, resources alone do not determine whether a health system functions well. Well-reasoned and flexible planning, reflection on priorities, and appropriate funding are all needed. More importantly, populations must be engaged and their specific needs and constraints (whether healthcare workers or patients) considered. We must continue to focus on the tangible needs of populations in crisis and ensure that they are helped today. Only by decreasing their vulnerabilities now can we increase the capacities to prevent and withstand shocks such as the Ebola epidemic.

Notes

1. For surgery see Bundu et al. 2016, blood transfusions Tapko and Kamno 2016, and mental health Grigoryan et al. 2016 or Van Bortel et al. 2016. Discussion on malnutrition can be found in various articles on maternal and child health during the crisis.
2. https://www.cia.gov/library/publications/the-world-factbook/rankorder/2223rank.html.
3. Various health indicators for a range of years can be downloaded, sorted, and ranked at http://data.worldbank.org/indicator/.
4. Fiscal space is an economic concept relating to the ability to use a country's income for budgeting and expenditure for public services. See Heller 2005.
5. For instance, a UNICEF survey of status of peripheral health units in Sierra Leone in August 2014 found that 4.1% were closed at the height of the epidemic (UNICEF 2014).
6. In most health facilities where Ebola infection incidents happened, all furniture was burned to avoid potential contamination.
7. WHO reference value is one to two hospitalization beds per 1,000 inhabitants.
8. See, for example, the WHO *Guidance for Immunization Programmes in the African Region in the Context of Ebola*, revised March 30, 2015, and the various announcements for restarting vaccination campaigns in mid-2015. "Liberia conducts first polio, measles immunizations since Ebola outbreak," Joint WHO/Liberian MOH statement, May 8, 2015, http://www.afro.who.int/en/liberia/press-materials/item/7654-joint-statement-from-the-ministry-of-health-and-social-welfare-liberia-the-cdc-unicef-and-the-who.html; "Sierra Leone wraps up four-day health and vaccination campaign," WHO, May 2015, http://www.who.int/features/2015/vaccination-campaign-sierra-leone/en/.
9. *Ibid.*
10. For a discussion of the issues involving pregnant women in distressed labor and Ebola, see Black 2015.
11. These centers were intended to care for Ebola patients only and were unable to provide the necessary care for patients suffering from other illnesses or for women in labor.
12. During the visit these were reported as the "usual" fees in JFK Hospital in Monrovia.
13. See João Nunes's chapter in this volume, Chapter 1.

References

ACAPS. 2015a. "Briefing paper: Ebola in West Africa—impact on health systems, 26 February 2015."

ACAPS. 2015b. "Thematic note—25 March 2015: Ebola outbreak in West Africa, impact on health service utilisation in Sierra Leone."

Barden-O'Fallon, J., Barry, M. A., Brodish, P. and Hazerjian, J. 2015. "Rapid assessment of Ebola-related implications for reproductive, maternal, newborn and child health service delivery and utilization in Guinea." *PLoS Currents*, 7; doi:10.1371/currents.outbreaks.0b0ba06009d d091bc39ddb3c6d7b0826.

BBC. 2014. "Ebola crisis: Sierra Leone health workers strike."

Black, B. O. 2015. "Obstetrics in the time of Ebola: Challenges and dilemmas in providing lifesaving care during a deadly epidemic." *British Journal of Obstetrics and Gynaecology* 122: 284–86.

Bundu, I., Patel, A., Mansaray, A., Kamara, T. B., and Hunt, L. M. 2016. "Surgery in the time of Ebola: How events impacted on a single surgical institution in Sierra Leone." *Journal of the Royal Army Medical Corps* 162(3): 212–6; doi:10.1136/jramc-2015-000582.

Check, Erica Hayden. 2014. "Ebola outbreak shuts down malaria-control efforts. Public-health experts fear that one epidemic may fuel another in West Africa." *Nature* 514: 15–16; doi:10.1038/514015a.

Connoly, Maire, and David Heyman. 2002. "Deadly comrades: War and infectious diseases." *Lancet* 360 (supplement). http://www.thelancet.com/pdfs/journals/lancet/PIIS0140673602118071.pdf.

Cooper, Catherine. 2015. *Minimum standard assessment at priority healthcare facilities in Montserrado, Ministry of Health and Social Welfare, Monrovia, Liberia.*

De Cock, Kevin M., and Wafaa M. El-Sadr. 2015. "A tale of two viruses: HIV, Ebola and health systems." *AIDS* 29: 989–91.

Delamou, Alexandre, et al. 2014. "Ebola in Africa: Beyond epidemics, reproductive health in crisis." *Lancet* 384(9960): 2105.

Drain, Paul K. 2015. "Ebola: Lessons learned from HIV and tuberculosis epidemics." *Lancet Infectious Diseases* 15(2): 146–47.

Dunn, A. C., T. A. Walker, J. Redd, et al. 2015. "Nosocomial transmission of Ebola virus disease on pediatric and maternity wards: Bombali and Tonkolili, Sierra Leone, 2014." *American Journal of Infection Control* 44(3): 269–72; doi:10.1016/j.ajic.2015.09.016.

Dynes, M. M., L. Miller, T. Sam, et al. 2015. "Perceptions of the risk for Ebola and health facility use among health workers and pregnant and lactating women—Kenema District, Sierra Leone, September 2014." *Morbidity and Mortality Weekly Report* 63(51): 1226–227.

Elston, J. W. T., A. J. Moosa, F. Moses, et al. 2015. "Impact of the Ebola outbreak on health systems and population health in Sierra Leone." *Journal of Public Health* 2015 Oct 27, pii: fdv158.

Epicentre. 2014. "Cross-sectional survey on health care capacity and utilization, safety and hygiene measures available in health structures, and attack rate among health facility staff during the Ebola outbreak, Monrovia, Liberia, August 2014." Final Report, Epicentre/MSF, September.

Evans, D. K., M. P. Goldstein, and A. Popova. 2015. "The next wave of deaths from Ebola? The impact of health care worker mortality." World Bank Policy Research Working Paper 7344.

GAVI. 2015. Report to the Board, 2–3 December 2015. Downloaded May 20, 2016, from http://www.gavi.org/about/governance/gavi-board/minutes/2015/2-dec/.

Government of Liberia, Ministry of Health. 2015. "Investment plan for building a resilient health system in Liberia 2015–2021." April 15.

Grigoryan, A., R. Bitsko, H. Y. Lee, et al. 2016. "Literature review of mental health and psychosocial aspects of Ebola virus disease. *Online Journal of Public Health Informatics* 8(1).

Heller, P. 2005. "Back to basics: Fiscal space: What it is and how to get it." *Finance and Development-English Edition* 42(2): 32–33.

Helleringer, S., and A. Noymer. 2015. "Assessing the direct effects of the Ebola outbreak on life expectancy in Liberia, Sierra Leone and Guinea." *PLoS Currents* 7. Outbreaks. 2015 Feb 19. Edition 1; doi:10.1371/currents.outbreaks.01a99f8342b42a58d806d7d1749574ea.

Hurum, Lindis. 2015. "Beyond Ebola: The collateral damage on the urban health care system and modelling excess mortality among pregnant women, Monrovia Liberia August 2014." Master's thesis, University of Copenhagen, School of Global Health.

IPC Partners Mapping. 2014. "December 4 presentation at Coordination meeting, Monrovia, Liberia."

Iyengar, P., K. Kerber, C. J. Howe, and B. Dahn. 2015. "Services for mothers and newborns during the Ebola outbreak in Liberia: The need for improvement in eemergencies." *PLoS Currents*, 7. http://doi.org/10.1371/currents.outbreaks.4ba318308719ac86fbef91f8e56cb66f.

Kieny, M. P., and D. Dovlo. 2015. "Beyond Ebola: A new agenda for resilient health systems." *Lancet* 385(9963): 91–92.

Kentikelenis, L. King, M. McKee, and D. Stuckler. 2015. "The International Monetary Fund and the Ebola outbreak." *Lancet* 3(2). http://www.thelancet.com/journals/langlo/article/PIIS2214-109X(14)70377-8/fulltext.

Kruk, M. E., M. Myers, S. T. Varpilah, and B. T. Dahn. 2015. "What is a resilient health system? Lessons from Ebola." *Lancet* 385(9980): 1910–912.

Leone, T., V. Cetorelli, S. Neal, and Z. Matthews. 2016. "Financial accessibility and user fee reforms for maternal healthcare in five sub-Saharan countries: A quasi-experimental analysis." *BMJ Open* 6: e009692; doi:10.1136/bmjopen-2015- 009692. http://bmjopen.bmj.com/content/6/1/e009692.full.pdf+html.

Leuenberger, David, Jean Hebelamou, Stefan Strahm, et al. for the IDEA West Africa Study Group. 2015. "Impact of the Ebola epidemic on general and HIV care in Macenta, Forest Guinea, 2014." *AIDS* 29(14): 1883–887.

Lori, J. R., S. D. Rominski, J. E. Perosky, et al. 2015. "A case series study on the effect of Ebola on facility-based deliveries in rural Liberia." *BMC Pregnancy and Childbirth* 15(1): 1.

Loubet, Paul, Guillaume Mabileau, Maima Baysah, et al. 2015. "Likely effect of the 2014 Ebola epidemic on HIV care in Liberia." *AIDS* 29(17): 2347–351.

McKenna, Maryn. 2015. "Ebola could cause thousands more deaths—by ushering in measles." *Wired*. May 15. http://www.wired.com/2015/03/ebola-measles/.

McLaughlin, Jenna. 2015. "Ebola's legacy: A potentially horrifying measles outbreak in West Africa." *Mother Jones*. http://www.motherjones.com/politics/2015/03/ebola-measles-vaccination-study-west-africa.

McPake, Barbara, et al. 2015. "Ebola in the context of conflict affected states and health systems: Case studies of Northern Uganda and Sierra Leone." *Conflict and Health* 9: 23; doi:10.1186/s13031-015-0052-7.

Minor Peters, Melissa. 2014. "Community perceptions of Ebola response efforts in Liberia: Montserrado and Nimba Counties." Oxfam GB, December 18.

Mobula, M. L., C. A. Brown, G. Burnham, and B. R. Phelps. 2015. "Need for reinforced strategies to support delivery of HIV clinical services during the Ebola outbreak in Guinea, Liberia, and Sierra Leone." *Disaster Medicine and Public Health Preparedness* 9(5): 522–526.

MSF. 2015. "Mission Exploratoire Guinée Forestière, Republique de Guinée." Final report of exploratory mission in Nzerekore region by Michele Telaro and Marie Laure de Séverac, MSF-OCB, November.

MSF. 2016a. "Out of focus: How millions of people in West and Central Africa are being left out from the global HIV response." April. http://www.msf.org/sites/msf.org/files/2016_04_hiv_report_eng.pdf.

MSF. 2016b. MSF Ebola response, Part 1: Medico-operational. OCB Ebola Review, Stockholm Evaluation Unit, MSF. http://evaluation.msf.org/evaluation-report/ocb-ebola-review-2016.

MSF. 2016c. MSF-supported research on Ebola, March 2016, Operational Centre Brussels, MSF. http://www.msf.org/en/article/report-msf-supported-research-ebola.

OCHA. 2015. Guinea Priority Needs Overview, July.

Parpia, A. S., M. L. Ndeffo-Mbah, N. S. Wenzel, and A. P. Galvani. 2016. "Effects of response to 2014-2015 Ebola outbreak on deaths from malaria, HIV/AIDS, and tuberculosis, West Africa." *Emerging Infectious Diseases* 22(3): 433.

Partners in Health, 2014. "Ebola: Countries need 'Staff, stuff and systems.'" http://www.pih.org/blog/for-ebola-countries-need-tools-to-treat-patients-in-their-communities.

Pellechio, Umberto. 2015. "Back to life: Report from the anthropological study on the risk perceptions during the decrease of the epidemic." MSF OCB internal report, Monrovia, Liberia, February.

Philips, M., and K. Derderian. 2014. "Health in the service of state-building in fragile and conflict-affected contexts: An additional challenge in the medical-humanitarian environment." *Conflict and Health*. https://conflictandhealth.biomedcentral.com/articles/10.1186/s13031-015-0039-4.

Philips, M., and Á. Markham. 2014. "Ebola: A failure of international collective action." *Lancet* 384(9949): 1181.

Philips M. 2015. Assessment of access to health care in Monrovia, Liberia. Debriefing visit January-February 2015. Internal report, MSF Brussels.

Plucinski, M. M., T. Guilavogui, S. Sidikiba, et al. 2015. "Effect of the Ebola-virus-disease epidemic on malaria case management in Guinea, 2014: A cross-sectional survey of health facilities." *Lancet Infectious Diseases* 15(9): 1017–23.

Ponsar, F., M. Van Herp, R. Zachariah, et al. 2011a. "Abolishing user fees for children and pregnant women trebled uptake of malaria-related interventions in Kangaba, Mali." *Health Policy Plan* 26(Suppl 2): ii72–83; doi:10.1093/heapol/czr068. http://www.ncbi.nlm.nih.gov/pubmed/22027922.

Ponsar, F., K. Tayler-Smith, M. Philips, et al. 2011b. "No cash, no care: How user fees endanger health—lessons learnt regarding financial barriers to healthcare services in Burundi, Sierra Leone, Democratic Republic of Congo, Chad, Haiti and Mali." *International Health* 3(2): 91–100; doi:10.1016/j.inhe.2011.01.002. http://www.ncbi.nlm.nih.gov/pubmed/24038181.

Rabkin, Miriam, and Wafaa M. El-Sadr. 2015. "Ebola: The real lessons from HIV scale-up." *Lancet Infectious Diseases* 15(5): 506.

Ribacke, K. J. B., A. J. van Duinen, H. Nordenstedt, et al. 2016. "The impact of the West Africa Ebola outbreak on obstetric health care in Sierra Leone." *PloS One* 11(2): e0150080.

Roll Back Malaria. 2013. "Key learning for malaria programme managers. AMFM Phase 1." http://www.rollbackmalaria.org/files/files/commodities_access/AMFm-Key-Learings-2013-en%281%29.pdf.

Rowden, Rick. 2014. "Health systems in Africa are ill-equipped to deal with Ebola. And that's partly the fault of IMF policies." *Foreign Policy*. October 30. http://foreignpolicy.com/2014/10/30/west-africas-financial-immune-deficiency/.

Save the Children. 2015. "Children's Ebola recovery assessment: Sierra Leone." June.

Suk, J. E., A. P. Jimenez, M. Kourouma, et al. 2015. "Post-Ebola measles outbreak in Lola, Guinea, January–June 2015." *Emerg Infect Dis* 22(6): 1106–8; doi:10.3201/eid2206.151652.

Takahashi, S., C. J. E. Metcalf, M. J. Ferrari, et al. 2015. "Reduced vaccination and the risk of measles and other childhood infections post-Ebola." *Science* 347(6227): 1240–242.

Tapko, J. B., and K. Tcheumagam Kamno. 2016. "Coping with Ebola crisis in transfusion services in West Africa." *ISBT Science Series* 11: 285–91; doi:10.1111/voxs.12224

Taylor, Marisa. 2015. "Child measles deaths set to soar in Ebola-hit countries." *Al Jazeera America*, March 12. http://america.aljazeera.com/articles/2015/3/12/measles-may-kill-more-than-ebola-in-west-africa.html.

Telaro, Michele, and Marie Laure de Séverac. 2015. "Mission Exploratoire Guinée Forestière, Republique de Guinée," MSF-Belgium exploratory mission report.

Telegraph. 2014. "Liberia health workers strike over Ebola 'danger money': Doctors, nurses and carers in worst-hit country demand 'danger money' to care for Ebola patients." http://www.telegraph.co.uk/news/worldnews/ebola/11159217/Liberia-health-workers-strike-over-Ebola-danger-money.html.

UNDG Western and Central Africa. 2015. "Socioeconomic impact of Ebola virus disease in West African countries: A call for national and regional containment, recovery and prevention."

Downloaded May 17, 2016, from http://www.africa.undp.org/content/rba/en/home/library/reports/socio-economic-impact-of-the-ebola-virus-disease-in-west-africa.html.

UNDP/Irish Aid. 2015. "Assessing sexual and gender-based violence during the Ebola crisis in Sierra Leone." October.

UNICEF. 2014. "Sierra Leone Health Facility Survey 2014. Assessing the impact of the EVD outbreak on health systems in Sierra Leone: Survey conducted 6-17 October 2014."

Van Bortel, T., A. Basnayake, F. Wurie, et al. 2016. "Psychosocial effects of an Ebola outbreak at individual, community and international levels." *Bulletin of the World Health Organization* 94(3): 210–14; doi:10.2471/BLT.15.158543.

Van de Pas, R., and S. Van Belle. 2015. "Ebola, the epidemic that should never have happened." *Global Affairs* 1(1): 95–100.

VSO. 2015. "Exploring the impact of the Ebola outbreak on routine maternal health services in Sierra Leone." Report commissioned by VSO and the Ministry of Health, Sierra Leone.

Walker, P. G., M. T. White, J. T. Griffin, et al. 2015. "Malaria morbidity and mortality in Ebola-affected countries caused by decreased health-care capacity, and the potential effect of mitigation strategies: A modelling analysis." *Lancet Infectious Diseases* 15(7): 825–32.

Whittall, J., M. Philips, and M. Hoffman. 2014 "Building resilience by deconstructing humanitarian aid." MSF-UK Opinion and Debate page. http://www.msf.org.uk/article/opinion-and-debate-building-resilience-deconstructing-humanitarian-aid.

WHO. 2014. "Information Note (Version Oct. 24/2014 rev): Guidance for immunization programmes in the African region in the context of Ebola." October 24. Ref: WHO/IVB/14.08

WHO. 2015. "Health worker Ebola infections in Guinea, Liberia and Sierra Leone, a preliminary report." May 21. Accessed May 26, 2016, from http://www.who.int/hrh/documents/21may2015_web_final.pdf.

Witter, S. et al., 2016. "The Sierra Leone Free Health Care Initiative (FHCI): Process and effectiveness review." Chapter 5.4 Human Resources for Health.

Witter, S., H. Wurie, and M. Bertone, M., 2015. The free health care initiative: how has it affected health workers in Sierra Leone? *Health Policy and Planning* 31: 2–91; doi:10.1093/heapol/czv006

Yates, R. 2009. "Universal health care and the removal of user fees." *Lancet* 373: 2078–81.

Zachariah, R., R. Ortuno, V. Hermans, et al. 2015. "Ebola, fragile health systems and tuberculosis care: A call for pre-emptive action and operational research." *International Journal of Tuberculosis & Lung Disease* 19(11): 1271–275.

Treating, Suffering, and Surviving Ebola

The Story of Prince as told to Patricia Carrick

PRINCE LAHAI AND PATRICIA CARRICK

In times of crisis and disaster they say ordinary people sometimes find in themselves extraordinary strength, courage, and generosity of spirit. On an evening in September 2014, toward the end of one of my first days working in MSF's Ebola Treatment Center (ETC) in Kailahun, Sierra Leone, I met just such a person—a young staff nurse named Prince. He told me he had been working for MSF since the ETC opened in July 2014, but I had not previously met him because he had been on sick leave. He had had Ebola. He had been treated in this very ETC. He had survived. This evening shift was his first time back to work after his weeks of illness and post-infection recuperation. I was stunned: after all he had endured, in the face of his own exhaustion and the fears of his family and friends, he had returned to do the relentless, heartbreaking, day-after-day work of caring for and comforting his dying countrymen and women.

That evening, we were performing our regular duties, heading toward the 8 p.m. patient handover. As the team of national and expatriate staff—nurses, community health officers, doctors, health promotors, water and sanitation experts, hygienists, and guards—all prepared for change of shift, there was a sudden uproar in the "convalescent" part of the confirmed wards. Although we were separated in the "low-risk zone" from all our inpatient wards by double barricades of plastic fencing plus a line of supply tents, dressing and undressing tents, feeding and laundry structures, we had a partial view into the open areas between the ward tents. These areas were lit by electric lights, and, on this evening, as usual, patients well enough to do so escaped the heat inside the tents to sit on chairs or lie on mats on the ground outside enjoying the evening air. Suddenly, dozens of patients began shouting and moving quickly, even running, through the open alleys toward our left. We could not tell what was going on. Many of us at our medical and nursing work centers in the low-risk area surged toward the fences, trying to see clearly what was happening. Staff called out to the patients to ask what was disturbing them.

Then we saw her, stumbling toward the others from our right: one of our convalescent patients, a tall, slim, young adult woman, was careening toward the others, walking quickly with angular limbs akimbo, gesticulating wildly, shouting and throwing her arms out, grunting harshly. We could not tell if she was angry, frightened, or in pain, having some kind of physical attack or psychotic break. Gradually our national staff, shouting over the barriers in local dialect, were able to glean that she felt her heart was "wrong" (palpitations? tachycardia?) and was having pain in the chest. Almost anything could have been happening. Because Ebola often manifests with many days of horrible stomach pain, nausea, and repeated vomiting and diarrhea, metabolic derangement is almost unavoidable and can result in any number of potentially fatal complications. We were not able to test for electrolyte abnormalities nor target them specifically in our setting, but we assumed them and relentlessly pushed oral rehydration salts (ORS) containing life-saving electrolytes that are ubiquitous in the treatment of the many dehydrating diseases (generic dysentery, cholera, malaria, HIV, and the viral hemorrhagic fevers, among others) that afflict poor countries.

Helplessly we watched, tried to gain the young woman's attention to communicate with her, understand her symptoms, calm her, and simultaneously reassure the frightened patients who had run from her, all by shouting from across our plastic fence barricades that MUST NOT be breached but that seemed suddenly so fragile, so flimsy. What if she in her agitation flung herself through the protective fencing? It was effective only by mutual agreement between those who were and those who were not infected. Since we did not wear the suits of personal protective equipment (PPE) except in the high-risk zone, all of us "outside" were vulnerable if that agreement broke down. Of course our impulse was to intervene and contain her, to protect the other patients, to assess, reassure, and treat her. But in the ETC two of us would have first had to dress in full PPE (a 5 to 10-minute process at minimum), then pass carefully through all the other wards (another 5 to 10 minutes) before we could have arrived at her side. Additionally, we had been trained that we must never knowingly place ourselves in proximity with a patient who was out of control. Our only safety was the integrity of our PPE, equipment that could be easily compromised by an aggressive or unpredictable patient; our only assurance as a team to prevent endangering ourselves and one another was to adhere absolutely to our protocols and procedures. So we restrained ourselves; we watched and shouted in to her and to the others, we waited and hoped she would not be driven through the barriers by whatever demons tormented her. Gradually she was able to respond more calmly. We threw a small packet of sedative and pain-relieving pills across the barriers and she was cajoled into taking them. The other patients drifted slowly from their hiding places in the darker corners of their ward. A plate of food was found for her. The other patients encouraged her, and she ate as she paced in her agitation steadily but ever more slowly back and forth.

As she calmed, others on my side of the barricade gradually returned to their end-of-shift tasks. I found myself watchfully monitoring the "inside" accompanied by only one other colleague—Prince—and that was when he told me his story. He described in a quiet, pragmatic voice what it was like to have worked in our ETC and suddenly to have found himself a patient there. He was at first terrorized by his illness and the high likelihood of death. He felt isolated and uncertain despite his familiarity with the setting. His mother was beside herself, sure he would die, and desperate because she could not be with him. Like our patient that night, perhaps, he felt like he was in a cage, surrounded by others on the outside who were separate, free, to whom he was suddenly not a colleague but a peril. Just as we could see "inside," he could see "outside," could see his friends moving about freely, leaving for home at the end of their shifts, laughing, joking, carrying on with their lives. He felt constrained and frustrated. It was his sickness that convinced him finally "I needed to be here, inside." His friends and colleagues took care of him—took *good* care of him, he asserted. He told me "my colleagues and my family gave me the hope and the strength I needed to become better." When he finally turned the corner from illness to a gradual return to health, it was his coworkers who encouraged and inspired him, who celebrated his triumph on the day of his discharge, and who then welcomed him back as comrade among them. His simple statement: "Kaiyengoma." Praise be to God.

While Prince recited his extraordinary story, we sat together in the dark observing our convalescent but still at-risk patients settling past their disruption into evening routines. Even in an Ebola ward, there were the daily routines people performed when they could—brush teeth, hold and comfort children, listen to the radio, visit and laugh, cherish companionship, worry for loved ones. All the time he spoke, Prince exuded a gentle calm, a sense of hope and gratitude that seemed to bathe me as I sat beside him and that seemed to stretch across the barricade to soothe our patients into the darkening quiet of night.

But that is not the end of Prince's story.

When Prince was discharged from the ETC he returned home to live with his mother, his partner, and their three children. Although this had been his home before his illness, now his home was infiltrated by tendrils of stigma and fear. When he was ill, his mother had "lost her senses", he told me, because she thought he would die. "I am the only educated son, and she lost her courage because she lost every hope. She ran into the bush." Upon his return, "She was afraid. She thought I was a ghost." It took days to cajole her back into the household. "My partner was also afraid. We did not share a bed for many months. We did not know what to expect. After five months, she accepted my coming around. But I never said bad about that. I knew I had to stay back."

People of the community were also afraid, hesitant to accept him again into community life. Even though he returned to work at the ETC, there were many weeks when he felt ostracized by friends and neighbors. As the number of survivors in the district increased, messages were disseminated that survivors could not infect others through casual contact. Radio announcements and informational programs began to sensitize the public. Local authorities gradually stepped in over time: fines were announced for those who indulged in overtly stigmatizing behavior. But it was a slow process and, through it all, Prince had to reassure himself and his own family, dress every day and go to work, push through his own discouragement and uncertainty.

Now, more than a year and a half later, Prince is still in Kailahun. He has regained strength after the initial months of debilitating fatigue and overwhelming weakness that characterize both Ebola infection and the subsequent recuperation period. He has survived bouts of post-Ebola headaches and generalized body pains, and these are much better. He has worried about some pain in his left ear, wondering if it will become permanent or affect his hearing. We know so little about post-Ebola syndrome. Everything is new and we are just beginning to learn what are predictable sequelae or complications for Ebola survivors. Daily, Prince faces one of the challenges faced by many Ebola survivors: the challenge of balancing a healthy awareness of his body's sensations while trying to distinguish which might be a sensation associated with the normal physical stresses of life versus a pathological or syndromic result of his devastating bout with infection, all in the context of the need to push on with "normal" life filled with its multitude of routine tasks and responsibilities. Many who experience serious illness of all kinds experience this dilemma, but added to that difficult but not unusual dilemma is all too unusual uncertainty of new symptomatology associated with this heretofore little-studied class of patients. We simply have never before had a cadre of Ebola survivors to observe, monitor, treat, and study, with whom to share what we do know and from whom to try to learn what we do not yet know.

For Prince, as for many in Sierra Leone, addressing these questions and making these distinctions is not so easy. There is no survivors' clinic in Kailahun. The District Medical Officer has assured district survivors that there is a facility for their needs, a "post-Ebola center" in Bo where care for any health condition is completely free for Ebola survivors. Assistance for the cost of transport and sustenance while seeking consultation is available as well. But Prince is trying to hold down a job, and Bo is an almost four-hour drive from Kailahun in the rainy season. Because our experience is so limited, because we know so little of the consequences of post-Ebola symptoms, Prince must weigh his risks every day. Is his symptom serious enough to warrant taking two or more days off work for consultation? If he ignores pain in his ear, does he risk deafness? If he does not address his back or joint pain, is there some sort of chronic inflammation that will constantly worsen without intervention?

Despite all this uncertainty, Prince has taken on a new leadership role for survivors in Kailahun District. This is a volunteer role in a volunteer organization. The Survivors' Group in Kailahun has an office space, an empty room donated by the District Medical Officer, but it cannot afford furniture or office supplies. Nonetheless, Prince travels to area chiefdoms, reaching out to identify other survivors, to inform them of available services and to offer support. He represents the survivors in his district at Survivors' Group meetings in Freetown. He sees this as a crucial role, to keep the suffering and challenges of survivors in the public eye, to help the public understand that surviving the initial infection is only the first step in a long road to recovery. But for Prince, "Sometimes I don't feel so good about my work. So many are illiterate and they do not understand. It isn't very much that I can do."

In the meantime, there is a final uncertainty, not biological but human, economic, and perhaps political that impacts Prince's well-being every day. Prince, a trained nurse with recognized nurse certification in Sierra Leone, does not have the "pin code" that would entitle him to work for the Ministry of Health. Like hundreds, maybe thousands of others who risked their lives to care for Ebola victims, before the epidemic he was working as a "volunteer" nurse for no pay. This is commonly done in Sierra Leone, as unemployed nurses seek to maintain their skills and demonstrate their worthiness for employment until opportunity opens. When the epidemic struck, the Government of Sierra Leone recognized this available pool of trained professionals and reached out to them, publicly promising that, if they would join in the fight against the disease, they would be granted pin codes and therefore secure employment for the Ministry when the epidemic was over. This agreement was overt and widely recognized; it was not implicit, and there were no other stipulations. Not every nurse leapt at the opportunity to put his or her life on the line, and not every nurse who did so did so out of altruism. Many took these chances with their own lives and those of their families because of the stated reward that was promised: stable, long-term, government employment. However, to this day, most of those who worked for over a year in the Kailahun ETC and in other Ebola-related services throughout the country, who suffered ostracism by frightened friends and neighbors, who sacrificed for months the warmth of physical interactions with their own children and spouses in order to protect them, who risked their lives time after time—most of these men and women have never yet received the promised recognition and pin codes. After all they have been through, even unto facing down the threat of death as Prince has done, this final disappointment seems intolerably unjust.

PATIENTS

6

How Did Médecins Sans Frontières Negotiate Clinical Trials of Unproven Treatments During the 2014–2015 Ebola Epidemic?

ANNETTE RID AND ANNICK ANTIERENS

In 2014, the world began to witness an unprecedented Ebola epidemic in West Africa. The epidemic was a "perfect storm"[1] that resulted from weak health systems after decades of war, distrust in national governments and the West, extensive mobility within and across national borders, and burial rites that involved close physical contact with the deceased. In equal measure, the epidemic was a perfect storm for the global health community that ignored early signs of alarm and was overall slow to respond.

Compared to other diseases, Ebola had not been a major global health issue before this epidemic. Previous Ebola outbreaks had a devastating impact on the affected communities, but were overall limited in scope: 29 documented outbreaks had claimed less than 3,000 lives cumulatively over four decades.[2] Given this, insight into the natural progression of Ebola and its treatment, and to a lesser extent its prevention, was very limited before 2014.[3]

Supported by governments of high-income countries who feared that the Ebola virus might be used as a biological weapon, several researchers were developing targeted treatments and vaccines against Ebola.[4] However, these interventions had not been tested in humans when the 2014–2015 epidemic struck. For example, ZMapp (Mapp Biopharmaceutical, United States)—a combination of monoclonal antibodies—was under study in primates when it was first administered to two U.S. citizens in July 2014 after they had contracted Ebola as volunteers in Liberia.[5]

Given the grim prospects that patients with Ebola Virus Disease faced, these experimental treatments and vaccines—along with other unproven therapeutic interventions—sparked immediate interest even though their potential benefits and harms were uncertain. Fatality rates had been as high as 90% in previous Ebola outbreaks, and at the beginning of this epidemic it was considered unlikely that supportive care—fluid replacement, broad-spectrum antibiotics, malaria treatment, anti-emetics, analgesics and antipyretics—would significantly improve the prospects of survival for patients with Ebola Virus Disease.[6] After the two U.S. citizens had received ZMapp, extensive international controversy arose as to whether and how unproven treatments and vaccines should be used in this epidemic.

Key points of controversy were (1) which of the available unproven interventions (if any) should be used; (2) whether they should be used only in clinical trials or on a "monitored emergency use" basis outside formal trials;[7] and (3) how trials should be designed and implemented. MSF took a clear stance toward these issues, agreeing to collaborate on clinical trials but only if certain conditions were met. Because MSF was treating two thirds of the patients with Ebola Virus Disease in the three most affected countries—Guinea, Liberia, and Sierra Leone—its views were highly influential in the debate.

This chapter traces how MSF negotiated trials of unproven Ebola treatments and shows how the organization's values and beliefs shaped key decisions about research priorities and clinical trial design. It sets the scene by summarizing how MSF approached research before the 2014–15 Ebola epidemic and then explains how the treatment trials conducted in this epidemic mark both a continuation and a departure from MSF's previous research practices. In particular, this was the first time that MSF engaged in clinical trials of interventions that were in the earliest stages of development for a disease. Moreover, given the high fatality of Ebola, MSF not only was willing to assume greater risks from unproven treatments than in previous research, but actually felt an obligation to maximize access to these treatments. This had important implications for how the trials were conducted. The chapter closes with some open questions for MSF on how the organization aims to approach the conduct of treatment trials during future epidemics of Ebola or comparable emerging infectious diseases.

Four important limitations need to be highlighted up front. First, the chapter draws extensively on the archive of Ebola-related documents and communications that were written or processed by MSF's Operational Center in Brussels and the MSF Investigational Platform for Experimental Ebola Products.[8] The latter was a platform of experts from different MSF sections that had the mandate to engage MSF in clinical trials.[9] Drawing on this archive means that communications of other MSF centers, units, or affiliates are not necessarily reflected. Moreover, many of the cited documents were written as working documents for internal purposes and not for external use. By necessity, these documents do not reflect the detail and nuance of MSF's deliberations and often omit critical information. In some cases, they may also represent views or decisions that were later changed.

Second, due to time constraints the authors were unable to conduct interviews with members of the Investigational Platform and others within MSF who played an important role in negotiating the use of unproven treatments for Ebola during this epidemic. This means that the chapter should be read as a first attempt to understand how the organization made key decisions about this matter; future work will be needed to add further context and detail.[10]

Third, MSF's involvement in clinical trials was extensive during the epidemic and a single paper cannot cover all relevant aspects. This chapter focuses on trials of unproven treatments that specifically targeted the Ebola virus because they were initially prioritized by MSF and—for better or for worse—because these trials raised the most controversy during the epidemic. As a result, the chapter does not cover a wide range of important research that MSF either led or contributed to, including clinical trials of experimental vaccines and new diagnostic tests as well as research on the characteristics and clinical outcomes of patients with Ebola Virus Disease, Ebola virus transmission, laboratory testing, and infection control and anthropological research on the understanding and perception of Ebola Virus Disease and interventions against the epidemic among patients and affected communities.[11] Readers should note, however, that MSF used the same process to decide about its involvement in all clinical trials, even though it ended up making different decisions about treatment trials when compared to vaccine trials. This means that the chapter's insights into MSF's decision-making process about treatment trials apply more generally, even though the organization's substantive decisions about vaccine trials differed.[12] Furthermore, the chapter focuses primarily on how MSF and the research consortium in which it took part made decisions between September and December 2014. Other time periods are only covered briefly, if at all.

Fourth, MSF had to take a position on whether and how the available unproven treatments should be used under extremely challenging circumstances. In particular, the organization had to make decisions at the height of the epidemic and navigate an acute sense of urgency to act, profound uncertainty about the outbreak and the available treatment candidates, major feasibility constraints in the field, as well as international ethical controversy around the clinical trials.[13] Much has been learned since, and it is difficult to appreciate the complexity of the situation at the time. In fact, it is difficult (if not impossible) to write or read about the events without the benefit of hindsight. Readers are asked to bear this in mind.

Finally, some notes on terminology. A large number of unproven treatments were proposed for compassionate or monitored emergency use, or investigation in clinical trials, and the existing data on their safety and effectiveness in humans varied greatly. Nearly all proposed treatments were untested in patients with Ebola Virus Disease; however, some had never been investigated in humans, while others were approved for clinical use, or in various stages of clinical testing, for diseases other than Ebola. Moreover, a range of laboratory data existed to support the proposed interventions' anti-Ebola effects—from experiments in cell cultures to tests in rodents or (non-human) primates to no laboratory data at all. This chapter uses "unproven treatments" as the overarching term for all treatments that were proposed for compassionate or monitored emergency use, or clinical trials, during the 2014–15 Ebola epidemic. The evidentiary base for particular treatment candidates is described as necessary when they are discussed. The term "experimental treatment" is reserved for interventions that had previously not undergone testing in humans. The chapter uses the term "2014–15 epidemic" because the epidemic—which officially lasted from December 2013 until June 2016—peaked during this time.

MSF Research Before the 2014–15 Ebola Epidemic

MSF is a medical humanitarian organization that is committed to responding directly to human suffering, irrespective of where or why it occurs and irrespective of the challenges of mounting a response.[14] The organization's core mission is clearly clinical and patient-centered. For example, reflecting on its work in 2014, MSF wrote that the Ebola epidemic highlighted global failures in the humanitarian aid and health systems, yet addressing these was beyond the organization's core mission:

> Ultimately MSF is a patient-focused organisation and our attention remains primarily on those in need of medical care and not on overhauling global systems. MSF concentrates on individuals and we are constantly striving to provide assistance to those who need it most. Our role is to save patients' lives, today, and we respond to crises with that at the forefront of our minds.[15]

What, then, is the role of research in a patient-centered humanitarian medical organization like MSF? Among such organizations, MSF is known for conducting a wide range of research studies—from qualitative studies and quantitative surveys to observational research, retrospective data analysis, and prospective clinical trials—in order to generate knowledge that has the potential to improve MSF's ability to save or improve the lives of patients in the future. For example, in 1987 MSF founded Epicentre, a satellite nongovernmental organization (NGO) dedicated to conducting clinical and epidemiological research in complex humanitarian emergencies.[16] In the 1990s, MSF began building a comprehensive operational research infrastructure for the organization and created—among others—an explicit research policy, research support units, a research registry, an ethics review board, an innovation fund, annual scientific days, and an online publications repository.[17] MSF is also one of the co-founders of a research and development organization that actively promotes and manages research in other institutions in order to develop new drugs for the world's most neglected diseases.[18]

As a medical humanitarian organization, MSF has important reasons for engaging in research. First and foremost, research is necessary for improving clinical care and preventive measures in humanitarian emergencies. The evidence to support humanitarian medical interventions is often limited,[19] and this can jeopardize MSF's fundamental commitment to providing "high-quality medical care to all patients."[20] For example, the clinical practice guidelines for Ebola contained only a handful of primary sources before the 2014–2015 epidemic.[21] Moreover, because many academic and private-sector researchers lack the infrastructure, networks, and incentives to conduct research in humanitarian emergencies, MSF and other humanitarian medical organizations have to actively promote or conduct research studies themselves.[22]

In addition, MSF engages in research—and in particular in quantitative studies that document population health—in order to bear witness and "bring attention to extreme need and unacceptable suffering."[23] Speaking out about abuse and violence is one of the hallmarks of MSF,[24] and research studies can be a particularly effective way of witnessing because, in the words of Peter Redfield, they translate "suffering into the institutionally potent language of numbers."[25] Finally, engaging in research has other benefits for MSF, such as greater credibility in the medical community, improved access to national and international decision makers, more effective advocacy in policy circles, and added rigor in the organization's program planning, implementation, and evaluation.[26]

Despite these important reasons for MSF to engage in research, scientific activity can raise concerns among the organization's members. Some within MSF question the value of clinical research in particular because they view it as an academically driven, top-down exercise with little or no relevance to communities or staff in the field. In their view, researchers aim to identify generalizable solutions while MSF needs localized, immediate problem solving.[27] Others are concerned that it can be difficult to maintain sound scientific standards during humanitarian emergencies, especially in clinical trials that require controlled conditions for evaluating new treatments or vaccines. For example, logistical constraints and a high turnover of clinical staff with often limited research skills can compromise the scientific rigor of clinical trials and thereby undermine their fundamental ethical justification.[28] Some MSF members also raise concerns that even valuable and scientifically sound research "diverts too much resources and attention from its [the organization's] core job of delivering care."[29] Finally, the conduct of research can conflict with MSF's patient-centered orientation. For example, clinical trials can require performing procedures that serve to answer research questions but have no potential clinical benefits for participants, such as research-specific blood draws.

MSF has adopted a number of operational and ethical requirements for the research it conducts in order to minimize such concerns. MSF's research policy requires that research studies be of direct, practical relevance for the organization and have no more than a limited impact on its routine operations.[30] Human and other resources have to be carefully assessed—and strengthened as necessary—so that research activities do not pose a significant burden on routine clinical care and operations; if a conflict between the two arises, the provision of care takes priority. Moreover, MSF's research ethics framework mandates scientific rigor for all research studies that the organization engages in and highlights that preserving and enhancing the well-being of participants is the "overarching imperative of any engagement in research."[31]

Consistent with these requirements, MSF has traditionally conducted research that has had at most a limited impact on research participants and the organization's routine operations. Most MSF research before the 2014–15 Ebola epidemic was descriptive or observational, involving, for example, retrospective analyses of routinely collected patient data, studies on routinely collected samples, and interviews or surveys that were conducted by dedicated MSF research teams or satellite organizations.[32] Interventional research was generally avoided and was conducted only when descriptive or observational studies could not address the given research question. As a result, MSF's past research activities comprise relatively few interventional clinical trials. Furthermore, consistent with the organization's patient-centered orientation, the interventional trials that MSF did conduct have generally aimed to promote participants' well-being by exposing them to very limited (if any) research-specific risks. Specifically, past MSF trials have typically tested clinical interventions whose risks and potential benefits were relatively certain and that had a high likelihood of benefiting participants, such as proven effective treatments or promising combinations of established therapies.[33] Moreover, research-specific procedures that have no prospect of clinical benefit to participants, such as research-related blood draws, were avoided in these trials in order to reduce research risks to them. As will become clear throughout this chapter, the treatment trials that MSF helped to conduct in the 2014–15 Ebola epidemic mark both a continuation of, and a departure from, the organization's prior research practices.

The First Use of Unproven Ebola Treatments in the Field

MSF had its first brush with unproven Ebola interventions in the field in July 2014. The organization had been working in Guinea since 2001 and began responding to the epidemic from its very beginnings, in Guinée Forestière, in

March 2014. MSF had responded to Ebola outbreaks in nine countries over the last 20 years and was therefore able to mobilize an international team of experts in a very short time. By the end of July 2014, MSF was one of the very few international aid organizations caring for patients with Ebola Virus Disease in Guinea, Liberia, and Sierra Leone, having built four Ebola treatment units (ETUs) and several smaller centers and transit units in these countries.[34] As such, MSF clinicians were the first to confront the possibility of using unproven treatments for Ebola in the field.

Several vaccines and targeted treatments for Ebola were in development when the 2014–2015 epidemic broke, mostly as part of the U.S. government's biodefense program after the terrorist attacks in New York on September 11, 2001. One of these experimental interventions—the already-mentioned anti-body cocktail ZMapp—had shown important survival benefits in primates in early 2014 but was untested in humans.[35] Three doses were brought to Sierra Leone later that year for stability testing in a tropical climate,[36] and at the end of July MSF had the opportunity to provide one of them to a renowned Sierra Leonean clinician (see Chapter 7 in this volume). MSF ended up deciding against using ZMapp in this case, primarily because it feared that the drug would do more harm than good and its use might stoke suspicion of Western medical institutions, thereby compromising efforts to contain the outbreak.[37] However, another humanitarian organization provided ZMapp to two U.S. volunteers who had contracted Ebola in Liberia shortly thereafter. While, sadly, the Sierra Leonean clinician died, both U.S. volunteers survived after being repatriated, and headlines such as "Why do two US missionaries get an Ebola serum while Africans are left to die?" quickly followed.[38]

The Decision to Engage in Clinical Trials

Extensive international controversy arose when details about the use of ZMapp in the field became known. Two questions quickly dominated the debate. First, was it ethically acceptable to use experimental treatments and vaccines that had shown promising laboratory results but were untested in humans? Second, if the answer was yes, under which conditions should such experimental interventions be used?

Less than two weeks after ZMapp was given to the two U.S. volunteers, the World Health Organization (WHO) convened an international panel of experts for advice on both questions.[39] The panel concluded that there was an "ethical imperative" to use experimental interventions, provided that they had shown promising results in the laboratory and in animal models and several additional conditions were met.[40] This position marked a clear deviation from standard practice, according to which experimental treatments and vaccines are first tested in a set series of clinical trials and used more widely only after they have been shown to be safe and effective. However, the panel argued that the exceptional circumstances of the 2014–2015 epidemic—notably the rapid spread of Ebola in numerous locations and the lack of targeted treatments or vaccines for a highly fatal disease—justified this deviation. At the same time, the panel called for scientifically sound and rigorous studies of the available experimental interventions. In particular, although "compassionate use" outside such studies was justified as an exceptional emergency measure, this should not preclude or delay more conclusive investigations. Moreover, data on the clinical outcomes of compassionate use should be collected and shared (this practice was later referred to as "monitored emergency use").[41]

Things then moved very quickly. WHO convened several expert groups to review the "pipeline" of potential Ebola treatments and vaccines and discuss the challenges of using or testing them in this epidemic.[42] Importantly, this discussion not only covered experimental treatments and vaccines that were untested in humans, but also considered numerous interventions supported by varying levels of laboratory and clinical evidence. MSF was involved in the discussions from the start and quickly received requests for collaboration from academic researchers as well as the private sector. This was unsurprising given MSF's extensive past experience in responding to Ebola outbreaks and, in particular, its unique role in the response to this epidemic. By the end of July 2014, shortly before the first WHO meetings were being held, MSF had admitted 891 of the 1,440 suspected or confirmed Ebola cases to ETUs in Guinea, Liberia, and Sierra Leone.[43] This made MSF the primary caregiver for patients with Ebola Virus Disease and, from a research perspective, the primary "gatekeeper" to potential participants in treatment trials.[44]

Establishing the Investigational Platform for Ebola Products

MSF decided to engage in clinical trials in mid-August 2014[45] and immediately made two important procedural decisions about how the organization should navigate the trials.

First, MSF decided that it would not take the lead on investigating a particular intervention and instead would join a larger research consortium.[46] As mentioned earlier,[47] the organization had traditionally conducted clinical trials of established interventions—or combinations thereof—that had a high likelihood of benefiting participants. By contrast, the safety and effectiveness of the unproven treatments and vaccines for Ebola were uncertain, even when they were approved for clinical use or in clinical testing for diseases other than Ebola. To ensure the appropriate conduct of clinical trials, MSF had to collaborate with researchers who had expertise in testing interventions that were in the earliest phases of development for Ebola. Moreover, MSF did not have the capacity to execute clinical trials on its own, and joining larger research consortia meant that the responsibility for trial-related activities would be shared among several partners.

Furthermore, working with other partners reduced MSF's institutional risks, most notably the risk of distrust by local communities and national authorities in the affected West African countries. Attitudes toward clinical trials varied between countries and locations in the 2014–15 Ebola epidemic and were generally difficult to gauge. In addition, time pressure initially made it difficult for MSF and its research partners to initiate systematic community engagement activities.[48] In some regions there were also unsolved questions about who was a legitimate community representative, and whether engaging fully with local populations about clinical trials was always desirable. For instance, Ebola survivors in Conakry feared that community engagement about a convalescent plasma trial could fuel stigma against them. This meant that considerable uncertainty prevailed as to how communities would receive the conduct of clinical trials.[49] MSF's hope was that engaging in research collaborations would enable it to "remain (co)-decisional on what we use (or allow to use) on patients under MSF care" and "able to pull out if [this was] better for patient care or acceptability",[50] while spreading the risk of conflict with local communities. MSF also hoped that entrusting the leadership of trials to other institutions would reduce its own institutional risks in the longer term. In particular, spearheading "experiments on Africans" in the midst of an epidemic could have tainted MSF's image and made future missions more difficult to implement—an outcome that the organization was eager to avoid.

Second, MSF created a clear focal point within the organization—the already-mentioned Investigational Platform for Experimental Ebola Products—that obtained the mandate to engage MSF in clinical trials. The Platform consisted of experts from different MSF sections, including the MSF affiliates Epicentre and the Access Campaign, and was co-chaired by the medical directors of two (and later three) of MSF's five operational centers.[51] An Investigational Platform manager coordinated the work of the group and convened weekly meetings to discuss, decide about, and manage the clinical trials in which MSF would engage. The Platform actively liaised with relevant MSF staff, such as working group leaders or field coordination teams, and provided input to the communications team. The Platform also gave regular internal updates to key MSF personnel, including the organization's executive and associative leadership, on the Platform's work. Moreover, the Platform led the discussion and negotiations with institutions and stakeholders outside of MSF.

In addition, MSF immediately made several important substantive decisions about the conditions under which the organization would engage with potential research partners.[52] These conditions are the topic of the remainder of this chapter.

Prioritizing Treatment Trials

In line with WHO's recommendation, MSF decided to prioritize clinical trials over monitored emergency use and focused its efforts almost exclusively on engaging in clinical trials.[53] This decision was supported by several reasons. First and foremost, there was a real possibility that the available unproven treatments would cause harm to patients with Ebola Virus Disease, and clinical trials would allow more effective identification and management of negative clinical outcomes than monitored emergency use. Conversely, positive clinical outcomes were likely more straightforward to measure in clinical trials. Moreover, monitored emergency use was a relatively new concept, and it was expected that working within a clinical trial framework would make it easier to engage with drug manufacturers, obtain the necessary regulatory authorizations and research ethics committee approvals, and import the available unproven interventions into the affected countries. Thus, engaging in clinical trials would enable faster access to potentially life-saving treatments during this epidemic than monitored emergency use.

In addition, the data gathered in clinical trials would be more robust than those that could be collected during monitored emergency use. This meant not only that it was easier to evaluate the merits of candidate treatments with data from clinical trials, but also that regulatory approval and registration of any proven effective interventions could be obtained more easily. Furthermore, because regulatory approval was a precondition for the large-scale production, reimbursement, and widespread clinical use of treatments, clinical trials were the most effective way to maximize access to any effective interventions in the longer term. MSF also estimated that it would take as much time to develop protocols for monitored emergency use as it would take to develop clinical trial protocols. However, because monitored emergency use would provide less robust data, clinical trials would make better-quality data available sooner. Finally, working within a clinical trial framework was also thought to reduce institutional risks for MSF in the event that the available unproven treatments proved less effective or more harmful than expected.[54]

Furthermore, as one of the main providers of care for patients with Ebola Virus Disease in West Africa, MSF initially decided to prioritize treatment trials over trials of other interventions, notably experimental vaccines or diagnostic tests.[55] The organization later broadened its remit to include vaccines and then diagnostics,[56] but its initial focus was firmly on testing and identifying potential therapeutics.

MSF's decision to prioritize trials of unproven treatments was supported by several reasons. As a patient-centered organization, MSF was particularly concerned about the lack of targeted treatments for a disease that—according to its own data—had a fatality rate of 40% to 60%.[57] Moreover, the experience from past outbreaks suggested that supportive care would not significantly improve the prospects of survival for patients with Ebola Virus Disease in a low-resource setting.[58] Indeed, limited evidence indicated that supportive care might lower fatality rates by no more than 5% to 10%.[59] Moreover, the volume of patients was so overwhelming when MSF decided to engage in treatment trials that some of its ETUs became temporarily unable to provide the standard supportive care. For example, MSF's largest ETU in Monrovia had to switch from individualized to standardized care and restrict or suspend intravenous fluids between August and October 2014 (see Chapter 8 in this volume).[60] The epidemic was also growing exponentially at the time, and some experts warned that more than a million people could require treatment for Ebola by early 2015 in Liberia and Sierra Leone.[61] This grim situation extracted an enormous emotional toll from MSF staff, "exacerbated by exhaustion from long working hours, extreme heat, the limitations of working in full protective suits, and concerns about their own health and safety. National staff had the additional burdens of infection risk in their communities, stigmatization, and grief over the loss of family and friends."[62] Plainly, there was a "desperate expectation for therapeutic solutions."[63]

Some MSF members also argued that treatment trials would help to contain the epidemic because the prospect of receiving a potentially effective treatment would give people an incentive to seek care. For example, one of the members of the MSF's Investigational Platform stated: "At the moment, our big problem is finding the patients in a timely way and convincing them to come to the treatment center . . . If you don't have a carrot to hang out there and bring people in, then you can't contain it."[64] This argument also resonated with some community members. ETUs were often seen as places to die rather than places to recover, and treatment trials were thought to change this perception. As one 49-year-old man in a small interview study in Monrovia said: "If you say you have the drugs now, a hundred persons will run to you!"[65] MSF also hoped that clinical trials of unproven treatments would help to sustain a dwindling workforce of health professionals who were at increased risk of contracting Ebola.[66]

In addition, MSF recognized its unique role in the epidemic response and the responsibility this entailed with respect to contributing to trials of unproven treatments.[67] Plainly, if MSF had decided against engaging in such trials, studies would have been extremely difficult to get off the ground. MSF not only had extensive past experience with treating Ebola, but—as mentioned above—it was also caring for the majority of patients with Ebola Virus Disease in this epidemic. As the primary caregiver, MSF had a special responsibility to try to improve patient outcomes.

It was also the main "gatekeeper" to potential participants in treatment trials. Moreover, MSF had only limited capacity to engage in clinical research, and other institutions could conduct trials of vaccines and diagnostics without MSF involvement. The organization's collaboration was therefore key to the success of treatment trials in this epidemic, especially in its early phases.

Finally, MSF was unwilling to engage in vaccine trials before safety data on the existing experimental vaccines were available from first-in-human (phase 1) trials. In September 2014, none of the existing vaccine candidates had been tested in humans or were being evaluated in phase 1 trials. By contrast, safety data from other patient populations were available for at least some of the available treatment candidates. Moreover, experimental vaccines would have to be administered to healthy individuals, while unproven treatments were to be given to patients with Ebola Virus Disease with a high risk of dying. This important difference in background risk justified accepting higher uncertainty about the risks and potential benefits of unproven interventions in treatment trials than in vaccine trials.

Internal Debate About Treatment Trials

MSF's decision to engage in treatment trials caused considerable debate within the organization. When the Investigational Platform's manager sent a briefing paper about the platform to some key figures in the MSF movement, she said, "it is [was] evident that a lot is being said and thought in the corridors about MSF engaging in trials."[68] A key point of discussion was whether the decision to prioritize clinical trials over monitored emergency use—or indeed compassionate use that involves no systematic collection and sharing of data on clinical outcomes—was justified for all of the available unproven treatments. Everyone agreed that clinical trials were needed to evaluate the safety of experimental treatments that were untested in humans. However, some MSF members argued that certain other treatments should be offered to all patients without formal testing in trials. Specifically, the proposal was to "repurpose"[69] treatments that were approved for clinical use or in clinical testing for diseases other than Ebola, provided they had shown anti-Ebola effects in preclinical studies or they had an antiviral activity likely to affect the Ebola virus. The underlying rationale was that repurposed treatments were more likely to be safe than experimental treatments, given that they had been tested in healthy individuals and other patients, and that their risks were justified considering the possibility of benefit and the high risk of dying that patients with Ebola Virus Disease faced.

The position on compassionate use is difficult to trace in the available early documents but was later summarized in an open letter to the MSF movement that dates from December 2014: "Though it seems debatable to test experimental drugs [that have not undergone safety testing in humans] . . . in the context of a major outbreak . . ., the use of drugs on an off-label or compassionate basis (i.e. drugs that have already been given to human beings and data on safety is available) is not only imaginable, but essential given the very high mortality rates."[70] According to the authors of this letter, numerous reasons supported the widespread use of repurposed treatments on a compassionate use basis: MSF's humanitarian and clinical duty to improve patient outcomes; its humanitarian duty to offer hope; the patients' right to decide about their treatment for a highly fatal disease; considerations of fairness, given that almost all patients with Ebola Virus Disease from high-income countries were receiving repurposed treatments on a compassionate use basis; and the fact that the WHO advisory panel had given "clearance" for compassionate use which, in any case, was very common in clinical practice.

The Investigational Platform responded to this open letter by arguing that it could not be assumed that the available repurposed treatments would improve patient outcomes and therefore advocated for clinical trials to evaluate their effects; that providing false hope was problematic; that patients had a right to make *informed* treatment decisions and making such decisions required robust data; that WHO had endorsed monitored emergency use, but not unmonitored compassionate use as the letter suggested; and that common clinical practices—including compassionate use—are not necessarily justified.[71] Moreover, it would have been very difficult to select one of the many repurposed treatment candidates, and even more difficult to define criteria to continue or abandon a selected treatment for another one. In fact, preclinical studies showed later in the epidemic that some of the most promoted treatment candidates seem to be ineffective against Ebola.[72]

Readers should note that the open letter caused itself fierce controversy within the organization and some signatories later retracted their position and issued an apology. It is also important to highlight that proponents of compassionate use and clinical trials within MSF shared the goal of maximizing access to potentially beneficial treatments for Ebola, but differed about how this goal should best be achieved. For reasons discussed in the previous section, the Investigational Platform favored clinical trials because they thought that trials were the fastest and most effective way of ensuring treatment access both in the shorter and the longer term. Those who advocated for compassionate use believed that treatment access could best be maximized outside clinical trials.

Selecting Treatments for Study in Clinical Trials

MSF's Investigational Platform quickly entered into its first research collaboration with the University of Oxford, which was leading a large consortium of both public and private partners. One of the first tasks for MSF and this consortium was to determine which of the numerous proposed treatments for Ebola should be tested in clinical trials; more than 120 unproven treatments had been suggested to WHO within weeks.[73] To prioritize the most promising agents for clinical trials and accelerate the launch of research projects, WHO established a scientific advisory committee to review the relative merits of the various proposed interventions.[74] This committee prioritized convalescent plasma and whole blood as well as nine unproven treatments and vaccines for testing in the field—or, more specifically, five antivirals, one antibody product, one immune modulator, and two vaccines.[75] The priority list was largely based on the interventions' predicted safety and effectiveness against Ebola.[76]

In September 2014, shortly after WHO's priority list had been issued, the research consortium led by the University of Oxford appointed a steering committee that included representatives from the three most affected West African countries, researchers from Africa and other continents, as well as representatives from MSF, WHO, and the Oxford-led International Severe Acute Respiratory and Emerging Infection Consortium. The steering committee met to validate WHO's priority list and select treatment candidates that the consortium should aim to study first. Although there was "no common agreement [within the group] . . . that WHO pre-selected products . . . give [gave] a certain level of credibility or guarantee safety,"[77] they were overall considered "sufficiently interesting" to test.[78]

General Criteria for Selecting Treatment Candidates

The predicted risk/benefit profile of WHO's prioritized treatment candidates varied, and the differences in their predicted safety and effectiveness against Ebola were an important consideration for the steering committee of the Oxford-led research consortium. For example, the antibody cocktail ZMapp and the antiviral TKM-130803 (Tekmira Pharmaceuticals, Canada) appeared to be very effective in primates, but safety data in humans did not exist or were still being collected. By contrast, such safety data were available for the antivirals brincidofovir (Chimerix, United States) and favipiravir (Toyama Chemical of the Fujifilm Group, Japan), even though their anti-Ebola effects had been demonstrated only in cell cultures or mice.[79]

However, treatment candidates could not be selected based on their predicted risk/benefit profile alone. Several candidates were not available in larger quantities when the steering committee convened and, as MSF noted at a later point, "running trials is [was] dependent on drugs' availability."[80] Overall, "all agreed . . . the best answer is [was] to start those [trials] with the fastest implementation possibilities . . . as soon as possible."[81] Immediate availability therefore became an important determinant of the committee's decisions about which treatments on WHO's priority list to study first.

In addition, the feasibility of implementing the short-listed treatments in the field influenced the committee's selection of treatment candidates for clinical trials. MSF was committed to testing treatments that had the potential to make an impact on patients in *this* epidemic. The organization's leadership and staff in the field were looking for "results with immediate impact on decision-making and improvement of patient care and survival, rather than . . . results that might potentially only support tackling the next outbreak."[82] MSF hoped that initial trial results would be available by the end of 2014 or early 2015, and that any treatment considered to be "safe and promising in terms of efficacy" could then be made available to all patients while larger-scale trials were continued.[83]

Given these priorities, the steering committee of the Oxford-led research consortium focused on treatment candidates that were (1) promising in terms of their predicted safety and effectiveness against Ebola; (2) readily available so that trials could be started as soon as possible; (3) feasible to implement under the challenging conditions of this epidemic; and (4) relatively easy to produce in larger quantities so that post-trial availability for future patients could be ensured if a treatment improved clinical outcomes.[84]

Reasons for Deprioritizing Specific Treatment Candidates

The above focus meant that the steering committee decided against five of WHO's prioritized treatment candidates at this time. Specifically, the antibody cocktail ZMapp and the two antivirals AVI-7537 (Sarepta Therapeutics, United States) and BCX-4430 (BioCryst Pharmaceuticals, United States) were not selected for clinical trials because their availability was very limited and deemed insufficient for conducting a successful trial. There was unconfirmed information that 30 to 100 treatment courses of ZMapp would be produced by early 2015. However, although this stock would have allowed conducting a clinical trial, ZMapp was still not selected because the projected production was insufficient to ensure post-trial availability to the drug.

The antiviral TKM-130803 was not chosen because it was awaiting modification and subsequent phase 1 testing in order to specifically target the Ebola virus strain that was causing the 2014–15 epidemic; this meant considerable delays. Moreover, TKM-130803 had to be administered in daily, six-hour-long infusions for a total of seven days, and this was considered a serious challenge in the field in case of high admission rates. It was also unclear how TKM-130803 production could be scaled up if positive trial results emerged.

Finally, immune modulators like interferons were not selected because treatments that attacked the Ebola virus directly were expected to have a greater chance of improving patient survival than treatments that targeted disease processes caused by the virus; interferon also had not improved outcomes in preclinical studies. In addition, a trial of interferon was already being prepared by another group of researchers.

Reasons for Prioritizing Specific Treatment Candidates

The steering committee of the Oxford-led consortium thus selected the three remaining treatment candidates for testing, namely convalescent plasma and the antivirals favipiravir and brincidofovir. The two antivirals were repurposed treatments that had been developed for diseases other than Ebola, but had shown anti-Ebola activity in cell cultures or animal experiments. The use of such repurposed treatments had several advantages.[85] First and foremost, large numbers of treatment courses were immediately available because the treatments were either already marketed (favipiravir) or in larger-scale clinical testing (brincidofovir) and production could be scaled up. Moreover, human safety data and results from large-scale clinical testing in other patients existed that allowed making some predictions about the treatments' safety. However, safety in patients with Ebola Virus Disease could not be guaranteed, and this was an important reason for conducting clinical trials. For example, favipiravir was estimated to require a doubling of the dose that was shown to be safe in healthy volunteers in order to be effective against Ebola.[86] It was unclear to what extent this doubling would result in toxicities, especially because many patients with Ebola Virus Disease had liver problems that were known to lead to increased drug levels. There were also concerns about toxicities from interactions between favipiravir and malaria drugs that patients with Ebola Virus Disease were receiving as part of their supportive care.[87]

At the same time, repurposed treatments had the disadvantage that the evidence to support their anti-Ebola activity could be limited. For example, brincidofovir—which was still undergoing clinical testing as a treatment for cytomegalovirus and adenovirus infections—had shown anti-Ebola effects only in cell cultures, and studies in primates were not feasible for this drug.[88] Weeks after the steering committee of the Oxford-led consortium had selected brincidofovir for evaluation in a clinical trial, disappointing results from studies in mice became available that raised "a lot of questions and concerns."[89] Given the care necessary for interpreting these data, a wider WHO-led working group of Ebola experts and researchers was brought together in early December 2014 to discuss their implications for the clinical trial that was in planning by then. The group concluded that brincidofovir should remain a candidate for testing in patients with Ebola Virus Disease, provided that safety was closely monitored.

Convalescent plasma was primarily selected because of its predicted safety and relative availability.[90] Moreover, national authorities in the affected countries supported convalescent plasma trials because they considered plasma transfusions to be readily available and sustainable, provided that clinical trials included the necessary capacity building and investments in infrastructure. In their view, convalescent plasma trials provided the local population with greater control than trials of internationally developed drugs that were subject to intellectual property rights. However, the fact that the "production" of convalescent plasma required the goodwill and collaboration of Ebola survivors sparked considerable discussion within MSF. In particular, the collection of plasma exposed survivors to physical risks and potential stigma; efforts to ensure adequate supplies could lead to "coercion to get survivors involved"; plasma was not fit for "mass production" and its collection was labor-intensive; and procuring and managing blood products could create tensions with communities, given the special meaning of blood for communities in the region.[91] Still, MSF considered convalescent plasma a reasonable option, especially for patient groups who might not qualify for inclusion in clinical trials or monitored emergency use of other unproven treatments in the short and medium term—notably pregnant women.[92]

Negotiating Treatment Trial Collaborations

Following the selection of treatment candidates, MSF decided to engage in a clinical trial of brincidofovir in one of its ETUs in Monrovia (Liberia) with the research consortium led by the University of Oxford. Moreover, by this time the French Institut National de la Santé et de la Recherche Médicale (INSERM) was in advanced negotiations about a trial of favipiravir with national authorities in Guinea as well as the drug manufacturer, and MSF quickly offered to collaborate on a trial of favipiravir in its ETU in Gueckedou. Similarly, the Institute of Tropical Medicine (ITM) in Antwerp had already constituted a research consortium, engaged with national authorities in Guinea, and obtained funding for a trial of convalescent plasma at this point. MSF thus decided to collaborate on a convalescent plasma trial with this consortium in its ETU in Conakry. Table 6-1 provides an overview of all clinical trials with MSF involvement, including vaccine trials that are otherwise not covered in this chapter.

The subsequent weeks were packed with negotiating how the agreed trials should be conducted, obtaining ethical and regulatory approvals, drawing up contracts between consortium partners, engaging with communities, addressing operational challenges in planning the trials' implementation, and coordinating research efforts with other groups.[93] All partners had an essential contribution to make to the trials' success. Research was not going to go forward without

Table 6-1. **Overview of All Clinical Trials with MSF Involvement.** Partners of the different research consortia may have had different understandings of the trials. This table reflects MSF's understanding. Protocols for monitored emergency use with MSF involvement are summarized in footnote 53.

Intervention	Manufacturer	Trial design	Trial arm(s)	Trial name	Key collaborators	Key funders	Location	Start	Comments
Unproven treatments									
Favipiravir	Toyama Chemical, Fujifilm Group, Japan	Single arm	Favipiravir + standard care vs. standard care in historical controls	JIKI (meaning "hope" in the Malinke language)	INSERM (sponsor), Government of Guinea , MSF, Alliance for International Medical Action (ALIMA), French Red Cross, French Military Health Service	EU Horizon 2020, Agence nationale de recherche sur le sida et les hépatites virales (ANRS), INSERM	Guinea	Dec. 14	• Goal: gather preliminary data to optimize design of future studies (proof-of-concept) and collect preliminary data on safety and effectiveness in reducing mortality and viral load
Brincidofovir	Chimerix, United States	Single arm	Brincidofovir + standard care vs. standard care in historical controls	RAPIDE	University of Oxford (sponsor), Government of Liberia, MSF, University of Lancaster	Wellcome Trust	Liberia	Jan. 15	• Goal: quickly evaluate whether brincidofovir was safe and very effective, promising or ineffective
Convalescent plasma	N/A	Single arm	Convalescent plasma + standard care vs. standard care in historical controls	Ebola-Tx	Institute of Tropical Medicine Antwerp (sponsor), National Blood Transfusion Centre (NBTC) Guinea, WHO, MSF, Belgian Red Cross Flanders (BRC), Unit of Biology of Emerging Viral Infections (UBIVE), Pasteur Institute, etc.	EU Horizon 2020, Bill & Melinda Gates Foundation, Flemish government	Guinea	Feb. 15	• Goal: evaluate safety, efficacy and feasibility

Experimental vaccines

Intervention	Manufacturer	Trial design	Trial arm(s)	Trial name	Key collaborators	Key funders	Location	Start	Comments
rVSV-ZEBOV	Public Health Agency of Canada and NewLink Genetics (licensed by Merck), United States	Cluster randomized controlled: ring vaccination	Immediate rVSV-ZEBOV vs. deferred rVSV-ZEBOV	Ebola ça Suffit (Ebola this is enough) - part A	WHO (sponsor), MSF Epicentre, Ministry of Health Guinea, Public Health Agency of Canada, Norwegian Institute of Public Health, Public Health England, London School of Hygiene and Tropical Medicine, University of Bern, University of Florida, University of Maryland	MSF, Research Council of Norway, Wellcome Trust, Public Health Agency of Canada, WHO	Guinea	March 15	• Groups/clusters of individuals at high risk of infection are identified (based on social or geographic connection to a known case) and randomly assigned to receiving immediate or deferred vaccination. • Deferred vaccination cluster serves as concurrent control. • Goal: evaluate safety, immunogenicity, & efficacy • Adult at-risk population: contacts of patients with Ebola Virus Disease
		Single arm	rVSV-ZEBOV	Ebola ça Suffit (Ebola this is enough) - part B	WHO (sponsor), MSF, Government of Guinea	MSF, Research Council of Norway, Wellcome Trust, Public Health Agency of Canada, WHO	Guinea	March 15	• Goal: evaluate safety & immunogenicity • Adult at-risk population: frontline workers

the collaboration of local populations and their representatives. MSF had the local networks, operational and clinical expertise, and infrastructure to run a medical humanitarian mission responding to the epidemic. Academic researchers provided scientific expertise and access to research networks and funders. And pharmaceutical companies had the selected treatment candidates and infrastructure for scaling up their production. The result were intense negotiations about each trial that would normally take years, but were now condensed into several weeks or months.

MSF was aware of its considerable leverage in the negotiation process. By the time the trials were being planned, it was still treating the majority of patients with Ebola Virus Disease in the three countries most affected by the epidemic. However, the pressure to enable treatment trials was gradually decreasing because other medical humanitarian NGOs had entered the field. This meant that MSF remained one of the key gatekeepers to patients with Ebola Virus Disease and potential trial participants while having the flexibility to be "more selective in terms of partners we want to engage with."[94] MSF's values and beliefs thus significantly shaped the planning and conduct of treatment trials during this epidemic.

Reducing the Impact of Treatment Trials on MSF's Routine Operations

In line with its previous approach to research, MSF sought to ensure that all treatment trials had a minimal impact on the provision of patient care and its routine operations.[95] One of the Investigational Platform's "paramount priorities" was that trials should be implemented "without affecting the HR [human resources] teams nor the running of the treatment centers."[96] It was of the "utmost importance that the trials do not add workload on the [clinical] teams . . . and don't destabilize treatment structures that are stable."[97] This meant that trials had to be feasible from a logistical point of view as well as acceptable to MSF staff and the affected communities. Both considerations pointed in the direction of simple trial designs.

In terms of feasibility, MSF required that all trials minimize the number and invasiveness of research procedures. Consistent with this requirement, MSF made it clear that the trials' outcome parameters had to be kept simple: survival after two weeks was the primary outcome in all treatment trials. "[B]lood drawing for the sake of the trials should be kept to a minimum . . . [and] any additional blood sampling would require negotiation."[98] Moreover, additional samples were deemed acceptable only if they resulted in direct clinical benefits for the participants. For example, MSF required that samples be linked to tests of blood biochemistry or viral levels that had an immediate impact on patient care.

MSF generally rejected placebo interventions, in part because they were seen to pose excessive risks to trial participants and staff.[99] Furthermore, staff should not have to manage the potential harms caused by placebos in addition to caring for their patients. MSF also opposed trial designs that would have required following potentially complex protocols.[100] In addition, research aims could not justify significantly longer admission periods because this meant that beds would be unavailable for new patients. Similarly, a more detailed clinical follow-up for research purposes was not deemed acceptable because it could potentially compromise patient care.[101] The logistical rationale for these requirements was straightforward and consistent with MSF's previous research practices: the simpler a trial, the more limited its impact on routine operations and patient care.

In terms of acceptability, MSF had to ensure that its clinical staff would be willing and able to implement the trials. This further supported the use of simple designs with a minimal number of research-specific procedures. Clinical staff were justifiably anxious about contracting Ebola and therefore likely to be reluctant to perform invasive procedures solely for research purposes, and MSF leadership was equally anxious that such procedures might transmit Ebola to its staff. Moreover, complex research designs could be expected to generate resistance because MSF staff were already struggling to meet patient needs when the trials were being planned. This concern particularly applied to individually randomized controlled trial (iRCT) designs, which randomly allocate participants to an unproven treatment and supportive care (intervention group) or supportive care alone (concurrent control group) in order to evaluate the unproven treatment's clinical effects.

Furthermore, the caseload in MSF's ETUs was overwhelming in the fall of 2014 and—as previously mentioned—there was a "desperate expectation for therapeutic solutions."[102] This fueled MSF's concerns that iRCT designs would not be accepted in the field because staff would object to withholding a potentially life-saving treatment from some trial participants. The concerns about the acceptability of iRCTs were most clearly articulated later in the epidemic:

> Even if an [i]RCT has the potential to do the greatest good if [it] reaches a conclusion that would allow wide use of . . . [the study drug] in a timely manner, this is of small comfort to the front-line providers who are placed in the position of not being able to give a medication of presumed efficacy to patients who [face a high fatality rate and] find themselves in the control arm. . . . Our discomfort with the [i]RCT is in large part derived from sympathy for the people caring for the Ebola patients [patient with Ebola Virus Disease]. However we may feel, this also represents a practical consideration. A study which is unacceptable to the field teams who have to implement it is a study that will not get off the ground.[103]

Finally, MSF had to ensure that trials would be accepted by patients as well as communities. Again, this was most likely when trials had a minimal impact on routine care and avoided an iRCT design. "Whatever the communication/information . . . the perception of patients . . . will remain that refusing to participate in a [i]RCT or being allocated to the control group corresponds to losing the chances to a potentially life-saving treatment."[104] Indeed, concerns about the acceptability of iRCT designs to communities motivated MSF to argue against trial designs that would have included a concurrent control group even though participants would *not* have been randomized. Specifically, the convalescent plasma trial was initially going to include a concurrent control of patients who could not be transfused because a matching blood product was not available for them. However, MSF argued that "for perception reasons it would . . . be better to use only historical controls."[105]

The Perceived Obligation to Provide Treatment Candidates to All Trial Participants

In addition to these continuities in how MSF approached research during the 2014–2015 epidemic, there were important discontinuities. Preserving and enhancing the well-being of participants remained MSF's "overarching imperative of any engagement in research";[106] however, the organization's understanding of this imperative changed during this epidemic. This change had important implications for how MSF negotiated the design of the treatment trials.[107]

In the past, MSF had taken a decidedly risk-averse interpretation of the requirement to promote participants' well-being. The focus was on exposing participants to very limited (if any) research-specific risks. Previous trials did not only minimize research procedures that had no prospect of clinical benefit for participants, such as blood draws performed purely for research purposes, but they also took very limited risks with respect to study interventions that had a prospect of benefit for participants. As discussed earlier, the vast majority of trials MSF had conducted before the 2014–15 Ebola epidemic compared proven effective treatments or tested promising combinations of established ones.[108] This meant that MSF could be relatively confident that the potential clinical benefits of these research interventions would outweigh their risks, and thus that participants would benefit.

During the Ebola epidemic, MSF accepted much greater risks in order to promote participants' well-being. MSF maintained its risk-averse stance toward research procedures that had no prospect of clinical benefit, not least to ensure the feasibility and acceptability of the trials.[109] However, given that patients with Ebola Virus Disease were facing a high risk of dying, MSF was willing to discount potentially significant risks from interventions that had a prospect of clinical benefit in order to potentially save their lives: "The higher the case fatality [rate], the more risks for severe adverse events become irrelevant."[110] All treatment candidates on WHO's priority list were unproven in patients with Ebola Virus Disease, but those that the steering committee of the Oxford-led research consortium had selected for clinical trials first—convalescent plasma, brincidofovir, and favipiravir—had shown only limited or no anti-Ebola effects in animal experiments. Moreover, even though some human safety data for these treatments were available, it was possible that they would make patients with Ebola Virus Disease worse off than they would have been without the treatment under study. This meant that there was considerable uncertainty as to whether the clinical benefits of these treatment candidates would outweigh the risks and participants would benefit.

Furthermore, not only was MSF willing to accept potentially significant risks from unproven treatments, it actually felt an *obligation* to provide these treatments to all participants in a trial if they so wished. As one member of the Investigational Platform put it: "Preclinical data do suggest hope for a good effect, as well as a reasonable expectation of safety. In the setting of a poor prognosis, withholding such a drug is problematic."[111] Importantly, this sense of obligation extended to all patients who were treated in an ETU where a given treatment would be tested. There was "an overall consensus [among members of MSF's Investigational Platform] that all patients in the treatment structures, beyond patients enrolled in the trials, should receive the experimental drugs."[112] Although the underlying rationale is not spelled out, this position was likely motivated by a commitment to treating all patients entering an ETU equally. It was not feasible to conduct trials in all of MSF's ETUs, but it was feasible to provide an unproven treatment to all patients in a given ETU.

Maximizing Access to the Treatments Under Study

The sense of obligation to provide all participants in a trial with the treatment under study—and indeed all patients in the ETU where the trial was conducted—meant that MSF tried to maximize treatment access in the trial negotiations. This had important implications for how the trials were ultimately designed.

First, in addition to rejecting iRCTs due to concerns about their feasibility and acceptability to local communities and clinical staff, MSF objected to iRCT designs on ethical grounds. As an internal document noted:

> While MSF believes [individually] randomised-controlled trials ([i]RCTs) provide robust evidence, and support their use where this is ethical and practical, we do not believe that either consideration is

likely to be satisfied in the context of this outbreak. Having a [concurrent] control group would mean that there would be an intervention arm of patients receiving a medicine and patients in a non-intervention arm who would receive either a placebo with the standard level of care or the standard level of care alone. Randomisation is ethical when there is genuine uncertainty that an untested treatment has benefits or risks that exceed those of conventional care. But when conventional care involves such a high probability of death . . . it is problematic to insist on randomising patients when treatment holds out at least the possibility of a benefit."[113]

As a result, MSF only accepted single-arm designs that provided the treatment under study to all participants and relied on historical control groups—that is, data about patient outcomes that were collected in the past—in order to evaluate its safety and clinical effectiveness.

Second, MSF tried to ensure "maximum inclusion" in the trials.[114] The ultimate aim was to be "as inclusive as possible, excluding only people who are not willing to participate or those who are terminally ill."[115] Some of MSF's requests in this respect were readily implemented, such as including all patients in an ETU on the first day of trials irrespective of when they had been admitted.[116] However, intense negotiations ensued in some trials about the inclusion of children and pregnant women.

In the convalescent plasma trial, both patient groups were eligible for inclusion from the beginning. However, the picture was more complex in the antiviral trials. While the brincidofovir trial enrolled children older than one month from the start, pregnant women were excluded. Moreover, children and pregnant women were initially not eligible for participation in the favipiravir trial.

The main reason for excluding these patient groups was that they were at increased risk of harm. In particular, it was feared that the unproven treatments could cause teratogenic effects in pregnant women, and that serious adverse events would be difficult to manage and mitigate in children. Yet both groups of patients had some of the highest mortality rates in this epidemic, and MSF wanted to provide them access to potentially beneficial interventions; this was in line with the organization's commitment to "always prioritize . . . vulnerable groups and look to find new ways to deliver better care."[117] Moreover, no fetus or newborn was known to have survived Ebola at the time, so concerns about teratogenic effects in pregnant women seemed misguided. Ebola also tended to occur in family clusters, and clinical staff and communities had difficulty accepting that some family members could not be included in clinical trials primarily because they were pregnant or had not reached the age of maturity.

After extensive discussion, children above one year of age ended up being included the favipiravir trial.[118] However, MSF was unable to negotiate the inclusion of pregnant women in either the favipiravir or the brincidofovir trial.[119]

Third, MSF urged that patients who could not participate in a trial would either be referred to another trial or receive an unproven treatment on a monitored emergency use basis. Such use followed a clearly specified protocol and required the patient's informed consent as well as approval by a research ethics committee. In the favipiravir trial, MSF's collaborators agreed that pregnant women were offered favipiravir on an emergency use basis. Because favipiravir cannot be metabolized in children under the age of one year, it was also discussed that children between two and 12 months would receive brincidofovir in the ETU where the favipiravir trial was conducted. But the idea was abandoned because of concerns that developing the respective monitored emergency use protocol would cause additional delays. In the brincidofovir trial, the drug manufacturer did not agree to the emergency use of brincidofovir in pregnant women. MSF therefore decided to refer pregnant women to a convalescent plasma trial in a nearby ETU.[120]

Fourth, MSF negotiated arrangements to ensure uninterrupted access to all study interventions as soon as a trial had been started. This had different implications for the trials in which the organization was engaged. In the brincidofovir and favipiravir trials, MSF's goal was to ensure that the drug manufacturers were committed to the continued production and supply of treatments after the trials ended, provided they had shown positive results. MSF made the continued post-trial availability of any promising treatments a condition for both projects to move forward.[121] If a treatment showed "some efficacy," the organization wanted to be in a position to provide the treatment to future patients in all of its ETUs and ideally enable the treatment's wider use.[122] Indeed, in the case of brincidofovir, MSF's negotiations about post-trial drug availability were protracted and at one point almost jeopardized the trial.[123] MSF also began lobbying drug developers more generally[124] and briefly considered creating a "fund of (several tens of millions of euros) that would be used to purchase large volumes of forthcoming vaccines, treatments and diagnostics, to ensure that they are made available quickly enough to significantly impact the current Ebola epidemic."[125]

In the convalescent plasma trial, MSF's goal was to ensure the availability of the study intervention both during and after the trial. The key challenge was that the supply of convalescent plasma depended on the goodwill of Ebola survivors and the efforts of those collecting plasma. Given this, MSF required that the ITM-led research consortium ensure excellent collaboration with Ebola survivor groups and a smooth running of transfusion centers to secure sufficient plasma supplies. MSF made it clear that it would have ended the collaboration if there had been signs of insufficient supplies. Moreover, MSF requested that a "plasma reserve prior to trial start [be built] . . . to ensure—at least in the beginning—that all patients included can receive the treatment."[126] MSF also objected to including a concurrent control of patients for whom no matching blood product was available because this could have created a perverse incentive for research teams not to collect sufficient plasma and thereby obtain a large enough control group. There was to be "very little pressure on [obtaining] concurrent controls and more focus on trying to get a maximum patients receiving [convalescent plasma]."[127] All these steps testify to MSF's commitment to maximizing access to the given treatments under study.

Negotiating Individually Randomized Controlled Trial Designs

A key point of international controversy in the 2014–15 epidemic was how trials of the existing unproven treatments should be designed, given the high fatality rate of Ebola, the great fear of the disease, and the limited exposure to clinical trials in the affected populations before this epidemic. Some argued that iRCTs with a concurrent control group—which would receive supportive care but not the treatment under study—represented the only scientifically valid approach to evaluate the unproven treatments in this epidemic.[128] Others—including MSF—argued that iRCTs were neither ethical nor feasible under the circumstances, and that it was possible to obtain robust trial results without including a concurrent control group.[129]

It is important to note that the controversy centered on what trial design would be appropriate in the context of *this particular* Ebola epidemic; it was not a controversy about how to design treatment trials in general. For example, some now wrongly claim that MSF is generally opposed to iRCTs, although the organization recognizes the full spectrum of trial designs.[130] Moreover, even though MSF generally discourages the conduct of iRCTs because "their complexity and time and resource demands usually make them impracticable for a service organisation,"[131] it conducts iRCTs under certain circumstances. In fact, there is dedicated MSF guidance on how to design and implement iRCTs.[132]

As described above, MSF initially rejected iRCTs of unproven treatments in this epidemic for ethical and feasibility reasons. However, the organization was well aware of the fact that this position required making some scientific tradeoffs. For example, one member of the Investigational Platform noted in a personal document:

> For me, this [the limitations of historical controls] is the strongest argument for an [i]RCT. We know well from our own data that the variations in case fatality rate between centers make the proposal of knowing "mortality under standard care" illusory. Even in the same center over time there is no stability. The reasons for this are not entirely clear, but

there is some evidence that it stems from changes in patient selection. That being said, for certain sub-groups there may be very stable case fatality rates under standard care—e.g. patients with a Ct [cycle threshold] under 18 [indicating a high Ebola viral load] who may be reliable controls.[133]

Historical control data also had limitations because routine clinical data collection and laboratory testing methods varied considerably between ETUs and over time and could be limited in terms of their accuracy;[134] however, these limitations could be addressed to some extent by using historical data from a single ETU and large numbers of patients as well as adjusting for time variations. Both measures were taken in the favipiravir and convalescent plasma trials.

Similarly, MSF recognized that treatments with small or moderate effects may not be identified in trials with historical controls and seems to have made a deliberate tradeoff in this regard when it rejected iRCTs in this particular epidemic. For example, the manager of the Investigational Platform later stated: "The most important question [during a similar epidemic] might be to rapidly identify the agents with a large positive effect and eliminate the agents that have no [little] or a negative effect, rather than to acquire knowledge on the exact % of efficacy."[135]

Importantly, MSF's position with respect to individually randomized controlled trials was more nuanced than is often assumed. The organization collaborated on a cluster randomized controlled trial of an Ebola vaccine, given the morally salient difference in background risk between patients with Ebola Virus Disease and healthy individuals at risk of contracting Ebola.[136] Moreover, MSF shifted its position vis-à-vis iRCTs of treatments later in the epidemic when the conditions for conducting treatment trials had changed. The epidemic was waning at this point and 60 to 70 doses of ZMapp had just become available; it was clear that an efficient trial design was necessary to gather meaningful data in the remaining time window before the epidemic ended.[137] Any new trial could recruit only a low number of participants under these circumstances. If an iRCT was now the only design to deliver results, then rejecting an iRCT design would have meant losing the opportunity to test a promising treatment for the benefit of future patients. Moreover, because the epidemic was waning, any trial—whether new or continuing—was conducted mostly for the benefit of patients in future epidemics and less so for the benefit of patients in this epidemic. This meant for some within MSF that an iRCT was more acceptable to conduct, even though concerns about withholding a potentially beneficial treatment from some participants persisted.

These considerations, together with ZMapp's strong signals of an anti-Ebola effect in preclinical experiments, swayed MSF to seriously consider a proposal by the U.S. National Institutes of Health (NIH) to collaborate on an iRCT. MSF still had "major ethical and operational [feasibility] considerations around the fact that there is zero post-trial availability and this study would use a control group,"[138] and it was concerned about "walking back from our previous publicly expressed position."[139] However, MSF was open to collaborating on an iRCT if an iRCT design was the only way to conclude a trial before the outbreak was over.

Moreover, in discussions around this trial MSF made the innovative proposal to conduct a three-arm iRCT that would have allocated participants to two intervention arms or a concurrent control arm based on their prognosis. Experience earlier in the epidemic had shown that the prognosis of survival was not the same in all patients with Ebola Virus Disease. In particular, patients with a high viral load, children younger than five years, pregnant women, and people older than 65 years had a very poor prognosis.[140] The proposal was to provide all participants with a very poor prognosis with supportive care and ZMapp (intervention group 1) because this would offer them some measure of hope with only limited compromises in terms of scientific validity, given that their clinical outcomes were less variable and the total number of participants in this group was likely to be small. All other participants would be randomly allocated to either ZMapp and supportive care (intervention group 2) or supportive care alone (control group). The proposal of such an iRCT that would have stratified patients based on their prognosis offered an interesting approach to balancing obligations to benefit participants with safeguarding the scientific rigor of a trial. But although the design was endorsed by the U.S. Food and Drug Administration,[141] the collaboration with NIH did not come to fruition.

Treatment Trials During Epidemics: Some Open Questions for MSF

MSF's efforts to get treatment trials off the ground—and those of everyone else involved in these trials—are truly impressive. The 2014–15 Ebola epidemic was an extremely challenging environment for conducting clinical research. Ebola was a highly fatal disease that stoked fear not only in the affected communities, but also among health workers and those responsible for managing them. Relatively little was known about the disease before 2014, and the available unproven treatments were in the earliest stages of development for Ebola. Moreover, the affected West African countries had little preexisting research infrastructure and generally weak health systems that further deteriorated during this epidemic. Local communities had also had little exposure to clinical research in the past, and there was reasonable concern that clinical trials could magnify the existing social and political tensions. Finally, the severe time pressure and unprecedented global cooperation between a wide range of actors led to unavoidable tensions in the negotiations about clinical trials. This unique constellation of factors posed tremendous scientific, operational, ethical, and political challenges for MSF and its research partners.

There is much to commend in how MSF navigated its engagement in trials of unproven Ebola treatments under the circumstances. Consistent with WHO's recommendations, MSF prioritized the conduct of clinical trials over monitored emergency use. Furthermore, the organization upheld its standard ethical criteria for research and generally resisted letting the urgency of the situation dominate its decision making. MSF also adhered to important procedural safeguards for ethical research, such as prospective research ethics review, while overall steering clear of unreasonable delays.

At the same time, some of the decisions MSF made about the treatment trials raise important questions for the organization. The treatment trials that were conducted in this epidemic—with or without MSF involvement—did not yield definitive results, not least because they could not be completed or started as planned when the epidemic fortunately took a turn for the better. This means that important questions about the treatment of Ebola remain unanswered and more clinical trials will be needed during the next epidemic. Because MSF is likely to remain a key responder to future Ebola outbreaks, it is likely to be involved in future trials of unproven treatments for Ebola. Equally, MSF is likely to be a key responder to emerging infectious diseases that are comparable to Ebola and require clinical research. The chapter therefore closes with some open questions about MSF's decisions in this epidemic that aim to stimulate debate with a view to preparing for similar trials in the future.

In the 2014–2015 epidemic, MSF's patient-centered orientation motivated many of the organization's decisions about how it approached the treatment trials. In particular, MSF was committed to testing treatments that had the potential to make an impact on patients in *this* epidemic and therefore aimed to start trials as early as possible. This meant that the organization and its research partners selected treatment candidates for testing in clinical trials at least partially based on whether they were immediately available and feasible to implement in this epidemic. Similarly, MSF aimed to maximize access to unproven treatments because it considered these interventions to be the best available option for patients who faced a high likelihood of dying. This had important implications for how MSF negotiated the trials; the goal of maximizing treatment access was a key reason for MSF to reject iRCT designs, to promote the inclusion of children and pregnant women, and to press for the post-trial availability of any promising treatments from the start.

These decisions were entirely reasonable for a patient-centered organization like MSF that is committed to saving lives or reducing suffering *today*. However, as some of MSF's own deliberations in this epidemic illustrate, a "therapeutic orientation"[142] to clinical trials can require making important scientific and ethical tradeoffs. For example, for trials to start as early as possible and make an impact on patients in this epidemic, treatment candidates have to be selected at least partially based on their immediate availability. However, the availability of investigational treatments does not necessarily correlate with their therapeutic promise. It is, of course, notoriously difficult to predict the promise of available treatment candidates and judge their relative merits—especially when the evidence on their effects is so heterogeneous, and of such variable quality, as it was in the 2014–15 Ebola epidemic. Moreover, what appears to be the most promising treatment candidate may become available only when an epidemic is waning, so it can be impossible to complete trials or obtain results in a timely fashion. Trials of seemingly less promising agents may also be finalized by the time the preferred candidates become available, in which case a choice between interventions may not need to be made. Still, a commitment to making an impact on patients in the current epidemic can require making compromises in the selection of treatment candidates that require further analysis and discussion.

Similarly, a commitment to maximizing access to the available unproven treatments can require making compromises with respect to the scientific rigor of a given trial. For example, as the discussion around iRCT designs and the limitations of historical control data in this epidemic showed, MSF was well aware of the fact that providing the treatment under study to all trial participants could mean that less robust data would be collected. Such potential compromises with respect to the scientific rigor of a trial are not solely a scientific matter but also have important ethical import. Exposing participants to research risks, and using limited resources to conduct research, is ethically justifiable only when research yields robust data.[143] Moreover, justifiable decisions about patient care and the allocation of scarce resources for healthcare depend on solid evidence on the effects of clinical interventions (even though solid evidence cannot guard against poor decision making and real-world decisions are often not based on evidence alone). The rigor of future research equally hinges on the quality of data that have been collected in the past. These considerations underscore the ethical importance of safeguarding the scientific rigor of clinical trials during epidemics of diseases like Ebola, whichever trial design is under consideration.

It is important to note that the scientific rigor of a given trial design is highly contextual and specific designs should be neither rejected outright nor always given priority. For example, iRCT designs with a concurrent control group have important scientific advantages when an infectious disease has highly variable clinical outcomes, as was the case in Ebola. However, these advantages may decrease in the context of a waning epidemic when the volume of potential trial participants dwindles. For instance, the iRCT of Zmapp that was eventually conducted without MSF involvement had to be run in several locations and over a relatively long period of time in order to recruit sufficient participant numbers as the 2014–2015 epidemic waned. The trial's geographic spread and long duration increased the risk of obtaining a relatively heterogeneous concurrent control group, thereby complicating comparisons with the intervention group. A carefully validated historical control group in a single arm trial may have been equally or more robust in this situation, especially as it could have included a larger number of patients. Moreover, a single arm trial would have provided all participants with ZMapp and therefore yielded more data on the drug's clinical effects. These considerations highlight that the scientific merits of different trial designs are highly contextual and require careful evaluation. They also highlight the importance of considering a wide range of designs, including innovative trial designs that could provide a bespoke approach in the given epidemic.

If compromises with respect to the scientific rigor of a clinical trial have to be made, they can (and should) be reduced. For example, if an iRCT is not considered ethical or feasible in the next Ebola epidemic, trials without a concurrent control can be strengthened by improving and standardizing routine data collection and thereby enhancing the quality of historical control data. Similarly, collecting a wider range of data points in a trial can help to interpret the results. Nonetheless, it is important to recognize that scientific compromises may need to be made if a commitment to maximizing access to unproven treatments is to be upheld. The questions surrounding this tension require further discussion.

Finally, especially if a patient-centered orientation to research requires making significant compromises with regard to the choice of treatment candidates or the scientific rigor of trials, MSF may need to set priorities between conducting clinical trials and focusing on other activities. While the organization's staff and infrastructure are not fungible, strategic decisions about where to focus a given mission and allocate resources can be required. For example, in the 2014–15 Ebola epidemic, MSF could have redirected some of its investments in clinical trials of unproven targeted treatments to efforts to improve routine data collection, more observational research,[144] interventional studies of supportive care for Ebola,[145] more community outreach and health promotion activities, or more treatment for diseases other than Ebola.[146] It is difficult to say how the organization's engagement in the conducted trials compared to these potential alternative investments in terms of how well they addressed patient needs, how much impact they had on the epidemic, the extent to which other actors could have taken on the given role, and so on. It also seems likely that the treatment trials had a positive impact on some of these activities, such as routine data collection, supportive care, and community engagement. Furthermore, some of these alternative activities may have been just as complex to implement as the treatment trials that MSF helped to conduct. For example, it was not evident what interventions research on supportive care should have targeted, whether such research would have necessarily been less risky for participants or more promising to conduct than trials of unproven targeted treatments, and whether it would have been easier to conduct than these trials.[147] Nonetheless, questions about the role of treatment trials in the response to future Ebola epidemics—or epidemics of comparable emerging infectious diseases—are critical to address.

Acknowledgments

The authors are indebted to Armand Sprecher for his invaluable input. We also thank Sokhieng Au, Chiara Lepora, Franklin Miller, and David Wendler who provided additional comments on an earlier version of this chapter; Guillaume Nanin for his expert assistance with the document search; and Thomas Palfinger who agreed to format our references at the last minute. Any errors of fact, interpretation, or argument remain the authors' alone.

Notes

1. Piot, Peter. 2014. "Ebola's perfect storm." *Science* 345(6202): 1221.
2. Feldmann, Heinz, and Thomas W. Geisbert. 2011. "Ebola Haemorrhagic Fever." *Lancet* 377(9768): 849–62.
3. Ibid.
4. Ibid.
5. Fauci, Anthony S. 2014. "Ebola—Underscoring the Global Disparities in Health Care Resources." *New England Journal of Medicine* 371(12): 1084–86.
6. Feldmann, and Geisbert. "Ebola."
7. The formal term was "monitored emergency use of unregistered and experimental interventions (MEURI)." This term was introduced to distinguish MEURI practices from "compassionate use." Compassionate use involves the use of an unproven intervention outside a clinical trial, for example because a patient is not eligible for any ongoing trials or there are no ongoing trials. By contrast, MEURI involves the use of an unproven intervention outside a clinical trial together with the systematic collection and sharing of data on clinical outcomes. The terms "compassionate use" and "monitored emergency use" were often used interchangeably during the 2014–15 Ebola epidemic. In this chapter, "monitored emergency use" refers to MEURI practices even when they may have sometimes been called "compassionate use." World Health Organization. 2014. "Ethical Issues Related to Study Design for Trials on Therapeutics for Ebola Virus Disease." WHO Ethics Working Group Meeting in October 20–21 2014. Accessed August 27, 2016, http://www.who.int/medicines/wg_ethics_ebola_interventions/en/.
8. The archive contained all Ebola-related documents and communications from March 2014 to the summer of 2015. The Operational Center Brussels (OCB) led MSF's Ebola response in the early stages, but other operational centers soon joined the effort. MSF's clinical research activities were initially managed jointly by OCB and the Operational Center Geneva (OCG) and later included other MSF centers, units, and affiliates. For reasons of simplicity we do not discuss the role of different MSF sections and institutions in this chapter but speak of MSF as a uniform organization. For a discussion of MSF's organizational structure and the (sometimes complex) relationship between different MSF sections and institutions, see, for example, Redfield, Peter. *Life in Crisis: The Ethical Journey of Doctors Without Borders.* Berkeley: University of California Press, 2013 and Fox, Renee. *Doctors Without Borders: Humanitarian Quests, Impossible Dreams of Médecins Sans Frontières.* Baltimore: JHU Press, 2014.

9. No author. 2014. "Ebola Set-Up: Thematic Worksheets." Unpublished internal PowerPoint presentation, September 2014.

10. The chapter reflects the collaboration of a research ethicist (Annette Rid) and the manager of MSF's Investigational Platform (Annick Antierens). Rid developed a first draft of the chapter after reviewing relevant documents from the Ebola archive, pertinent gray and academic literature, as well as selected additional MSF documents provided by Antierens. Both authors then worked on several revisions of the draft and obtained extensive additional input from another member of the Investigational Platform (Armand Sprecher). Unless otherwise noted, any factual statements about how MSF made decisions about unproven treatments are based on Antierens' recollection of the events.

11. For more information, see: Médecins Sans Frontières. 2016. *MSF-Supported Research on Ebola.* Geneva: Médecins Sans Frontières. Accessed August 27, 2016, http://www.msf.org/sites/msf.org/files/msf_ocb_ebola_research_en_web.pdf.

12. As will become clear throughout this chapter, MSF decided to participate in several treatment trials early in the epidemic, in mid-August 2014, and initially rejected individually randomized controlled designs for these trials because such designs were deemed neither feasible nor acceptable. By contrast, MSF participated in just one vaccine trial—the Ebola ça Suffit ("Ebola, this is enough") trial in Guinea—that began recruiting in March 2015 and used a cluster randomized controlled design. Henao-Restrepo Ana M., Ira M Longini, Matthias Egger, Natalie E. Dean, John Edmunds, Anton Camacho, Miles W. Carroll, Moussa Doumbia, Bertrand Draguez, Sophie Duraffour, Godwin Enwere, FWACP, Rebecca Grais, Stephan Gunther, Stefanie Hossmann, Mandy Kader Kondé, Souleymane Kone, Eeva Kuisma, Myron M. Levine, Sema Mandal, Gunnstein Norheim, Ximena Riveros, Aboubacar Soumah, Sven Trelle, Andrea S. Vicari, Conall H. Watson, MFPH, Sakoba Kéïta, Marie Paule Kieny, and John-Arne Røttingen. 2015. "Efficacy and Effectiveness of an rVSV-Vectored Vaccine Expressing Ebola Surface Glycoprotein. Interim Results From the Guinea Ring Vaccination Cluster-Randomised Trial." *The Lancet* 86(9996): 857–66.

13. Rid, Annette "(How) Should Experimental Vaccines and Treatments for Ebola Be Used?" In *Ebola's Message: Public Health and Medicine in the Twenty-First Century*, edited by Nicholas G. Evans, Tara C. Smith, and Maimuna. S. Majumder, 183–200. Cambridge, MA: MIT Press, 2016.

14. Redfield, *Life in Crisis*, in particular 64–66.

15. Médecins Sans Frontières. 2014. "International Activity Report 2014." Geneva: Médecins Sans Frontières, 7. Accessed August, 27, 2016, http://cdn.msf.org/sites/msf.org/files/msf_international_activity_report_2014_en.pdf.

16. Brown, Vincent, Philippe J. Guerin, Dominique Legros, Christophe Paquet, Bernard Pécoul, and Alain Moren. 2008. "Research in Complex Humanitarian Emergencies: The Médecins Sans Frontières/Epicentre Experience." *PLoS Medicine* 5(4): e89. Accessed August 28, 2016, 10.1371/journal.pmed.0050089.

17. Zachariah, Rony, Nathan Ford, Bertrand Draguez, Oliver Yun, and Tony Reid. 2010. "Conducting Operational Research Within a Nongovernmental Organization: The Example of Médecins Sans Frontières." *International Health* 2(1): 1–6.

18. Pécoul, Bernard. 2004. "New Drugs for Neglected Diseases: From Pipeline to Patients." *PLoS Medicine* 1(1): e6. Accessed August 28, 2016, http://dx.doi.org/10.1371/journal.pmed.0010006.

19. Blanchet, Karl, Vera Sistenich, Anita Ramesh, Severine Frison, Emily Warren, James Smith, Mazeda Hossain, Abigail Knight, Chris Lewis, Nathan Post, Aniek Woodward, Alexander Ruby, Maysoon Dahab, Sara Pantuliano, Bayard Roberts. 2013. "An Evidence Review of Research on Health Interventions in Humanitarian Crises." Accessed August, 27, 2016, http://www.elrha.org/wp-content/uploads/2015/01/Evidence-Review-22.10.15.pdf.

20. Médecins Sans Frontières. "MSF Charter and Principles." Accessed August, 27, 2016, www.msf.org/en/msf-charter-and-principles.

21. World Health Organization. 2014. *Clinical Management of Patients with Viral Haemorrhagic Fever: A Pocket Guide for Front-Line Health Workers: Interim Emergency Guidance—Generic Draft for West African Adaptation.* Geneva: World Health Organization. Accessed August, 27, 2016, http://apps.who.int/iris/bitstream/10665/130883/2/WHO_HSE_PED_AIP_14.05.pdf; Médecins Sans Frontières. 2008. *Filovirus Haemorrhagic Fever Guideline.* Barcelona: Médecins

Sans Frontières. Accessed August, 27, 2016, http://www.slamviweb.org/es/ebola/FHFfinal. pdf.

22. Delisle, Hélène, Janet H. Roberts, Michelle Munro, Lori Jones and Theresa W. Gyorkos. 2005. "The Role of NGOs in Global Health Research for Development." *Health Research Policy and Systems* 3:3. Accessed August 27, 2016, http://health-policy-systems.biomedcentral.com/articles/10.1186/1478-4505-3-3.

23. Médecins Sans Frontières. "MSF Charter and Principles."

24. In contrast to MSF, many other humanitarian organizations believe that impartiality and neutrality—widely recognized political principles for humanitarian aid—can only be achieved without a commitment to bearing witness. See, for example, Slim, Hugo. 2015. *Humanitarian Ethics: A Guide to the Morality of Aid in War and Disaster.* Oxford: Oxford University Press.

25. As Redfield also notes, however, parts of MSF remain skeptical of the "illusionary certainty that it [quantitative data] can project on volatile field situations". Redfield, *Life in Crisis,* 116–117.

26. Zachariah et al. "Conducting Operational Research Within a Nongovernmental Organization."

27. Ibid.

28. Ibid. It is widely recognized that exposing research participants to risks, and using limited resources for conducting research, is justifiable only when a study is likely to yield robust data in response to socially valuable research questions. See for example Emanuel, Ezekiel J., David Wendler, and Christine Grady. 2000. "What Makes Clinical Research Ethical." *JAMA* 283(20): 2701–11.

29. Zachariah et al. "Conducting Operational Research Within a Nongovernmental Organization.", 6, and Zachariah, Rony, Anthony D. Harries, FRCP, Nobukatsu Ishikawa, Hans L. Rieder, Karen Bissell, Kayla Laserson, Moses Massaquoi, Micheal Van Herp, and Tony Reid. 2009. "Operational Research in Low-Income Countries: What, Why, and How?" *The Lancet* 9(11): 711–17.

30. MSF Operational Research Unit, and OCB Luxembourg. 2010. *Operational Research Policy Framework.* Brussels: Médecins Sans Frontières, 9 and 14–15. Accessed August 27, 2016, http://fieldresearch.msf.org/msf/bitstream/10144/190889/1/OR%20Policy%202010.pdf.

31. MSF Ethics Review Board. 2013. *MSF Research Ethics Framework: Guidance Document.* Geneva: Médecins Sans Frontières. Accessed August 27, 2016, http://fieldresearch.msf. org/msf/bitstream/10144/305288/5/MSF+Research+Ethics+Framework_Guidance+ document+%28Dec2013%29.pdf.

32. For illustration, consider three prominent examples: (1) MSF's retrospective analysis of routinely collected data revealed that a major outbreak of pellagra—a vitamin deficiency— among Mozambican refugees was due to a shortage of groundnuts. Groundnut supplies were then purchased and the outbreak was controlled within months; (2) MSF's research on routinely collected blood samples helped to develop a rapid diagnostic test for meningitis that was suitable for use in humanitarian emergencies; (3) MSF conducted a large survey of Rwandan refugees in the 1990s and operational centers used the results for planning purposes and as advocacy material. See Brown et al. "Research in Complex Humanitarian Emergencies."

33. Two prominent examples for illustration: (1) MSF conducted a randomized clinical trial that compared several proven effective antibiotics for meningitis and demonstrated their continued clinical relevance when production was going to be stopped; (2) MSF tested promising combinations of established malaria treatments in a randomized trial and identified new therapeutic pathways for the disease. See Brown et al. "Research in Complex Humanitarian Emergencies."

34. Médecins Sans Frontières. 2015. *An Unprecedented Year: Doctors Without Borders/Médecins Sans Frontières' Response to the Largest Ever Ebola Outbreak.* Geneva: Médecins Sans Frontières. Accessed August 27, 2016, https://www.doctorswithoutborders.org/sites/usa/files/ebola_accountability_report_us_version_7-8-15.pdf.

35. Xiangguo Qiu, Gary Wong, Jonathan Audet, Alexander Bello, Lisa Fernando, Judie B. Alimonti, Hugues Fausther-Bovendo, Haiyan Wei, Jenna Aviles, Ernie Hiatt, Ashley Johnson, Josh Morton, Kelsi Swope, Ognian Bohorov, Natasha Bohorova, Charles Goodman, Do Kim,

Michael H. Pauly, Jesus Velasco, James Pettitt, Gene G. Olinger, Kevin Whaley, Bianli Xu, James E. Strong, Larry Zeitlin, and Gary P. Kobinger. 2014. "Reversion of Advanced Ebola Virus Disease in Nonhuman Primates With ZMapp." *Nature* 514(7520): 47–53.

36. Although the first Ebola cases had already been diagnosed in Sierra Leone at the time, Gary Kobinger- the responsible researcher from the Public Health Agency Canada- said he had "no idea that it [ZMapp] would be used." Preston, Richard. "Ebola Wars: How Genomics Research Can Help Contain the Outbreak." *The New Yorker*, October 27, 2014. Accessed August 27, 2016, http://www.newyorker.com/magazine/2014/10/27/ebola-wars.

37. No author. 2014. "Experimental Ebola Drug: an Impossible Dilemma," unpublished internal document, August 2014; Pollack, Andrew. "Opting Against Ebola Drug for Ill African Doctor." *The New York Times*, August 12, 2014. Accessed August 27, 2016, http://www.nytimes.com/2014/08/13/world/africa/ebola.html?_r=1. See also Timothy O'Dempsey, "Failing Dr. Khan," Chapter 7 in this volume.

38. Till, Brian. "Why Did Two U.S. Missionaries Get an Ebola Serum While Africans Are Left to Die?" *New Republic*, August 6, 2014. Accessed August 27, 2016, https://newrepublic.com/article/118983/ebola-outbreak-2014-shows-worlds-inequality-disease-treatment.

39. World Health Organization. 2014. *Ethical Considerations for Use of Unregistered Interventions for Ebola Viral Disease: Report of an Advisory Panel to WHO*. Geneva: World Health Organization. Accessed August 27, 2016, http://apps.who.int/iris/bitstream/10665/130997/1/WHO_HIS_KER_GHE_14.1_eng.pdf.

40. The panel listed the following conditions: "transparency about all aspects of care, . . . trust, fair distribution, . . . cosmopolitan solidarity, informed consent, freedom of choice, confidentiality, respect for the person, preservation of dignity, and involvement of the community" as well as "a moral obligation to collect and share all the scientifically relevant data generated, including from treatments provided for "compassionate use." World Health Organization. "Ethical Considerations."

41. World Health Organization. "Ethical Issues Related to Study Design for Trials on Therapeutics for Ebola Virus Disease." See also footnote 7.

42. The groups presented their findings at an international consultation three weeks after the initial WHO advisory panel had made its recommendation to use the available unproven interventions. See World Health Organization. 2014. *Meetings Summary of Consultation on Potential Ebola Therapies and Vaccines*. Geneva: World Health Organization. Accessed August 27, 2016, http://apps.who.int/iris/bitstream/10665/136103/1/WHO_EVD_Meet_EMP_14.1_eng.pdf?ua=1.

43. Médecins Sans Frontières. *An Unprecedented Year*.

44. MSF maintained this position throughout the epidemic. It admitted more than 5,200 confirmed Ebola cases in the 2014–15 epidemic alone, which means that "no other national, international or non-governmental organisation has cared for more patients with Ebola than MSF." Médecins Sans Frontières. *MSF-Supported Research on Ebola*.

45. Draguez, Betrand, Mica Serafini, Annette Heinzelmann, Sid Wong, Judith Herrera, and Myriam Henkens. 2014. "Information Memo From the Medical Directors Regarding MSF Involvement in the Use of Experimental Products in Response to [the] Ebola outbreak." Unpublished internal document, September 4, 2014.

46. Ibid. See also: Unknown author. 2014. "Experimental Ebola Treatments Trials Communications: Internal MSF Q&A to Help Answer Questions From Media." Unpublished internal document, December 14, 2014.

47. See the section "MSF Research Before the 2014–15 Ebola Epidemic."

48. For example, a strategic plan for communication with local communities and staff at MSF's first treatment trial site—Gueckedou in Guinea—was drawn up only in the second half of November 2014. Investigation Platform for Experimental Ebola Products. 2014. "Minutes of the Meetings—Meeting 6, Tuesday 24 November 2014." Unpublished internal document.

49. The uncertainty about community views resulted from a paucity of systematic information. Moreover, the information that did exist sometimes pointed in opposite directions. For example, MSF commissioned an interview study in Monrovia in November 2014, before it had made any official communications about clinical trials in the community. In this study, everyone was "extremely enthusiastic about the potential of a new drug being brought . . .

even when it was explained . . . that any benefits would not yet be known." As one interviewee said: "Anything that can work, we want it! Anything that can help us. We're desperate." Emilie Venables. 2014. "'If they bring it, we will take it.' Community perceptions of clinical trials for Ebola in Monrovia, Liberia." Unpublished internal report, December 2014. At the same time, there were widespread rumors about human experimentation, harvesting of organs, and misuse of blood that suggested communities could meet clinical trials with hostility.

50. Draguez et al. "Information Memo From the Medical Directors".

51. Unknown author. "Ebola Set-Up." The Platform included around 20 experts in viral hemorrhagic fevers, laboratory and research methods, anthropology and ethics, as well as members from the MSF Ebola Taskforce and MSF's communications team. It was co-chaired by the medical directors of the operational centers in Brussels (OCB) and Geneva (OCG) and later Amsterdam. Additional members were added when the Platform's remit was extended to vaccines and diagnostics.

52. The following conditions were immediately decided upon: ". . . a study should . . . not have [a] negative impact on patient care . . . all epxerimental treatments will be further explored, unregistered drugs as well as off-label use of some products . . . scaling up possibilities and post-trial access [are an] . . . a-priori commitment . . . placebo-controlled [trials] cannot be accepted . . . as much as possible [make an] 'equal offer' to patients within the [trials' inclu- sion] criteria . . . space for compassionate use . . . simple protocol . . . simple outcome [mea- sures], not requiring more [blood] sampling than striclty needed . . . take into consideration community perception and links with potential security issues . . . preferably no military or pharmacy money . . . rapid result[s] allowing rapid adaptation/roll out acccording to results . . . priority to the treatment product investigation, without closing doors to other research questions". Draguez at al. "Information memo from the medical directors."

53. MSF developed three monitored emergency use protocols in the 2014–15 epidemic, but two of these were closely linked to clinical trials and one was not implemented. The first moni- tored emergency use protocol enabled pregnant women to access the unproven antiviral favipiravir (Toyama Chemical of the Fujifilm Group, Japan) because they were excluded from enrolling in the respective clinical trial. The second protocol enabled access to convalescent plasma after the trial of this intervention had been concluded. The third protocol aimed to provide access to the monoclonal antibody cocktail MIL 77 (MabWorks, China) and was not implemented due to lack of authorization from the authorities.

54. "[T]he implementation of compassionate use on a large scale isn't that simple, risk-free and swift as we think." Investigation Platform for Experimental Ebola Products. 2014. "Minutes of the Meetings—Meeting 2, Monday October 20th 2014." Unpublished internal document. See also: Unknown author. "Experimental Ebola Treatments Trials Communications."

55. Draguez et al. "Information Memo From the Medical Directors."

56. MSF began considering vaccine trials in the second half of November 2014. It became involved in diagnostic research in mid-December 2014.

57. Bah, Elhadj Ibrahima, Marie-Claire Lamah, Tom Fletcher, Shevin T. Jacob, David M. Brett-Major, Amadou A. Sall, Nahoko Shindo, William A. Fischer, Francois Lamontagne, Sow M. Saliou, Daniel G. Bausch, Barry Moumié, Tim Jagatic, Armand Sprecher, James V. Lawler, Thierry Mayet, Frederique A. Jacquerioz, María F. Méndez Baggi, Constanza Vallenas, Christophe Clement, Simon Mardel, Ousmane Faye, Oumar Faye, Baré Soropogui, Nfaly Magassouba, Lamine Koivogui, Ruxandra Pinto, and Robert A. Fowler. 2015. " Clinical Presentation of Patients with Ebola Virus Disease in Conakry, Guinea." The New England Journal of Medicine 372(1): 40–7. Chertow Daniel S., Christian Kleine, Jeffrey K. Edwards, Roberto Scaini, Ruggero Giuliani, and Armand Sprecher. 2014. " Ebola Virus Disease in West Africa: Clinical Manifestations and Management." The New England Journal of Medicine 371(22): 2054–57.

58. Feldmann, and Geisbert. "Ebola." 849–62.

59. Sprecher, Armand, personal communication, June 8, 2016 and Sprecher, A. 2008. Patient care in filovirus outbreaks. Presented at the 6th Congress of the International Federation of Shock Societies (IFSS) and the 31st Annual Conference on Shock (U.S. Shock Society). July 28–July 2, Cologne, Germany. As Sprecher notes, similar evidence was gathered in the 2014–15 epidemic. For example, one of MSF's ETUs had to significantly reduce intravenous fluids for a period of time due to staffing problems, and when it resumed the provision of fluids the case-fatality rate was unchanged. Grandesso, Francesco. 2015. "MSF EPI-Bulletin

Ebola Epidemic in West Africa, Week 51, update edited on 8 January 2015." Unpublished internal document.

60. Médecins Sans Frontières, and Stockholm Evaluation Unit. 2016. *OCB Ebola Review. Part 1: Medico-Operational.* Geneva: Médecins Sans Frontières. Accessed August 27, 2016, http://cdn.evaluation.msf.org/sites/evaluation/files/attachments/ocb_ebola_review_medop_final_2.pdf. See also Armand Sprecher, "Finding an Answer to Ebola's Greatest Challenge," Chapter 8 in this volume.

61. Meltzer, Martin I., Charisma Y. Atkins, Scott Santibanez, Barbara Knust, Brett W. Petersen, Elizabeth D. Ervin, Stuart T. Nichol, Inger K. Damon, and Michael L. Washington. 2014. "Estimating the Future Number of Cases in the Ebola Epidemic: Liberia and Sierra Leone, 2014–2015." *Morbidity and Mortality Weekly Report* 63(3): 1–14.

62. Marchbein, Deane. "The Response to Ebola - Looking Back and Looking Ahead: The 2015 Lasker-Bloomberg Public Service Award." *JAMA* 314(11): 1115–16, 1115. See also Josse, Evelyne. 2015. "Humanitarian Workers Confronted with Ebola: When the Masks Fall." *Journal of Forensic Medicine* 58(3): 195–203.

63. Antierens, Annick. "Therapeutic Trials During Epidemic Emergencies: From the Caregivers' and Medical Aid Agencies' Perspective." Unpublished PowerPoint presentation of a talk delivered at a public workshop of the National Academies of Sciences, Engineering and Medicine Committee on Clinical Trials During the 2014–2015 Ebola Outbreak, London, March 23, 2016.

64. Pollack, Andrew. "Ebola Drug Could Save a Few Lives. But Whose?" *The New York Times*, August 8, 2014. Accessed August 27, 2016, http://www.nytimes.com/2014/08/09/health/in-ebola-outbreak-who-should-get-experimental-drug.html?_r=0. Similarly, the Investigation Platform stated that "trials will . . . be an incentive to get people to seek treatment (by having the community understand that coming early to treatment centers will increase their chance of survival)." Investigation Platform for Experimental Ebola Products. 2014. "Minutes of the Meetings—Meeting 1, Friday October 10th 2014." Unpublished internal document.

65. Venables. " 'If they bring it, we will take it.' "

66. "A vaccine and experimental treatments are necessary to sustain the response to this unprecedented outbreak (i.e. for frontline workers asap)". Investigation Platform. "Minutes of the Meetings—Meeting 2."

67. Médecins Sans Frontières. *MSF-Supported Research on Ebola.* It is interesting to note that MSF's Ebola experts recognized the organization's important role in clinical research during an outbreak well before the 2014–15 epidemic. See in particular Bausch Daniel G., Armand G. Sprecher, Benjamin Jeffsc, and Paul Boumandoukid. 2008. "Treatment of Marburg and Ebola Hemorrhagic Fevers: A Strategy for Testing New Drugs and Vaccines Under Outbreak Conditions." *Antiviral Research* 78(1): 150–61; Calain, Philippe, Nathalie Fiore, Marc Poncin, and Samia A. Hurst. 2009. "Research Ethics and International Epidemic Response: The Case of Ebola and Marburg Hemorrhagic Fevers." *Public Health Ethics:* phn037. Accessed August 27, 2016, doi:10.1093/phe/phn037.

68. Antierens, Annick. "What is the Platform for Experimental Ebola products." E-mail message to a group of key figures in the MSF movement, October 1, 2014.

69. The term "repurposed treatment" normally refers to treatments that have achieved regulatory approval for clinical use in one condition and are then used or tested in another condition. Here, the term also denotes treatments that are still in clinical testing and therefore have not been approved as safe and effective for the first condition.

70. Balasegaram, Manica, Emmanuel Baron, Jean-Hervé Bradol, et al. "Ebola: A Challenge to Our Humanitarian Identity. A Letter to the MSF Movement." Unpublished internal document, December 4, 2014. The letter was signed by prominent MSF figures, including the executive directors of the MSF Access Campaign, the Drugs for Neglected Diseases Initiative, Epicentre, and the Centre de Réflexion sur l'Action et les Savoirs Humanitaires (CRASH), as well as the presidents of the MSF operational centers in Paris and Geneva. The letter was later published in the French newspaper *Libération* in conjunction with an interview with one of the letter's signatories: Christian Losson, "Rony Brauman: Contre Ebola, 'Le Traitement Symptomatique a Parfois Été Négligé, Voire Oublié." *Liberation*, February 3, 2015. Accessed August 27, 2016, http://www.liberation.fr/terre/2015/02/03/parfois-le-traitement-symptomatique-a-ete-neglige-voire-oublie_1194960.

71. Sprecher, Armand, personal communication, July 4, 2016.

72. Hensley, Lisa E., Julie Dyall, Gene G. OlingerJr, Peter B. Jahrling. 2015. "Lack of Effect of lamivudine on Ebola virus replication [letter]." *Emerging Infectious Diseases* 21(3): 550–552.

73. World Health Organization. "Scientific and Technical Advisory Committee on Ebola Experimental Interventions." Meeting of STAC-EE at the WHO Headquarter, Geneva, Switzerland November, 11–12, 2014. Accessed August 27, 2016. http://www.who.int/medicines/ebola-treatment/2014-1111_Agenda-STAC-EE_Final.pdf.

74. Ibid. The initial mandate of the committee was to make recommendations on experimental vaccines, treatments, and diagnostics for Ebola. However, as the committee's own work and that of other WHO working groups progressed, STAC-EE ended up focusing primarily on potential therapeutics and vaccines. Annick Antierens, the manager of MSF's Investigation Platform and co-author of this chapter, was one of 15 STAC-EE members.

75. World Health Organization. 2015. "Categorization and Prioritization of Drugs for Consideration for Testing or Use in Patients Infected with Ebola." Geneva: World Health Organization. Accessed August 27, 2016, http://who.int/medicines/ebola-treatment/2015-0116_TablesofEbolaDrugs.pdf. Readers should note that the earliest publicly available priority list dates from January 15, 2015, and no longer includes vaccines and convalescent plasma because both were by then discussed in other fora. See also World Health Organization. 2014. *Use of Convalescent Whole Blood or Plasma Collected From Patients Recovered From Ebola Virus Disease for Transfusion, as an Empirical Treatment During Outbreaks*. Geneva: World Health Organization. Accessed August 27, 2016, http://apps.who.int/iris/bitstream/10665/135591/1/WHO_HIS_SDS_2014.8_eng.pdf; World Health Organization. "Essential Medicines and Health Products, Ebola Vaccines." Accessed August 27, 2016, http://www.who.int/medicines/ebola-treatment/emp_ebola_vaccines/en/.

76. World Health Organization. "Scientific and Technical Advisory Committee;" And World Health Organization. "WHO Meeting of the Scientific and Technical Advisory Committee on Ebola Experimental Interventions – Briefing note." Accessed August 27, 2016, http://www.who.int/medicines/ebola-treatment/scientific_tech_meeting/en/.

77. Questions also remained regarding products that were not included in WHO's priority list. Investigation Platform. "Minutes of the Meetings—Meeting 1."

78. Sprecher, personal communication, June 8, 2016.

79. Ibid. Judging solely on the basis of risk and potential clinical benefit, MSF would have been most interested in testing ZMapp and TKM-130803 at the time.

80. Investigation Platform for Experimental Ebola Products. 2014. "Minutes of the Meetings—Meeting 5, Monday 17 November 2014." Unpublished internal document.

81. The goal in mid October was to start trials in the second half of November 2014. Investigation Platform. "Minutes of the Meetings—Meeting 2."

82. Antierens, Annick. 2016. "Trial Designs in Epidemic Emergencies: The Perspective of Caretakers and Aid Workers, Based on the Experience in the 2014–2015 Ebola Outbreak." Unpublished document submitted as evidence to the National Academies of Sciences, Engineering and Medicine Committee on Clinical Trials During the 2014–2015 Ebola Outbreak.

83. Unknown author. "Experimental Ebola Treatments Trials Communications."

84. Minutes of the Investigational Platform record that the treatment candidates on WHO's priority list were evaluated "from the perspective of combined feasibility, relevancy, access & supply (trial and post-trial)". Investigation Platform. "Minutes of the Meetings—Meeting 2."

85. The following points mirror some of the arguments in the debate about whether MSF should prioritize clinical trials over monitored emergency use for all of the available unproven treatments. See the section "Internal Debate About Treatment Trials."

86. Sissoko, Daouda, Cedric Laouenan, Elin Folkesson, Abdoul-Bing M'Lebing, Abdoul-Habib Beavogui, Sylvain Baize, Alseny-Modet Camara, Piet Maes, Susan Shepherd, Christine Danel, Sara Carazo, Mamoudou N. Conde, Jean-Luc Gala, Géraldine Colin, Hélène Savini, Joseph Akoi Bore, Frederic Le Marcis, Fara Raymond Koundouno, Frédéric Petitjean, Marie-Claire Lamah, Sandra Diederich, Alexis Tounkara, Geertrui Poelart, Emmanuel Berbain, Jean-Michel Dindart, Sophie Duraffour, Annabelle Lefevre, Tamba Leno, Olivier Peyrouset, Léonid Irenge,

N'Famara Bangoura, Romain Palich, Julia Hinzmann, Annette Kraus, Thierno Sadou Barry, Sakoba Berette, André Bongono, Mohamed Seto Camara, Valérie Chanfreau Munoz, Lanciné Doumbouya, Souley Harouna, Patient Mumbere Kighoma, Fara Roger Koundouno, Réné Lolamou, Cécé Moriba Loua, Vincent Massala, Kinda Moumouni, Célia Provost, Nenefing Samake, Conde Sekou, Abdoulaye Soumah, Isabelle Arnould, Michel Saa Komano, Lina Gustin, Carlotta Berutto, Diarra Camara, Fodé Saydou Camara, Joliene Colpaert, Léontine Delamou, Lena Jansson, Etienne Kourouma, Maurice Loua, Kristian Malme, Emma Manfrin, André Maomou, Adele Milinouno, Sien Ombelet, Aboubacar Youla Sidiboun, Isabelle Verreckt, Pauline Yombouno, Anne Bocquin, Caroline Carbonnelle, Thierry Carmoi, Pierre Frange, Stéphane Mely, Vinh-Kim Nguyen, Delphine Pannetier, Anne-Marie Taburet, Jean-Marc Treluyer, Jacques Kolie, Raoul Moh, Minerva Cervantes Gonzalez, Eeva Kuisma, Britta Liedigk, Didier Ngabo, Martin Rudolf, Ruth Thom, Romy Kerber, Martin Gabriel, Antonino Di Caro, Roman Wölfel, Jamal Badir, Mostafa Bentahir, Yann Deccache, Catherine Dumont, Jean-François Durant, Karim El Bakkouri, Marie Gasasira Uwamahoro, Benjamin Smits, Nora Toufik, Stéphane Van Cauwenberghe, Khaled Ezzedine, Eric Dortenzio, Louis Pizarro, Aurélie Etienne, Jérémie Guedj, Alexandra Fizet, Eric Barte de Sainte Fare, Bernadette Murgue, Tuan Tran-Minh, Christophe Rapp, Pascal Piguet, Marc Poncin, Bertrand Draguez, Thierry Allaford Duverger, Solenne Barbe, Guillaume Baret, Isabelle Defourny, Miles Carroll, Hervé Raoul, Augustin Augier, Serge P. Eholie, Yazdan Yazdanpanah, Claire Levy-Marchal, Annick Antierrens, Michel Van Herp, Stephan Günther, Xavier de Lamballerie, Sakoba Keïta, France Mentre, Xavier Anglaret, Denis Malvy, JIKI Study Group. 2016. "Experimental Treatment with Favipiravir for Ebola Virus Disease (the JIKI Trial): A Historically Controlled, Single-Arm Proof-of-Concept Trial in Guinea." *PLOS Medicine* 13(3): e1001967. Accessed August 27, 2016, http://dx.doi.org/10.1371/journal.pmed.1001967.

87. World Health Organization. "Categorization and Prioritization of Drugs."
88. Ibid.
89. Investigation Platform for Experimental Ebola Products. 2014. "Minutes of the Meetings— Meeting 4, Friday 7 November 2014." Unpublished internal document.
90. The effectiveness of convalescent plasma was contested and predicted to be low by many experts, based on negative results from a study in primates and inconclusive data from a small study in humans. Sprecher, Armand, personal communication, June 15, 2016.
91. For these reasons, MSF only engaged with blood donation centers for the trial through their partner ITM. Investigation Platform. "Minutes of the Meetings—Meeting 2"; Investigation Platform for Experimental Ebola Products. 2014. "Minutes of the Meetings—Meeting 3, Monday 29 [27] October 2014." Unpublished internal document; Investigation Platform for Experimental Ebola Products. 2015. "Minutes of the Meetings—Meeting 9, Wednesday 7 January 2015." Unpublished internal document.
92. Investigation Platform. "Minutes of the Meetings—Meeting 2."
93. The operational challenges of ensuring adequate staffing and trial infrastructure were numerous, but securing laboratory support was the "real bottleneck" in planning clinical trials. Investigation Platform for Experimental Ebola Products. 2014. "Minutes of the Meetings— Meeting 7, Friday 05 December 2014." Unpublished internal document.
94. Investigation Platform. "Minutes of the Meetings—Meeting 1."
95. See the section "MSF Research Before the 2014–15 Ebola Epidemic."
96. The other two priorities listed in the respective document were testing a "product we believe in" and conducting trials "in the most relevant sites." Investigation Platform. "Minutes of the Meetings—Meeting 1."
97. For example, to reduce the impact of trials on routine care, the Investigation Platform required that medical staff with experience in treating Ebola should not be allocated to support trials. Investigation Platform. "Minutes of the Meetings—Meeting 1."
98. Investigation Platform. "Minutes of the Meetings—Meeting 2."
99. For example, in the convalescent plasma trial a placebo arm would have involved several hours of saline infusion to participants many of whom had bleeding disorders. In the favipiravir trial, participants would have had to ingest large numbers of placebo pills that could have precipitated additional vomiting. Antierens. "Trial Designs in Epidemic Emergencies."

100. Investigation Platform. "Minutes of the Meetings—Meeting 2."
101. Antierens, Annick. "The Ebola Field Reality for Conducting Clinical Trials." Presentation delivered at the 9th European Congress on Tropical Medicine and International Health, Basel, Switzerland, September 7, 2015. Accessed August 27, 2016, http://www.ebolatx.eu/wp-content/uploads/2015/09/Annick-Antierens-MSF_Ebola-field-reality-to-conduct-trials.pdf.
102. Antierens. "Therapeutic Trials During Epidemic Emergencies."
103. Investigation Platform for Experimental Ebola Products. 2015. "Minutes of the Meetings—Meeting 12, Tuesday 3 February 2015." Unpublished internal document. Readers should note that this statement refers to a potential iRCT of Zmapp that MSF considered later in the epidemic. See section "Negotiating Individually Randomized Controlled Designs".
104. Antierens. "Therapeutic Trials During Epidemic Emergencies."
105. Investigation Platform. "Minutes of the Meetings—Meeting 6."
106. MSF Ethics Review Board. *MSF Research Ethics Framework.*
107. For reasons of space, this section and the following two sections focus on clinical trial design because this issue was particularly controversial during the epidemic. For a broader overview of how MSF approached treatment and vaccine trials, see, for example, Antierens. "The Ebola Field Reality."
108. See the section "MSF Research Before the 2014–15 Ebola Epidemic."
109. See the section "Reducing the Impact of Treatment Trials on MSF's Routine Operations."
110. Antierens, Annick. "Trial Designs in Epidemic Emergencies."
111. Sprecher, Armand. Undated. "Pro's and Con's of RCT as Argued in the Medical Journals." Unpublished personal document.
112. Investigation Platform. "Minutes of the Meetings—Meeting 2."
113. Sprecher. "Pro's and Con's of RCT."
114. Antierens. "Therapeutic Trials During Epidemic Emergencies." And elsewhere: "inclusion criteria will be very broad (i.e. exclusion criteria will be patients who can only receive palliative care)." Investigation Platform. "Minutes of the Meetings—Meeting 2."
115. Unknown author. "Experimental Ebola Treatments Trials Communications."
116. Investigation Platform. "Minutes of the Meetings—Meeting 7."
117. Médecins Sans Frontières. *MSF-Supported Research on Ebola.*
118. Because favipiravir had never been given to children, there was no established dosage regimen for this patient group. INSERM and the drug manufacturer then modeled the dosage for children more than one year of age, following a request from MSF. Children below the age of one were excluded from the trial because their metabolic system had been shown to be too immature to allow their safe participation. Bouazza, Naïm, Jean-Marc Treluyer, Frantz Foissac, France Mentré, Anne-Marie Taburet, Jérémie Guedj, Xavier Anglaret, Xavier de Lamballerie, Sakoba Keïta, Denis Malvy, and Pierre Frange. 2015. "Favipiravir for Children with Ebola." *The Lancet* 385(9968): 603–04.
119. The trial insurance for the favipiravir trial refused to cover pregnant women. In the brincidofovir trial, the drug manufacturer did not agree to include pregnant women.
120. Investigation Platform. "Minutes of the Meetings—Meeting 3."; Investigation Platform. "Minutes of the Meetings—Meeting 9."
121. MSF ensured including in the "research agreement's rules of engagement a point on the necessity to ensure access of the African patients to the drugs tried should they prove efficient" but abandoned the idea out of concerns about feasibility and delays. Investigation Platform. "Minutes of the Meetings—Meeting 3."
122. Investigation Platform. "Minutes of the Meetings—Meeting 4"; Investigation Platform. "Minutes of the Meetings—Meeting 5."
123. According to MSF, the drug manufacturer of brincidofovir (Chimerix) was able to scale up drug production but was "hiding behind potential demands of stock piling and availability for other indications." Investigation Platform. "Minutes of the Meetings—Meeting 6." MSF ended up abandoning its negotiations about post-trial availability of brincidofovir in the medium and longer term in order to focus on securing sufficient supplies for monitored emergency use immediately after the trial. It was trying to commit Chimerix to a certain number of doses: "we'll try 20,000 [doses], but [we] will not go below 5,000, or we call it off as we can't have patients showing up after the trial inclusion cohort is reached and [we] have no

drug available anymore." Investigation Platform. "Minutes of the Meetings—Meeting 7." The negotiations caused some tensions in the relevant research consortium, as some "seem[ed] to think that MSF's requests ... were unreasonable ... 'delaying' the trial start and wasting weeks." Investigation Platform for Experimental Ebola Products. 2014. "Minutes of the Meetings—Meeting 8, Friday 12 December 2014." Unpublished internal document.

124. The goal of MSF's lobbying efforts was "to ensure production supply and availability in the quantities needed to tackle the outbreak in West Africa, provided clinical research would demonstrate efficacy and safety." Unknown author. "Experimental Ebola Treatments Trials Communications."

125. Investigation Platform. "Minutes of the Meetings—Meeting 3."

126. Investigation Platform. "Minutes of the Meetings—Meeting 7."

127. As discussed in the section "Reducing the Impact of Treatment Trials on MSF's Routine Operations," another reason for rejecting a trial design that did not randomize participants to a concurrent control group, but included a control of patients who could not be transfused due to a lack of matching blood products, was that it might not be accepted by communities. Investigation Platform for Experimental Ebola Products. 2015. "Minutes of the Meetings—Meeting 10, Friday 16 January 2015." Unpublished internal document.

128. The key argument was that patient outcomes varied so significantly that any treatment effects could not be detected without including a concurrent control group. See for example: Goodman, Jesse L. 2014. "Studying 'Secret Serums': Toward Safe, Effective Ebola Treatments." *New England Journal of Medicine* 371(12): 1086–89; Joffe, Steven. 2014. "Evaluating Novel Therapies During the Ebola Epidemic." *JAMA* 312(13): 1299–1300; Cox, Edward, Luciana Borio, and Robert Temple. "Evaluating Ebola Therapies: The Case for RCTs." *New England Journal of Medicine* 371(25): 2350–2351; Shaw, David. "Randomisation is Essential in Ebola Drug Trials." *The Lancet* 384(9955): 1667.

129. See for example: Adebamowo Clement, Oumou Bah-Sow, Fred Binka, Roberto Bruzzone, Arthur Caplan, Jean-François Delfraissy, David Heymann, Peter Horby, Pontiano Kaleebu, Jean-Jacques Muyembe Tamfum, Piero Olliaro, Peter Piot, Abdul Tejan-Colé, Oyewale Tomori, Aissatou Toure, Els Torreele, and John Whitehead. 2014. "Randomised Controlled Trials for Ebola: Practical and Ethical Issues." *The Lancet* 384(9952): 1423–24; Caplan, Arthur L., Carolyn Plunkett, and Bruce Levin. 2015. "Selecting the Right Tool For the Job." *The American Journal of Bioethics* 15(4): 4–10; Caplan, Arthur L., Carolyn Plunkett, and Bruce Levin. 2015. "The Perfect Must Not Overwhelm the Good: Response to Open Peer Commentaries on 'Selecting the Right Tool For the Job.'" The American Journal of Bioethics 15(4): W8-W10. Note that ethical debates about how unproven treatments for patients with highly fatal infectious diseases and no or limited treatment options should be tested go back at least to the HIV/AIDS epidemic. See, for example, Schuklenk, Udo. *Access to Experimental Drugs in Terminal Illness: Ethical Issues*. Boca Raton: CRC Press, 1998.

130. MSF Operational Research Unit, and OCB Luxembourg. *Operational Research Policy Framework*.

131. Zachariah et al. "Conducting Operational Research Within a Nongovernmental Organization."

132. McConnell, Rebecca; Stephanie Roll, Saskia van der Kam, Leslie Shanks, Sarah Venis, Philipp du Cros, Ruby Siddiqui, Jane Greig. 2012. "Randomised Controlled Trials: How to do them in MSF." Geneva: Médecins Sans Frontières. Accessed August 28, 2016, http://fieldresearch.msf.org/msf/bitstream/10144/213311/1/RCT.pdf.

133. Sprecher. "Pro's and Con's of RCT."

134. For example, because there was no standardized way to collect routine clinical data, each MSF ETU set up its own data collection system. In some ETUs, the results of ward rounds also had to be shouted from the high-risk zone to the low-risk zone because paper records could not be carried between zones due to infection control measures—an approach that was prone to error. Médecins Sans Frontières, and Stockholm Evaluation Unit. *OCB Ebola Review*. 13 and 26.

135. Antierens. "Trial Designs in Epidemic Emergencies."

136. Specifically, because healthy individuals are not faced with a high risk of dying and they have alternative means for preventing an Ebola infection than receiving an unproven vaccine, the

perceived obligation to provide them with that vaccine seems much weaker than the perceived obligation to provide patients with Ebola Virus Disease with a potentially beneficial treatment.

137. Investigation Platform. "Minutes of the Meetings—Meeting 12."
138. Investigation Platform. "Minutes of the Meetings—Meeting 9."
139. Investigation Platform. "Minutes of the Meetings—Meeting 12."
140. Médecins Sans Frontières. *MSF-Supported Research on Ebola.*
141. Investigation Platform for Experimental Ebola Products. 2015. "Minutes of the Meetings—Meeting 20, Tuesday 31st of March 2015." Unpublished internal document.
142. A therapeutic orientation to clinical trials means that trials are conceived from the perspective of the patient–clinician relationship rather than from the perspective of the participant–researcher relationship. See Miller, Franklin G., and Donald L. Rosenstein. 2003. "The therapeutic orientation to clinical trials." *New England Journal of Medicine* 348(14): 1383–85.
143. Emanuel, Wendler, and Grady. "What Makes Clinical Research Ethical."
144. MSF conducted important observational research, but more could have been achieved if a dedicated structure like the Investigation Platform for Experimental Ebola Products had enabled and coordinated MSF's operational research. Médecins Sans Frontières, and Stockholm Evaluation Unit. *OCB Ebola Review.* 52.
145. Many within MSF believed that supportive care would reduce mortality by no more than 5% to 10% (see footnote 59). However, others had higher hopes for the clinical impact of supportive care. For example, Paul Farmer of Partners in Health asked at one point in the epidemic: "What if the fatality rate isn't the virulence of disease but the mediocrity of the medical delivery?" McNeill, Donald G. "Ebola Doctors Are Divided on IV Therapy in Africa." *The New York Times,* January 1, 2015. Accessed August 28, 2016. http://www.nytimes.com/2015/01/02/health/ebola-doctors-are-divided-on-iv-therapy-in-africa.html?_r=1. See also Roberts, Ian, and Anders Perner. 2014. "Ebola Virus Disease: Clinical Care and Patient-Centred Research." *The Lancet* 384(9959): 2001–02. Unfortunately, little systematic research on supportive care was conducted in this epidemic, and one report concluded that "the evidence base with respect to patient care and staff protection has not significantly grown and still relies largely on expert opinion." Médecins Sans Frontières, and Stockholm Evaluation Unit. *OCB Ebola Review.* 59.
146. The burden of disease from insufficient care for infectious diseases other than Ebola and pregnancy-related complications is considered to have been greater than the burden of disease from Ebola in this epidemic. Médecins Sans Frontières, and Stockholm Evaluation Unit. *OCB Ebola Review.* 59.
147. Sprecher, personal communication, June 15, 2016.

7

Failing Dr. Khan

TIM O'DEMPSEY

In July 2014, Sierra Leone was in the grip of a rapidly escalating epidemic of Ebola virus disease (EVD). The virus, having emerged in Guinea in December 2013, was detected in Sierra Leone in May 2014 following the death and unsafe burial of a traditional healer in Kailahun District, which resulted in numerous transmission chains and alone gave rise to an estimated 365 deaths.

The first case of EVD in Sierra Leone was confirmed at the Lassa Fever Unit Laboratory in Kenema Government Hospital on May 23, 2014. The Lassa unit rapidly filled with cases of EVD, mainly from Kailahun District, and it was necessary to commandeer a nearby hospital building for use as a ward for suspect and probable cases and to construct a temporary ward for the growing number of confirmed cases. This became the Kenema Ebola Treatment Center (ETC). On June 26, MSF opened a purpose-built ETC outside Kailahun Town; compared to the Kenema ETC, it was well staffed, well organized, and well supplied.

Transmission in eastern Sierra Leone continued relentlessly. By mid-July, the Kenema ETC was severely overcrowded, with upward of 60 patients, 25% of whom were healthcare workers, among them several senior staff, including the head nurse of the Lassa unit. The ETC was poorly maintained and disorganized, with grossly inadequate attention to infection prevention and control (IPC) procedures; evidence of numerous structural and procedural breaches; and catastrophic standards in hygiene, sanitation, and management and disposal of medical waste and corpses. Essential treatment supplies for patients and personal protective equipment (PPE) for staff were woefully inadequate and only haphazardly available. Staff morale was at an all-time low; the nurses were on strike and the few staff willing to care for EVD patients had to endure stigmatization by their communities and, as they witnessed increasing numbers of their colleagues fall ill and die, a growing sense of inevitability that they would be next.

And so it was with Dr. Sheik Humarr Khan, the physician in charge of Kenema Government Hospital's Lassa fever program and Sierra Leone's leading expert on viral hemorrhagic fevers. On the morning of Saturday, July 19, standing out-side the ETC, Dr. Khan told me that he was feeling unwell and would be unable to join a visit to the MSF ETC in Kailahun planned for the following day. Over the weekend he self-treated for malaria without any improvement. On July 21 he decided to have himself tested for Ebola. The result was positive. Rather than remain in Kenema and be admitted to the overcrowded ETC alongside his ailing colleagues, he arranged to be transferred to the MSF ETC in Kailahun, where he hoped to find greater privacy, and, one imagines, better care than he anticipated would be available in Kenema.

On hearing that Dr. Khan had tested positive for EVD, the WHO clini-cians working in the Kenema ETC asked the WHO field coordinator whether WHO would be arranging for Dr. Khan to be evacuated from Sierra Leone for treatment in Europe. The response was an emphatic "no"; Dr. Khan was not a WHO employee and therefore was not eligible for evacuation under WHO's auspices. The first, and perhaps the best, opportunity to save Dr. Khan had been missed.

On July 23, news reached the WHO clinicians in Kenema that the Canadian laboratory team, co-located with and providing diagnostic services for the MSF ETC in Kailahun, had a limited supply of an experimental therapeutic that had been previously tested with some success in Ebola-infected non-human primates in a laboratory setting. The therapeutic agent was ZMapp. The Canadians were willing to offer this to MSF for treatment of Dr. Khan. Neither this, nor any simi-lar therapy, had previously been used to treat a human being with EVD. At that time there had been no trials whatsoever of this therapy in humans. Not only were there no data on the efficacy of this therapy in treatment of EVD in humans, there were no data on the safety, side effects, or appropriate dosing in humans.

Clearly, the decision whether or not to treat Dr. Khan with an experimen-tal therapy was one that the MSF team caring for him did not wish to take lightly. Therefore, with the endorsement of the WHO country representative, MSF invited me, as the senior clinician on WHO's team in Kenema, to meet with the MSF team in Kailahun to discuss this difficult and complex clinical and ethical issue.

Let us pause for a moment and consider the circumstances in which this dis-cussion took place. Any analysis of the decisions made around Dr. Khan's care is incomplete without consideration of the larger sociopolitical, economic, and epidemiological situation that prevailed at that time. By the latter half of July 2014, the Ebola epidemic in West Africa was spiraling out of control. Incidence rates were rising exponentially. Health ministries in the region were finding it impossible to confine the epidemic to the less populated rural areas; the virus was spreading relentlessly throughout the region and was now gaining a foot-hold in major urban populations. This unprecedented and potentially explosive situation was of grave international concern. There were only a handful of ETCs in the entire region. In Sierra Leone there were just two: MSF's in Kailahun, and the Ministry of Health's unit supported by WHO in Kenema. By now these centers were receiving EVD patients from all over Sierra Leone, most of whom were critically ill by the time they reached the treatment facility. Many did not survive the long journey. It was common to discover one or more corpses on opening the door of an ambulance on arrival at the ETC.

Members of the general public were repeatedly informed that this was a disease where nine out of 10 of those affected were expected to die, a statistic widely quoted by various "experts" and the media. Over and over again it was reported that "there is no treatment for Ebola." Nevertheless, communities were urged, encouraged, even coerced, into coming forward with individuals with Ebola-like symptoms, whereupon their loved one, neighbor, colleague would be taken away by masked strangers clad in weird clothing, never to be seen again. There were whispers of secret experimentation and the harvesting of organs. Traditional burial practices that included the ritual washing of corpses and anointing of mourners, essential for the spiritual well-being of the deceased and their community, had been deemed unsafe and were banned by the government of Sierra Leone. Meanwhile, even among affected communities, there was still widespread denial that Ebola was "real." Rumors abounded that the disease was caused by witchcraft or that it was something introduced by Western agencies intent on undermining and exploiting the people of Sierra Leone.

The impact of the epidemic on healthcare workers was devastating. Of the 60 or so patients being treated at the Kenema ETC in the latter half of July 2014, 15 were healthcare workers. The MSF ETC in Kailahun was also treating healthcare workers, some of whom were from Kenema.

On the morning that Dr. Khan was informed that his test for Ebola was positive, the clinical team in the Kenema ETC were struggling to save the life of Sr. Mbalu Fonnie, the Lassa unit's head nurse and a woman of high standing in the community. An agitated crowd of around 200, mainly women, gathered in the hospital compound intent on removing her from the treatment center. Fortunately, they were persuaded to disperse. An hour or so later, Sr. Mbalu died.

The scene was uglier a few days later when hundreds of Kenema residents gathered outside the ETC angrily complaining that they had never been consulted about locating the ETC in the hospital grounds and that the ETC was now attracting patients with Ebola from all over the country, placing the population of Kenema at greater risk and deterring access to the general hospital, the wards of which were mostly deserted. The crowd threatened to attack and destroy the ETC but were dispersed by Sierra Leone armed forces using tear gas.

And so it was, late on July 23, amidst this highly volatile atmosphere of nationwide fear, mistrust, and misinformation, that the discussion took place to determine the most appropriate course of action for Dr. Khan's care at the MSF ETC in Kailahun. The discussion began privately among senior MSF staff at the ETC. In the meantime, I visited Dr. Khan to ask how he was feeling. He looked remarkably well, smiling and inquiring about the staff and the situation in Kenema. Apart from fever, headache, and body pains, he had few complaints. He was eating and drinking and asked for "jelly water" (milk from young coconuts), which he favored as part of oral rehydration for patients with EVD in Kenema.

After about an hour of internal discussion, I was invited to join the discussion with the MSF team. A senior member of the MSF team explained that the Canadian lab team had revealed that there was a limited supply of ZMapp in the lab, which could be made available for treatment of Dr. Khan if required. MSF expressed the following concerns:

1. ZMapp was an experimental therapeutic that had never been used before in humans. MSF policy precluded the use of experimental treatments in humanitarian emergencies.
2. Dr. Khan was one of many patients, including other healthcare workers, being treated for EVD in the unit. It was not equitable to single him out for special treatment in preference to other patients.
3. Should Dr. Khan suffer adverse effects from treatment with ZMapp, MSF did not have the resources to escalate care, nor could they provide anything more than rudimentary monitoring. For example, the constraints of PPE limited the frequency of monitoring vital signs, there were no means of monitoring biochemistry, and there was no equipment for providing life support in the event of organ failure.
4. Were Dr. Khan to die following treatment with ZMapp, whether as a result of treatment with ZMapp or as a consequence of EVD, MSF ran the risk of being accused of experimenting on him. This might jeopardize their mission not only in Kailahun but possibly elsewhere in the region, and would reduce the likelihood that MSF would be in a position to escalate their response in Sierra Leone or elsewhere. Given that MSF was the only nongovernmental organization (NGO) engaged in the clinical response at that time, this would have a devastating impact on efforts to contain the epidemic and provide care for victims of Ebola.
5. At that time, Dr. Khan was clinically stable, ambulatory, and tolerating oral therapy. Other care options should be considered—for example, medical evacuation to a center outside Sierra Leone where he could be optimally managed and, if deemed appropriate, could receive ZMapp or another experimental therapy with better and more appropriate levels of monitoring and life support than available in Kailahun.

Several of the MSF staff involved in the discussion were particularly adamant that to offer Dr. Khan preferential treatment would be inequitable and unethical. They said they would resign from the mission if such a decision were made.

The official WHO position was that WHO did not support the use of experimental treatments in the Ebola epidemic region at that time. To obtain more information about the experience with the experimental use of ZMapp in non-human primates, I called the head of the research group in Canada, explained the situation in Kailahun, and asked whether, if in Dr. Khan's predicament, he would want to be treated with ZMapp. "Absolutely" was the reply.

Advocating on behalf of Dr. Khan, I put forward the following points:

1. Although there were no data on the use of ZMapp in humans, there were data from experiments in non-human primates that the therapy was effective, particularly if given at a relatively early stage in the disease.
2. Regarding the possibility of adverse effects, the experimental studies had not indicated these to be a major problem.
3. The lead researcher involved in the animal studies felt strongly that the potential benefit far outweighed the possible risks of treating Dr. Khan with ZMapp.
4. Dr. Khan should be informed that ZMapp was available. He should be provided with as much information as possible and should be given the opportunity to make an informed choice with regard to his treatment.

The MSF team members were opposed to informing Dr. Khan of the availability of ZMapp because they were not willing to administer the treatment. The MSF doctor leading discussions on behalf of the MSF team reiterated concerns about the possibility of triggering a severe adverse reaction were ZMapp to be used. I arranged for the MSF doctor to discuss his concerns with the Geneva-based clinical team lead for the physicians deployed by WHO to Sierra Leone. The WHO clinical team lead was unable to alleviate the MSF doctor's concerns.

I asked whether the MSF team would allow me to take personal responsibility for administering the ZMapp to Dr. Khan and supervise his subsequent management. The MSF team members were opposed to this as they regarded the administration of ZMapp as an undesired medical act. They stressed that it would not be possible for me as a single clinician to administer the treatment alone, and, if I were to do so, they would not be willing to be involved in any aspect of Dr. Khan's subsequent care. A number of those present reiterated that, were Dr. Khan to be singled out for "special" treatment, they would resign from the mission.

To understand the fundamental basis for their reluctance to administer or support the administration of the ZMapp for Dr. Khan, I proposed a hypothetical situation. What if a drug were available that was known to be effective in treating EVD, with no appreciable side effects, but was available only in sufficient quantity to treat one patient? Would the MSF team be willing to administer this to Dr. Khan? The team members said they would not be prepared to do so as this would be inequitable; they had a duty to treat all patients on the basis of clinical need rather than social or other status. It would be unethical to single out Dr. Khan for special treatment.

The final decision was that Dr. Khan would not be offered treatment with ZMapp, nor was he to be informed that ZMapp was available. The following morning I visited Dr. Khan and tried to persuade him to return to Kenema for ongoing care on the basis that (a) it might be possible to offer him treatment in Kenema that was not available in Kailahun and (b) given the distance from Kailahun to Lungi Airport and the dreadful condition of the road between Kailahun and Kenema, it would be better for him to be in Kenema if medical evacuation became possible. Dr. Khan insisted that he wanted to remain in Kailahun, as this would provide him greater privacy. I returned to Kenema alone.

Attempts to save Dr. Khan now shifted to mobilizing a medical evacuation. MSF made it clear that WHO would have to take full responsibility for arranging and managing Dr. Khan's evacuation. WHO Geneva contacted International SOS, the designated company for medical evacuation of WHO international staff, and instigated the process to evacuate Dr. Khan from Sierra Leone. More than 72 hours elapsed between initiating this process and the arrival of the SOS aircraft at Lungi Airport in Sierra Leone. On arrival, the crew were obliged by aviation regulations to rest for 12 hours prior to making a further flight.

In the meantime, MSF staff were updating me in Kenema on a daily basis. Dr. Khan's condition had begun to deteriorate. He had developed diarrhea and vomiting. International SOS said they were not equipped to manage EVD patients with diarrhea or vomiting and refused to evacuate Dr. Khan. Numerous calls took place between myself in Kenema, International SOS, and WHO Geneva, but International SOS refused to change its position.

On July 26, the WHO country representative for Sierra Leone asked me to return to Kailahun and personally assess Dr. Khan. In the few days that had passed, Dr. Khan's condition had significantly deteriorated. He still insisted that he wanted to remain at the MSF ETC in Kailahun. Given the condition of the road and the likelihood that he was developing a bleeding tendency to further complicate his illness, it was unlikely that he would have tolerated the four-hour journey in the back of an ambulance over the bumpy, muddy road to Kenema. A helicopter would be required for the journey to Lungi Airport should international evacuation become possible.

By now, Sierra Leone's minister of health was in regular contact with me. Both she and Sierra Leone's president were growing increasingly anxious about the deteriorating condition of Sierra Leone's leading physician in the fight against Ebola. I asked the minister whether she would be able to arrange for Dr. Khan to be evacuated by government means or by an alternative agency. She said this was not possible.

On the evening of July 26, I received a call from a colleague in Kenema that one of the WHO doctors had sustained a penetrating injury to his finger while opening a glass vial in the "red zone." He was immediately evacuated (on a commercial flight, as he posed no risk to others) to Geneva for 21 days of observation. With only one doctor and a handful of nurses remaining in the Kenema ETC to care for around 60 EVD patients, I was obliged to return to Kenema. Early the following morning, prior to leaving Kailahun, I went in to see Dr. Khan and explain the situation. Dr. Khan asked me to remain in Kailahun but accepted that the need was much greater in Kenema. Before departing I discussed Dr. Khan's further management with the MSF doctors and left a detailed written plan for escalation of care, including recommendations for intravenous fluids and intravenous antibiotics. Dr. Khan was a strong and determined man, and there was still hope that he might pull through.

Dr. Khan's preference for remaining under the care of MSF in Kailahun was understandable given the further deterioration in conditions at the ETC in Kenema. The MSF ETC in Kailahun had numerous doctors, nurses, clinical officers, and hygienists providing care in well-organized shifts. In contrast, while the citizens of Kenema celebrated the festival of Eid on July 28, the other remaining WHO clinician and I struggled to attend to the patients on the dreadfully overcrowded wards of the Kenema ETC without nursing assistance for almost the entire day. At the end of a second six-hour shift in the "red zone," our final task was to remove the corpses of patients who had died the previous night. Given the conditions in Kenema, it is questionable whether Dr. Khan's chances of survival would have been better there, with or without ZMapp.

Dr. Khan's final call to me was on the morning of July 29. He said he was feeling very weak. He said he had not received intravenous fluids or intravenous antibiotics the previous day. He asked me to return to Kailahun. Given the dire situation and staff shortages in the Kenema ETC, this was impossible.

News of Dr. Khan's death reached us in Kenema later that afternoon. The International SOS plane left Sierra Leone the following day. A profound sense of loss, grief, and shock descended on the people of Kenema and throughout Sierra Leone. Many have since remarked that the death of Dr. Khan was the pivotal point at which the majority of the population began to believe that Ebola was real.

Let us now reflect on some of the dilemmas and decisions I have presented. Although Dr. Khan may have died whatever decisions were made or whatever resources were available, his death highlights technical, procedural, and ethical issues that require further discussion.

Medical Evacuation

It is likely that Dr. Khan's best chance of survival would have been if, as soon as he was confirmed to have EVD, he had been evacuated to a country outside Sierra Leone where he could receive comprehensive clinical care and could be given the option of receiving experimental therapy in a highly controlled and monitored setting. No agency or government was willing to support this initially. However, two days after his admission to the MSF ETC in Kailahun, following discussion at a senior level in Geneva, WHO initiated the process for Dr. Khan's evacuation by International SOS, a well-established medical evacuation agency designated by WHO to provide specified WHO staff and their eligible dependents with the opportunity to secure essential medical care or treatment for a severe illness requiring medical intervention if it was locally unavailable or inadequate.

Although Dr. Khan was not working for WHO, the WHO team in Geneva went to considerable effort to initiate the process of medical evacuation and identified a European country (Germany) that was willing and able to provide Dr. Khan with specialist medical care. Under the circumstances, this was commendable. However, what followed exposed major shortcomings in International SOS's capability to evacuate individuals with EVD and revealed a failure on WHO's part to anticipate the needs of individuals with EVD requiring medical evacuation.

Evidently, the medical evacuation process and facility offered by International SOS was not adequate for the purpose of evacuating symptomatic patients with EVD. Diarrhea and vomiting are early symptoms, yet International SOS refused to evacuate Dr. Khan at a relatively early stage in his illness when his general condition was good because he had developed diarrhea and vomiting. It is absurd that International SOS was engaged as the preferred operator for the medical evacuation of patients with EVD if the company was inadequately equipped to transport such patients. Furthermore, the process involved a series of what should have been predictable procedures that delayed and ultimately prevented Dr. Khan's evacuation. Given the delays associated with mobilizing a suitably equipped air ambulance, crew, and medical team; delays in obtaining various permissions to transport a patient with EVD through different international airspace zones; and the necessity for the crew to rest for 12 hours following arrival, it seems highly improbable that by the time the plane was ready to depart the patient would still be considered suitable for evacuation (according to the International SOS's criteria) even if the company had been notified at the very onset of the patient's symptoms. WHO subsequently switched to a different provider for medical evacuation of patients with EVD, one capable of transporting individuals with diarrhea and vomiting.

Ethics and the Use of Unregistered Interventions

Experimental therapies and vaccines were known to be in existence and available, albeit in limited quantities, prior to the onset of this epidemic. It was also widely known that such interventions would be offered to (evacuated) international staff if they became infected and developed symptoms of EVD. However, at the time of Dr. Khan's illness, WHO maintained that it was unethical to offer experimental interventions to people within the affected countries, a view shared by MSF. It was not until August 11, 2014, two weeks after Dr. Khan's death, as international concern and controversy grew regarding the withholding or use of such treatment, that WHO convened an emergency meeting of medical ethicists and other experts. After this meeting the recommendations were changed in favor of use under specified circumstances.

Opinion was divided regarding the criteria for the selection of particular groups or individuals for prioritization and allocation of investigational interventions (WHO 2014):

> As the number of candidate interventions was currently limited and doses of the most promising interventions were in extremely short supply, choices would have to be made, not only about who would receive the intervention but also which country would get what and on the basis of what criteria. It was agreed that the principles used for setting priorities in resource-constrained settings should be applied to make such choices. Some of the criteria mentioned were:
>
> i. distributive justice: fairness between countries and among populations within countries;
> ii. reciprocity and social usefulness: Although the panel was not unanimous, many members proposed that health care workers be considered of high priority, including for access to therapy. This proposal is based on two ethical principles: reciprocity (they put their life at risk to care for others) and social usefulness (they are instrumental to controlling the outbreak). The same principles

should apply to other workers providing supportive services (such as sanitation and burial services) and to relatives who provide care to patients. Other panel members advocated that patients in the community should have the same priority as the groups mentioned above, particularly for therapy;

iii. likelihood of a positive impact on both individual and public health outcomes;

iv. clinical stage of the disease;

v. the characteristics of the unregistered medical product.

The "reciprocity and social usefulness" argument clearly favors a recommendation to offer ZMapp to Dr. Khan, although, like many of the MSF staff in Kailahun, some ethics panel members opposed this position on grounds of inequity. Based on animal studies, it could be argued that the "clinical stage of the disease" and "the characteristics of the unregistered medical product" also would have favored a recommendation to offer ZMapp to Dr. Khan early in his admission to the MSF ETC in Kailahun. There is greater uncertainty regarding the "likelihood of a positive impact on both individual and public health outcomes."

We should also consider two additional guiding principles proposed by the panel:

Families and communities must be involved, to the extent possible, in decisions on priority allocation.

The ultimate choice of whether to receive the experimental intervention must rest with the patient, if the patient is in a condition to make the choice.

However, among the essential considerations prior to use of unregistered interventions stipulated by the panel is the following:

Capacity should be available to administer the experimental therapy in conjunction with the necessary supportive treatment, to monitor and manage any side-effects and to monitor the progress of treatment, including, at a minimum, measuring when possible appropriate surrogate outcomes, such as disease and immune response markers.

Additional guiding principles state:

Standard supportive care must be provided when the unregistered product in question is used as a therapeutic agent;

Minimal infrastructure and equipment to administer the experimental therapy, monitor its efficacy and treat any severe adverse effects appropriately must be available.

Thus, even if WHO had called the meeting of ethicists at an earlier stage in the epidemic, neither the MSF team in Kailahun nor the WHO team working with the Ministry of Health in Kenema would have been in a position to comply with these requirements.

Although it would have been practically impossible to involve all the families and communities of all the EVD patients in the MSF facility in the decision on priority allocation, clearly Dr. Khan would have been in a position to make an informed choice had he been made aware that ZMapp was available. No one can be certain what his choice would have been. Perhaps he would have declined on the basis of inequity or concerns that the risks outweighed the benefits. Perhaps he would have opted for treatment. If so, the MSF and WHO clinicians, whether in Kailahun or Kenema, would still have been faced with the challenges of providing adequate monitoring and supportive care and of maintaining patient confidentiality while ensuring that Dr. Khan's decision and subsequent progress were appropriately communicated, particularly given the risk of accusations of experimentation were he to die, or of providing preferential treatment were he to survive. In the volatile and precarious circumstances that gripped Sierra Leone at the time, not one but many lives were at stake.

The Value of a Life

The processes and policies concerning medical evacuation and the ethical principles guiding the use of unregistered interventions in extreme circumstances could have been explored, if not before the epidemic became established, certainly at an earlier stage in its evolution. Anticipation of scenarios around international medical evacuation and earlier discussion concerning the ethics of offering unregistered treatment would have led to more appropriate and less costly decisions.

The people of Sierra Leone, Liberia, and Guinea suffered the consequences of a weak, delayed, reactive, and inadequate international response. National, regional, and international preparedness planning would have led to earlier and more effective interventions that would have shortened the epidemic by months and saved many lives. The epidemic not only exposed and exploited the fragility of health systems in West Africa but also highlighted major deficiencies in the capability and capacity of international organizations to respond in a proactive, timely, and effective manner.

It is impossible to say with any confidence that Dr. Khan's life could have been saved. Dr. Khan was one of 38 health workers from Kenema, one among 221 Sierra Leonean healthcare workers, one among 3,956 Sierra Leoneans, who died of Ebola during the epidemic. His death had an impact way beyond the borders of Sierra Leone, exposing glaring inequalities, failures in forward thinking, institutional inertia and rigidity and revealing how self-interest blinds us to the reality of our fear, prejudice, and personal frailty: we do not hold every human life to be of equal value.

Just ask yourself: How have I lived the last 24 hours of my life?

Reference

"Ethical considerations for use of unregistered interventions for Ebola viral disease. Report of an advisory panel to WHO." WHO/HIS/KER/GHE/14.1. Geneva: WHO, 2014.

8

Finding an Answer to Ebola's Greatest Challenge

ARMAND SPRECHER

The sum of all our answer is but this:
We would not seek a battle as we are,
Nor, as we are, we say we will not shun it.

Henry V, *Act 3, Scene 6*

On June 14, 2014, at the general assembly of MSF-Brussels, Dr. Moses Massaquoi, a senior member of the Liberian Ministry of Health and Social Welfare (MHSW) and also a member of MSF, asked the assembled members when MSF was going to come to the aid of Liberia, as the first cases of Ebola had recently been found in the capital, Monrovia. The response to Moses' request was that help would not be coming from MSF anytime soon, as current Ebola operations in West Africa already stretched the organization to its limits.

Nevertheless, two months later, in Monrovia, MSF would open the largest Ebola Treatment Unit (ETU) that anyone had ever operated. This would be known as ELWA3, as it was the third ETU to be built on the grounds of the Eternal Love Winning Africa (ELWA) ministry. The unit could not be sufficiently staffed, so its coordinators struggled to find the right way to deliver care with the limited human resources they had. Each morning, patients were admitted until the available beds were filled, and then the gates to the unit were closed for the rest of the day. The patients who were admitted did not receive the full extent of MSF's usual care for Ebola patients. The compromises that had to be made did not please anyone, especially not those who had to make them.

While this was going on, the epidemic raged. What had started as a handful of cases in Monrovia became thousands, at one point accumulating at a rate of over 250 new cases per week. In August 2014, the West African Ebola outbreak that had been simmering for several months began to boil. The epidemic began its phase of exponential growth that would result in the majority of its nearly 29,000 cases occurring in the ensuing months, and it began in full view of the world in the capital of Liberia, where MSF had one understaffed ETU trying to cope with a situation no one had prepared for.

How Did This Happen?

In July 2014, MSF decided to do something in Monrovia despite its engagements elsewhere, but this assistance was limited to sending a few people to provide technical assistance to the health authorities. MHSW was not entirely unprepared to deal with Ebola, and it was felt that its existing capacity would be sufficient to manage the epidemic if given sufficient support. Back in March, four cases of Ebola had been detected in Lofa County, in northern Liberia, across the border from the epicenter of the outbreak in southeastern Guinea (Nyenswah et al. 2014). This immediately raised concern about spread of the epidemic to Monrovia. In April 2014 an MSF team was briefly present in Monrovia and set up an ETU in a former cholera treatment unit adjacent to the John F. Kennedy (JFK) Medical Center, the country's main tertiary referral hospital. Staff there were then trained in the appropriate treatment and infection control procedures and provided with materials. By the end of June the Liberian health authorities had gained a small amount of experience with Ebola control in responding to the cases in Lofa County.

By the first week of July, the Liberian government had put into place in Monrovia all of the necessary outbreak control activities: an alert hotline, case investigation teams, safe patient transport, safe burial teams, a laboratory capable of testing blood specimens for Ebola, a social mobilization system, countywide reinforcement of infection control in health structures, an ETU, and a coordination body to manage the overall response. The last remaining piece, albeit a critical one, a contact tracing system, was set up during the second week of July (Sprecher 2014a).

Unfortunately, none of these services was of sufficient scale to meet the massive demands of the epidemic. Not all the reported cases could be investigated, not all the suspected cases could be transported to the ETU, and not all the bodies could be buried in a timely manner. Already in July 2014 money and material to help the Liberians combat Ebola provided by international donors were flowing into the country, but transforming these resources into a robust response exceeded the absorptive capacity of the health authorities. Thus the epidemic began to grow. How and where it was growing, and how big it had become, was not immediately apparent, as it spread out of sight of the outbreak control managers. By early August, cases were being found across all of Monrovia. This was an especially disturbing sign because it hinted at the magnitude of what was going on out of view.

When Ebola reaches a large city, an early concern among those unfamiliar with the virus is that it will spread like wildfire through the population. This belief stems from more familiar epidemics of airborne and diarrheal diseases, diseases for which the population at risk is large because of the nature of transmission— anyone can be sneezed upon or drink unsafe water. For Ebola, transmission is not so haphazard, as it is primarily transmitted through direct contact—that is, to those who care enough about the sick person to provide care or to attend their funeral (Brainard 2016). Because of this focused transmission, the vast majority of a large urban population is at little immediate risk of exposure, though there is an important exception to this: healthcare facilities.

Cities are where large hospitals are found. The poor infection control not uncommon in Central African healthcare settings makes hospitals good disease amplifiers, as many people can be infected by unwashed hands or unsafe injection practices. Hospitals are also excellent ways of bringing Ebola to new social groups, allowing whole new communities to be exposed when patients are sent home incubating the virus or when exposed healthcare workers go home from work.

The initial arrival of Ebola in Conakry, Guinea, in March 2014, several months earlier than the outbreak in Monrovia, raised concerns that the city would quickly be overrun by Ebola. However, it resulted in only dozens of cases, as the spread was limited to a small number of transmission chains that were put under surveillance and controlled. The size of the Ebola outbreak when it arrived in Conakry was not proportional to the city's population of almost two million people. This may be because the hospitals involved did not cater to a broad range of social groups, perhaps they had better-than-average infection control practices, or perhaps the style of healthcare delivery in Conakry involved minimal contact with the patient. In any case, the small scale of the early outbreak in Conakry may have created a false sense of security among outbreak control agencies by showing that the arrival of Ebola in a large city did not necessarily result in a large number of cases.

Monrovia would prove to be different for some unknown reason. Perhaps the social networks in the city were denser or more interconnected. Maybe the disease amplification caused by hospitals was greater. There is some suggestion of this from the large number of healthcare workers among the early cases (MSF 2014). There may have been some novel means of transmission at work. Perhaps all of these were occurring.

Whatever the cause, the large number of locations throughout the city where cases were being found, however many cases there were, indicated that there were many active chains of transmission. This is important because two cases of Ebola virus disease (EVD) within a social group may not expose many more people than one if they share the same care providers or likely funeral attendees. Two cases in two different networks may double the number of people exposed. This is why the distribution of cases across Monrovia in early August was so concerning, as it implied many chains of transmission and a much larger population at risk of the disease than if the cases had been more tightly clustered in just one part of the city.

As the ETU run by Liberian health workers at JFK, the only one in Monrovia, had only about 25 beds, and because of limited safe patient transport capacity, some hospitals in the city had to hold patients suspected of having Ebola more than 24 hours before they could be transferred to the JFK ETU. One hospital, ELWA, supported by the medical charitable organizations Serving In Mission (SIM) and Samaritan's Purse, created a dedicated place for these patients in one of its chapels, which became a de facto five-bed ETU.

The JFK ETU was handicapped by its lack of experience with managing Ebola patients, meager resources, and suboptimal infrastructure. The ELWA hospital ETU had the benefit of Samaritan's Purse having operated an ETU in Foya, Liberia, with assistance from MSF. This ELWA chapel facility was, however, too small to allow the staff to fully exploit their experience. The MHSW and the ELWA team, led by Samaritan's Purse, decided to join forces and jointly run an ETU that would be well staffed, under experienced management, and sufficiently resourced, in a facility that was well designed for care of EVD patients. As had been the case in Foya, MSF's role would again be to support Samaritan's Purse, who would take the lead in managing the new ETU.

In July 2014, this facility, the ELWA 2 ETU, was opened in a former kitchen and laundry facility upon which Samaritan's Purse had done significant reconstruction work to serve for care of Ebola patients. The plan was to move the MHSW staff from the JFK ETU to staff an ETU in the ELWA 2 facility under the guidance of experienced Samaritan's Purse staff. However, shortly after this move was made, two Samaritan's Purse international staff members, Kent Brantly and Nancy Writebol, became ill with EVD and Samaritan's Purse withdrew from Liberia (McKay 2014). (See also Lindis Hurum's contribution in this volume, Vignette 1.) MSF had insufficient staff in country to manage an ETU. This deprived the MHSW staff in ELWA 2 of the assistance of experienced supervision.

Another lurking problem was that ELWA 2 was built within the concrete walls of the former kitchen and laundry facility. Its original 20 beds were increased to 40 by expansion into an adjacent building, but that was the limit of the potential for growth imposed by the wall. This facility also sat on low ground with poor drainage, which made it a bad choice for placement of additional bed capacity. For this reason, it had already been decided even before opening ELWA 2 that

MSF would begin construction of ELWA 3 on open ground higher up within the ELWA compound. Designed to have a 120-bed capacity, the new larger ETU would receive the staff and patients from the existing ELWA 2 when competed. While ELWA 3 was in preparation, the capacity of ELWA 2 was quickly filled, and then over-filled.

ELWA 3, like most of the ETUs set up during the West African Ebola outbreak, was made up of a collection of tents. These allowed the designers to place them in a configuration that optimized the patient and staff flows for infection control and provided adequate spacing to limit cross-contamination due to crowding. Such a treatment unit should be set up quickly, but there were delays caused by community resistance, as the people living and working nearby were not enthusiastic about having an Ebola treatment facility in their neighborhood. Eventually their concerns were addressed and the work was completed. ELWA 3 was scheduled to take on the patients and staff from ELWA 2 in mid-August.

While ELWA 3 was in preparation, ELWA 2 was not doing well. The staff were trying to care for nearly twice as many patients as they had beds for. Because the same overtaxed safe burial system that was failing to pick up the bodies accumulating around Monrovia was responsible for removing the patients who died in ELWA 2, the dead bodies began accumulating there as well. Staff deprived of experienced supervision by the departure of Samaritan's Purse were unable to keep order as stressed and unhappy patients opened back doors to let in friends, family, and more patients. Patients hoping to gain entrance to a facility that had room for no more died waiting outside the gates. When an ELWA 2 staff member was found drowned in one of the unit's septic tanks, the strong suspicion of suicide added to the feeling that ELWA 2 was approaching a breaking point.

At the point when ELWA 3 was nearly operational, it seemed that the solution it offered had been overtaken by events. Following the original plan to move the staff and patients from ELWA 2 to ELWA 3 would have meant filling two thirds of the available beds immediately. The press of new patients also needing beds at that point would have taken up the remaining capacity within a few days. Proceeding as planned would quickly have placed ELWA 3 into the same predicament as ELWA 2. As bad as things were inside ELWA 2, things were no better outside. Patients were dying to get in, literally. They died while waiting outside the closed gates, hoping for a bed to open. They died while seeking shelter under nearby trees. They died waiting in the backs of the abandoned cars that brought them, their drivers having fled. These were only the people with Ebola that the team could see; there were many more elsewhere in the city.

The MSF team made a difficult decision to leave the ELWA 2 patients and staff where they were and to open ELWA 3. ELWA 2 would be closed to new admissions, relieving the staff there of any increase in their patient care burden and allowing them to complete the care for the patients they had until they died or recovered. ELWA 3 would open with just the staff MSF had available at that time. This was not an easy decision. As MSF had planned merely to support the Liberian medical staff, not to run its own ETU, the available medical manpower was meager—one doctor and one nurse, neither with experience in treating Ebola patients. This would place severe limitations on what could be done for the patients who were to be admitted to ELWA 3, and it would not be nearly enough to provide a full package of care for the patients. However, it would at least provide them with a bed and a clean and comfortable environment in lieu of the deplorable conditions in which they currently suffered. As the patient care burden declined in ELWA 2, more MHSW staff could be moved to ELWA 3—or at least that was the plan—and MSF would hire and train its own staff to increase the patient care capacity of ELWA 3. If the MSF team were to care for patients, it needed people right away.

Comprehensive care for EVD patients is labor intensive. It involves presumptively treating for malaria and bacterial infections, in case the patient has these instead of, or along with, EVD. The patient's discomfort from pain, nausea, vomiting, or anxiety should be treated. The patients also need to eat and drink, and they are often so weak that they require assistance for this. EVD patients may also need fluid therapy, either orally or intravenously, to replace what they have lost from their vomiting or diarrhea, as well as to support their circulation, as shock is a frequent feature of the later stages of EVD.

Further complicating the care of EVD patients is the protective gear the healthcare workers caring for them must wear. The fluid-resistant materials that cover the wearer from head to toe do not allow for sweat to evaporate. The user can wear the protective clothing for only 45 minutes to an hour before it needs to be removed to prevent the wearer from overheating. As most staff would dress to enter the part of the ETU where the patients were cared for, the high-risk zone, only two or three times a shift, the amount of patient contact time they had available to them was greatly reduced from what it would otherwise be.

With little in the way of medical staff, and with that staff limited in the time they could spend with their patients, the patients who were admitted to ELWA 3 would have to receive only the most essential care. The first therapeutic interventions to be put aside were the most time- and labor-intensive ones—providing assistance with eating and drinking and providing intravenous fluid therapy. The latter also had the disadvantage of being a hazardous intervention, as needlestick injuries have historically been one of the ways to get Ebola (Edmond et al. 1977; anonymous 2004).

Opening ELWA 3 with so few staff members available would have been foolish if there had not also been a few water and sanitation (watsan) engineers. The watsans are the secret ingredient of ETU management. They create and maintain the safe environment for the healthcare staff to work in and for the patients to receive care in. The sad experience of Ebola over the years has been that when doctors and nurses care for EVD patients in an unsafe environment, more cases result among the healthcare staff themselves. This is of little benefit to the patients. The ETU is a safe place to care for EVD patients, and for patients suspected of having EVD but who turn out not to have it, because of strict infection control that is engineered into the environment and the work practices of those within it. With the support of the watsans, ELWA 3 could be at least be a safe place.

The new plan was challenged almost immediately, as things turned out to be much worse than had been thought. The MSF epidemiologist had been given a copy of the MHSW database containing the list of the suspected Ebola cases the investigation teams encountered. With this, he was able to compare what the investigation teams had found with the information MSF had on the patients coming to the ELWA ETUs. The two lists did not match up as well as they should have, and this was a bad sign.

There is a technique that epidemiologists borrow from ecologists who are trying to estimate the size of an animal population called "capture–recapture." An ecologist first traps a number of animals and marks them in some manner, whereupon they are released back into the environment. Sometime later, a sample of the same animal is trapped again and the proportion of marked animals allows an inference to be made about the size of the total population. For example, someone wanting to know the number of rabbits living on an island sets out some traps and captures 100 rabbits, each of which has its ear tagged and is released. A week later the traps are reset, and 100 rabbits are again captured. Noting that ten rabbits among the second hundred have tags on their ears, it may be estimated that there are about 1,000 rabbits on the island, as it is assumed that the proportion of captured animals bearing tags is the same as the proportion of tagged animals in the total population.

An epidemiologist who has access to two different ways of counting cases of a disease may compare which patients are in both groups to draw conclusions about the total number of cases of disease in the population—the individuals on the second group who were also found in the first being analogous to the tagged rabbits in the example. In Monrovia the two ways of counting Ebola cases were the list from the investigation teams and the list of patients coming to the ELWA ETUs. The first group had 227 patients and the second 99. Only 25 names were the same on both lists. This meant that there had been approximately 876 cases of EVD in Monrovia in the preceding 2.5 months. Thus, we were pretty sure that there had been between 608 and 1,143 cases (Gignoux et al. 2015). For comparison, the largest Ebola outbreak ever prior to the West African outbreak had 425 cases. Thus, the epidemiologist's estimate came as a shock, as up until that point we were under the impression that there had been only a couple hundred cases. The MSF team had just found out that the epidemic in Monrovia was three times larger than they had thought it was. There were some assumptions made in the use of capture–recapture to estimate the true number of cases, but if these assumptions failed to be true, our estimate would be an undercount, not an overcount.

There is a scene in the 1975 movie *Jaws* where Roy Scheider first sees the size of the shark he is hunting, and he tells Robert Shaw, "You're gonna need a bigger boat." We needed a bigger boat. MSF immediately started looking into how far ELWA 3 could be expanded given the space available around it. After much deliberation, scaling up to a 450-bed unit was considered reasonable. "Reasonable" here only meant that the planned additional structures would not be so crowded as to cause problems. Building an ETU 10 times larger than any that had been built prior to the West African outbreak was decidedly ambitious, even intimidating. Preparations for expansion began.

ELWA 3 quietly received its first patients on August 16, 2014. No announcement was made, but 11 patients hoping for admission to ELWA 2 who had been huddling under a tree for protection from the rain were admitted to ELWA 3 and given beds in clean tents out of the rain, food and drink, and some presumptive treatment for other possible illnesses. The official opening of ELWA 3 was announced on Monday, August 18, and by the end of the day there were 30 patients. There was also a collection of trucks, bulldozers, and graters hard at work preparing the space adjacent to ELWA 3 for expansion.

Once word spread that ELWA 3 was open, the ambulances started coming. Often several arrived at once, carrying multiple patients. Patients were sent from all over. Those who came were the sickest sort. Monrovia did not yet have laboratory diagnostic capacity to test all of the people who might have Ebola, so it was mostly those patients who were well into their course of illness, and so sick that they could easily identified as likely cases, who were sent to ELWA 3. Many of these patients died shortly after admission; some even died in transit to ELWA 3. As the patients arrived, the small team manning ELWA 3 evaluated them to be sure that they should be brought inside the unit, and then the patients were, like the others, given a bed, food and drink, and some medicines.

The beds began to fill up, and the staff did what they could: distributing bottles of oral rehydration solution, distributing food, moving suspect patients to the confirmed area when their test results came back positive, bringing pain medications to those in need, putting the patients who had died into body bags and moving them to the morgue. This was no one's idea of how MSF should take care of Ebola patients, but it was what was possible.

A week after it opened, ELWA 3 had admitted 198 patients, of whom 61 had already died, and all of its 120 beds were filled. Fortunately, the team that opened ELWA 3 was no longer alone. MSF had worked in Liberia in the past, and when it was announced that MSF needed staff for its ETU, its former employees quickly returned to work for the organization. MSF's national staff, wherever they work, have ever been the backbone and the true workforce of the organization. These former MSF employees were brought on board and quickly trained in the proper procedures for working in an ETU. Additional MSF international staff began to arrive, among them a doctor and some nurses. The nurses quickly began to organize the delivery of care, and something more like MSF's usual care began to emerge.

The notable exception to this was that the team was not ready yet to provide intravenous fluid therapy. They tried, but it took time to place the intravenous catheters in the patients, to hang the one-liter bags of solution, to replace the catheters that some patients pulled out, to monitor the patients while the fluid ran in, and to replace the empty bag with another when warranted. While doing this, more patients arrived. It soon became clear that continuing to provide such a labor-intensive treatment with the staff that was available would mean leaving patients in need outside with no care at all. Furthermore, ensuring that intravenous fluid therapy was administered safely and properly for the patients who needed it would require a well-controlled environment as well as sufficient patient contact time. Neither sufficient time nor an appropriate environment was available, and the team decided to discontinue intravenous fluid therapy until the situation changed to better help the patients coming to them.

A few days after opening, ELWA 3 gained a valuable partner when the U.S. Centers for Disease Control and Prevention (CDC) and the National Institutes of Health set up a joint field diagnostic laboratory adjacent to the treatment unit. Having this lab next to the treatment unit would be invaluable, as it allowed the ETU staff to reduce the time needed to determine if someone had Ebola from a day or two to just hours. This would allow them to more quickly move the patients they knew had Ebola away from those they were still unsure about, and to send home those patients whom they determined did not have, or no longer had, the Ebola virus. This separation made ELWA 3 a safer place for the patients and freed up beds more quickly than when the patient specimens had to be sent to the national laboratory for testing.

The lab staff were quickly surprised to find that every test they ran came back positive. This provoked concern about the quality of their assays. There was, however, nothing wrong with their test: all one had to do was look at these first patients to know what was wrong. In some ways, Ebola causes a very vague disease that is difficult to differentiate from other common diseases. Patients with EVD have nonspecific symptoms like fever, headache, weakness, and body aches. However, a couple of days into their illness they have a characteristic profound weakness that is almost diagnostic during an outbreak. Most of the patients who were the first arrivals at ELWA 3 were barely able to walk, and many could not even manage that. Looking at the patients arriving at ELWA 3, we did not need polymerase chain reaction tests to know they had Ebola.

It usually takes about two weeks to survive Ebola; it takes much less time to die of it. The bodies of the patients who died in ELWA 3 in the first week had begun to fill the morgue. Monrovia sits on ground not far above the water table, and in most locations throughout the city a freshly dug grave quickly fills up with water. The government, faced with the need to safely dispose of the bodies of those who died of Ebola, had turned to mass cremation. The crematorium, like so many other services tasked by the outbreak, was insufficient to the demands placed upon it. It could cremate 20 bodies a day, and so, to resolve its problem with the accumulation of deceased patients, MSF added to its construction plans an expansion of the crematorium.

In late August, amidst the uncertainty surrounding the mounting challenge of the Ebola outbreak, CDC quietly dropped a bombshell. Though not yet officially published, the CDC's forecast of what was in store for West Africa was discussed discreetly ahead of its scheduled release with those who needed to know. Perhaps this was done because the CDC was aware of the implications of the MSF capture–recapture study. The mathematical model created by CDC epidemiologists, which was an extrapolation of the trends in effect in late August and assumed no significant changes, predicted a possible 21,000 cases in Liberia and Sierra Leone by the end of September and 1.4 million cases by the end of January 2015 (Meltzer et al. 2014).

This had a profound impact on everyone's planning. Whatever staff had been working on before, focus now shifted to preparing for the coming storm. Earlier, in mid-August, CDC had made it quite clear that community care centers and holding centers, places where suspected cases of Ebola might be placed until ETU space was available for them, were a bad idea. A week later, after the results of the predictive model were available, they were endorsing the idea they had previously rejected and pushing for a rapid scale-up to have 1,000 beds available for EVD patients in Monrovia. Representatives from the U.S. Agency for International Development were proposing that the U.S. Defense Department be engaged to construct ETUs throughout the city. Coping with a large number of patients became everyone's priority—or almost everyone's.

Despite the attention on the volume of care that needed to be provided, the quality of that care remained an issue. Much consternation arose from MSF's decision not to give intravenous fluid therapy. For those who saw this as a lifesaving intervention, MSF's decision was viewed as a failure to ensure the well-being of its patients. One group that saw things this way was the Liberian Medical and Dental Council. It complained about MSF's failure to provide intravenous therapy to the national Ebola incident management system and in meetings with WHO. It would not be the last group to make its displeasure known.

The belief that intravenous fluids might save the lives of patients with EVD stems in part from some of the disease's common symptoms: vomiting and diarrhea. There is not often great loss of body fluids due to these gastrointestinal disturbances, though this does occasionally occur, and patients who are able to drink oral rehydration solutions may be able to compensate for these losses. However, even when nausea and vomiting are controlled, Ebola often leaves its victims weak and apathetic, making oral rehydration difficult. In more advanced stages of the disease, it is not clear that there is sufficient blood flow to the gut to allow for good absorption of oral fluids. This is part of the rationale for intravenous fluid therapy.

In the medical literature, there is support for the idea that the immunology and molecular biology of Ebola is similar to that of sepsis (Bray and Mahanty 2003), an overwhelming inflammatory syndrome that usually occurs when the body is experiencing a serious bacterial infection (although it has other causes as well). Intravenous fluids are part of the usual package of interventions for patients with sepsis, although their importance has been diminishing somewhat, as they appear to be less effective than previously thought (Marik and Bellomo 2016).

As intravenous fluids are the mainstay of care of critically ill sepsis patients, and as patients with EVD are often critically ill and often have fluid losses due to gastrointestinal symptoms, the use of intravenous fluids is considered a standard practice for many Ebola patients. The limited clinical experience with Ebola over the years has meant that our treatment protocols are based upon principles and analogy rather than on evidence, however.

The effectiveness of intravenous fluid therapy for patients with EVD is unknown, even though it has been given since MSF began taking care of Ebola patients in 2000. As Ebola was a rare disease, not enough experience had been accumulated, even over such a lengthy period, with which to judge its effectiveness. Intravenous fluid therapy is certainly not dramatically effective, as it can be in patients with cholera or severe dengue fever, as such effectiveness would have been obvious with even a few patients in prior outbreaks. It may have little to no effect, as is the case with severe yellow fever. A very crude measure of the effect of MSF's care for Ebola patients over the years, in which intravenous fluids have usually played a role, would be that the survival rate among those patients who come to the ETU is usually around 5% to 10% higher than that in the outbreak as a whole (Sprecher 2008). However, this comparison assumes that the group of people coming to the ETU is similar to all EVD cases in the community outbreak as a whole. This is probably not a valid assumption, as many milder cases of Ebola in the community are likely missed, especially early in the outbreak. This would underestimate the overall survival rate, and so overestimate the effect of MSF's care.

Opinion on whether or not to provide intravenous fluids has swung like a pendulum over the years. Going into the outbreak in Gulu, Uganda, in 2000, when MSF started providing medical care for EVD patients, intravenous fluid therapy was simply a normal part of care for the severely ill. With the high death toll among healthcare workers during that outbreak, some within the Ebola clinical community began to call for restricting support to oral fluid only to protect staff from life-threatening needlestick injuries. Nevertheless, intravenous fluid has always been a part of MSF's care for Ebola patients (Baert 2001). Over time, as confidence in the ability to safely deliver intravenous therapy grew, this risk aversion waned, and intravenous fluid therapy has taken on a greater role in the care of EVD patients (Sterk 2008; Sprecher 2014b). The publication of a case report of one of the first international staff with EVD evacuated to Europe for care highlighted the significant volume of fluids he lost, peaking at 10 liters per day (Kreuels et al. 2014). Many clinicians during the 2014 epidemic latched onto this anecdote and decided that replacement of lost fluids was the key to saving Ebola patients.

Since they were first written in 2001, MSF's clinical guidelines for Ebola have had intravenous fluid therapy as a part of treatment, assuming the prerequisites were in place: a safe, well-controlled, well-staffed, and well-lit working environment where the basic aspects of care had already been put into place and could be ensured (Baert 2001; Sterk 2008; Sprecher 2014b). This was the norm for MSF. There were exceptions from time to time, however, and the situation in ELWA 3 in August 2014 was one of these.

The balancing act between the demand for care of EVD patients generated by the outbreak and what the ELWA 3 staff was able to provide was dramatically upset less than a month into ELWA 3's operation. One of the MSF international staff, a French nurse, became ill. The fever and headache that appeared on September 15 was confirmed to be Ebola the next day. She was evacuated to a hospital in Paris, where she, like all of the international medical staff who were brought out of West Africa to hospitals in Europe and North America for care of their EVD, received the best that modern medicine had to offer. Ultimately, she survived, but her illness was a severe shock to the MSF team in Monrovia. Hers was the first-ever case of EVD among international staff in MSF's 20-year experience with Ebola. It also meant that there was a gap in the protective measures MSF had in place. Though the source of her infection was never definitively determined, it was believed to be a result of the lack of control in the area where newly arriving patients were brought into the ETU. Many patients congregated there, and while still outside the high-risk zone of the ETU, the staff were not in full protective gear and the environment was not well engineered to control exposure risks. The so-called triage area was then revised to minimize the risks to the staff working there, but the damage had been done.

As the limited size of the staff in the face of a large, growing, and uncertain number of patients was the reason to provide less than MSF's usual package of care, the availability of more staff and the slowing rate of new cases occurring in Monrovia would ordinarily signal the moment to revise the clinical procedures to provide a normal level of care. However, making this decision required an expectation that things would go well and a certain degree of risk tolerance. In the wake of watching their colleague contract Ebola and depart for care in Europe, the team members in ELWA 3 were not ready to take on intravenous fluid therapy.

In December 2014 an open letter from a group of senior MSF medical staff not involved in the response to the Ebola outbreak was circulated throughout the organization (Losson 2015). This letter was a strong criticism of MSF's medical care of Ebola patients, based in no small part upon the visits of a few of the authors to Liberia and ELWA 3. The letter noted that MSF core principles, which include the provision of quality medical care to victims of humanitarian emergencies, had been neglected. The discontent was not limited to the lack of provision of intravenous fluids, but that was the primary example of what was portrayed as a lack of willingness to do all that could be done to save each individual patient.

Needless to say, the circulation of the open letter had a devastating effect on the morale of many in MSF operations. Faced with patients whose need exceeded the means available, the MSF team had sought to provide the best possible assistance. The accusation of "institutionalized non-assistance" hurt many who had made the difficult decision to give compassionate care to as many as they could instead of MSF's usual standard of care to but a few. Although the letter acknowledged that the situation in Monrovia in August and September had been difficult, the authors assumed that the compromises in patient care had been made to pursue a strategy of containment, rather than to maximize the number of patients who could be given some comfort with the limited means available.

By the time the open letter was circulated, the issues that it had raised were already slipping into the past. That month MSF would launch in ELWA 3 its first-ever clinical trial of an experimental therapeutic agent for Ebola, brincidofovir (MSF's lack of engagement with novel therapies was another concern cited in the letter). Not only by then had the use of intravenous fluid therapy been put into place, but the clinicians in ELWA 3 also had access to biochemistry testing—yet another concern in the open letter. By December, however, the epidemic wave had crested and broken. Just as Monrovia had had an explosive growth in the number of cases occurring in August and September, the decline was equally abrupt, and the brincidofovir trial launched in December had to be cancelled, only enrolling ELWA 3's last five EVD patients.

Given all the handwringing, the concerns over the quality of the care provided, and the accusations of disregard for the patients' welfare, did the decision to provide a limited package of care to a larger number of patients, for whatever reason, cause harm? Did more patients die or suffer than would otherwise have been the case? It is very likely that there will never be a definitive answer to this question. We still know too little about the most effective Ebola therapies to know for sure. With the advent of new therapeutic agents for Ebola, it may well be hoped that our care in the next outbreak will be different from what it was, and so this question may not be answered in the future either.

Nevertheless, there is indirect evidence to allow some reasoned speculation. The proportion of patients who survived their stay in ELWA 3 is known. The trend of this proportion over the last five months of 2014 varied from 40% to 65% (Grandesso et al. 2015). These proportions and their variability were not especially different from the other ETUs MSF was operating at this time. In one ETU in Foya, patients also received little in the way of intravenous fluid when the epidemic overmatched the staff of the ETU in much the way it did in Monrovia. Once additional staff arrived, the provision of intravenous fluids resumed. An analysis of survival rates before and after the resumption of intravenous fluid therapy found no significant difference in patient outcomes (Grandesso et al. 2015). None of this proves that no harm was done or that intravenous fluid therapy is without effect; it merely suggests that if there is an effect, it is not a dramatic one. Thus, if harm was done, it was not great harm.

Care is not only about improving patients' chances of survival. Ebola patients suffer. Patients who die in a bed in some comfort inside a treatment unit and those who die alone outside the gates of a treatment unit while hoping to get in are both dead, but in the long run we are all dead. How we die is of some importance. Providing a clean bed, food and drink, relief from discomfort, and a measure of human dignity is of no small value. The ELWA 3 team decided to open before they were ready to relieve the suffering of those they saw dying under the trees, outside the gates, and in the backs of the abandoned taxis that had brought them. This allowed ELWA 2 some breathing room to bring the deplorable situation there under control. Though the planned movement of the staff of ELWA 2 to ELWA 3 never occurred, ELWA 2 recovered and operated independently, safely, and effectively for the rest of the outbreak.

ELWA 3 ultimately never needed to expand beyond 250 beds. It closed at the end of March 2015. Nearly 2,000 patients were admitted there, of whom 1,241 were confirmed to have Ebola. This is more than any other ETU and represents nearly a quarter of all the Ebola patients MSF treated in the West African outbreak (MSF 2015). If the much-hoped-for advancements in Ebola care and prevention that novel therapies and vaccines offer render future outbreaks small and quickly managed, an ETU the likes of ELWA 3 may never be seen again, and the difficult decisions and compromises that had to be made may never need to be repeated.

References

Anonymous. 2004. Russian scientist dies after Ebola lab accident. *Science* 304: 1225b. http://science.sciencemag.org/content/304/5675/1225.2/.

Baert, B. 2001. "Ebola briefing." Médecins Sans Frontières (unpublished MSF guideline).

Brainard, J., L. Hooper, K. Pond, K. Edmunds, and P. R. Hunter. 2016. "Risk factors for transmission of Ebola or Marburg virus disease: A systematic review and meta-analysis." *International Journal of Epidemiology* 45(1): 102–16. doi:10.1093/ije/dyv307. [Epub Nov. 20, 2015]

Bray, M., and S. Mahanty. 2003. "Ebola hemorrhagic fever and septic shock." *Journal of Infectious Diseases* 188(11): 1613–617. [Epub Nov. 14, 2003]

Emond, R. T., B. Evans, E. T. Bowen, and G. Lloyd. 1977. "A case of Ebola virus infection." *British Medical Journal* 2: 541–44.

Gignoux, E., R. Idowu, L. Bawo, et al. 2015. "Use of capture–recapture to estimate underreporting of Ebola virus disease [letter]." *Emerging Infectious Diseases* 21(12): 2265–67. doi:10.3201/eid2112.150756.

Grandesso, F., E. Gignoux, and I. Ciglenecki. 2015. "MSF Epi-Bulletin Ebola Epidemic in West Africa—week 51, 2014." Médecins Sans Frontières, January 8 (unpublished internal MSF report).

Jaws, directed by Steven Spielberg. USA: Universal Pictures, 1975.

Kreuels, B., D. Wichmann, P. Emmerich, et al. "A case of severe Ebola virus infection complicated by gram-negative septicemia." *New England Journal of Medicine* 371(25): 2394–401. doi:10.1056/NEJMoa1411677. [Epub Oct. 22, 2014]

Losson, C. 2015. Rony Brauman: contre Ebola, «le traitement symptomatique a parfois été négligé, voire oublié». *La Liberation*, Feb. 3. http://www.liberation.fr/terre/2015/02/03/parfois-le-traitement-symptomatique-a-ete-neglige-voire-oublie_1194960

Marik, P., and R. Bellomo. 2016. "A rational approach to fluid therapy in sepsis." *British Journal of Anaesthesia* 116(3): 339–49. doi:10.1093/bja/aev349. [Epub Oct. 27, 2015]

McKay, Betsy. 2014. "Peace Corps, aid groups evacuate personnel from Ebola-hit West Africa." *Wall Street Journal*, July 31, 2014. http://www.wsj.com/articles/u-s-missionary-group-plans-partial-evacuation-from-ebola-hit-liberia-1406747747.

Médecins sans Frontières. 2014. Monrovia ELWA Ebola Treatment Center, August 24 (unpublished data).

Médecins sans Frontières. 2015. MSF Internal Ebola Response Update #92, December 3 (unpublished internal MSF report).

Meltzer, M. I., C. Y. Atkins, S. Santibanez, et al. 2014. "Estimating the future number of cases in the Ebola epidemic—Liberia and Sierra Leone, 2014–2015." *Morbidity and Mortality Weekly Report (Suppl.)* 63(3): 1–14.

Nyenswah, T., M. Fahnbulleh, M. Massaquoi, et al. 2014. "Ebola epidemic—Liberia, March–October 2014." *Morbidity and Mortality Weekly Report* 63(46): 1082–86.

Sprecher, A. 2008. *Patient care in filovirus outbreaks.* Presented at the 6th Congress of the International Federation of Shock Societies (IFSS) and the 31st Annual Conference on Shock (U.S. Shock Society). July 28–July 2, Cologne, Germany.

Sprecher, A. 2014a. *Draft filovirus field manual.* Médecins Sans Frontières. https://www.evernote.com/pub/agsprecher/FilovirusFieldManual

Sprecher, A. 2014b. *Montserrado County outbreak control system.* Médecins sans Frontières, July 15 (unpublished MSF field visit report).

Sterk, E. 2008. *Filovirus haemorrhagic fever guideline.* Médecins sans Frontières (unpublished MSF guideline).

Children in the Ebola Treatment Centers

ALLIE TUA LAPPIA AND PATRICIA CARRICK

Ebola was cruelest in the way it attacked so fiercely the most vulnerable and dependent among us—the children. For those of us working in the treatment wards, the epidemic became a litany of profound tragedies played out in small bodies. There were, of course, an overwhelming multitude of challenges in every aspect of the delivery of care, in the practical and diagnostic and ethical decisions we faced from moment to moment, day after day. But one of the greatest difficulties of all was the separation of parents from their children, and the terrible obstacles to comforting the youngest victims as they were torn from their families, placed in the care of health staff in strange plastic suits, separated from the intimate human contact that had been a constant in their life's experience, an unshakable basis of family culture in Sierra Leone.

Ibrahim came to us in the arms of his mother, his older brother Lamin walking at her side. He was a little more than a year old on arrival. We couldn't be sure of his age exactly and his mother did not know. The father had died the preceding week at home, of uncertain causes. We tested all three, mother and two children, and, while they stayed with us awaiting test results, little Ibrahim's bright spirit crept into the hearts of many of our staff. Mother was confirmed positive, but the two boys were both negative. They could not stay with their mother, who, after her positive test, was moved from our "suspect" wards to our "confirmed" wards to be cared for separately from those who only *might* have Ebola. In order to protect the boys from risk, they were taken to a small orphanage that MSF supported, with the hope that they might be returned to their mother if she survived.

The orphanage was also to care for "Ebola orphans"—children who suffered the loss of both parents—until the Ministry of Social Services, stretched thin by the overwhelming losses generated by the epidemic, could make other provisions for placement.

In the treatment center, Ibrahim's mother grew weaker day by day. Two days later both Ibrahim and his brother were brought back to the treatment center because orphanage caregivers feared they were not well. However, they both seemed quite robust and both test results returned negative for the second time. Their mother in the meantime seemed to turn a corner; she began to gain strength. Although she could not be allowed to leave the confirmed area of the treatment center to be with her children, we made her completely aware of the children's readmission and their second negative tests. We could only imagine her relief. For our part, we were thrilled to send these endearing fellows back to the orphanage together for safekeeping, anticipating now their reunion with their recuperating mother once her viral load subsided.

Then Ibrahim was returned to us for the third time. His sweet, cheerful spirit persisted, but we admitted him immediately for testing—again. This time, his Ebola test result returned positive. Now known to be infected, Ibrahim could be transferred to the confirmed ward to be reunited with and cared for by his own, steadily improving mother.

Ibrahim deteriorated over the following three days and died in the treatment center in the care of his mother. She was later discharged cured to join her remaining son, to return to a home empty of husband and second child.

Who knows why Ibrahim died and his brother lived? Ebola was ruthless in attacking those who were the closest, the most dependent. Perhaps he died because he was younger, carried close to the warmth of his mother more often. Perhaps at the onset of his mother's illness he was still breastfeeding. Perhaps, being a smaller child, he just did not have as strong or developed an immune system. In the end, the reason didn't matter: he was gone, and his mother had to live with constant terror for the well-being of her only remaining son and the gift and guilt of her own survival.

One skinny 11-year-old boy proudly announced to us when his father brought him to the Ebola Treatment Center, "I am in Form 5." He held his school book tightly, refusing to relinquish it on entry to the Center, unwilling to give up a moment of his studies. He told his father, "You must take me back home. My exams are coming." His father had attended the funeral of a neighbor. The boy's test was positive, as was his father's. They were placed together in the confirmed ward, side by side, where MSF gave the boy toys to occupy him as his sicker father fought for his life. But the boy spurned the toys, clinging to his school book, bowing over it, trying to study, day after day, even as his father weakened. Every day we Ebola workers would ask him, "How many sentences did you read?" But then he could not read any more because of the sickness. As our Sierra Leonean colleague described it, "After his father died, it happened that he died too."

Issah was a six-year-old whose mother had died at home. Like so many others, he was admitted to the Ebola Treatment Center with his remaining parent, his father, who was very ill. The father tested positive upon admission and was transferred to the confirmed ward, where he gradually succumbed to illness, while Issah initially tested negative and was held in the suspect ward for retesting. He was anxious, eager to know about his father, repeatedly interrogating staff in their "space suits" as they passed through his ward, "Where is my papa? Is my papa alive? Where is he?" On the third day, Issah was retested and found to be positive. He didn't really understand the ramifications of his positive test and was excited, overjoyed to be transferred to the confirmed ward where he was reunited with his father who, despite being desperately depleted, embraced his child quietly. As the days passed, Issah faded relentlessly. His father died beside him. As long as he could walk, Issah could be found stumbling through the confirmed wards, falling, crying. "Papa, papa, are you alive? Where are you?" Even when weakness finally overwhelmed him, he continued to seek rescue for his beloved Papa, hallucinating airplanes coming to carry them both away, until finally he himself was carried away.

We all remember one little boy who drove us completely nuts. He was a vigorous 11- or 12-month-old who was admitted with his mother. She tested positive and had to be moved to the confirmed wards, but his first blood test was negative, so we had to hold him behind in the suspect ward while we awaited completion of his second test. But he could faintly hear his mother's voice in the open-air setting of our tent hospital. He seemed to be able to pick it out from the cacophony of other voices and other sounds—murmurs, cries, moans, laughter, shouts, music from radios, croaking of hundreds of frogs, distant thunder—all the sounds that characterize life in Sierra Leone, whether within or outside the Ebola ward. Between trips into the suspect ward by nursing staff who repeatedly replaced him into his bed and fed and comforted him, every time he was unattended he clambered out of the bed and crawled through the contaminated soup of dirt, gravel, and puddles that were the alleys between our wards, making his way under our precious orange net fence dividers, relentlessly homing in on the sound of his mother's voice. We would find him under the beds, crawling through the shallow drainage ditches that kept us from floating away when the rains came. We would find him on the edge of the low-risk zone, where his presence threatened the staff who were unprotected by the personal protective equipment (PPE) that provided our life-saving barrier to infection when worn in the high-risk zone. We would find him on his way toward the confirmed wards, where his risk of infection was multiplied unbearably. We were all upset by his pure desperation and at a loss as to how to provide for his safety and our own. We appealed to our logisticians, the magicians and life's blood of every MSF mission. They built him a beautiful playpen/crib out of a huge plastic barrel bottom, cut off about two and a half feet high, with our orange plastic netting above to form a see-through barrier from just below his eye level to well above his head. The whole thing was constructed with the durable, unmistakable red-and-white strapping tape that is ever-present wherever MSF is found, the tape that literally holds us together in the field. When we placed him into his playpen, all of us who worked in the high-risk zone heaved a communal sigh of relief. Here we could care for him, keep track of him, contain him between nursing rounds in PPE when we could not be present with him.

It took him less than one shift to clamber between the edges of the barrel and the netting and renew his solitary, endlessly single-minded quest. His second blood test was positive. Given the time frame, his infection was not likely the result of any exposure while he was in our Center, but probably was transmitted from his mother. It was no consolation. Although once we knew he was positive he could then be placed with his mother, within a matter of a few days this little fellow with the dauntless spirit of a warrior was dead.

In any normal hospital setting, pediatric patients are continuously attended. When would any of us have tolerated an unaccompanied infant crawling on the floor of a hospital ward? When would we have allowed a desperate six-year-old to agonize over his father uncomforted? Never before. Not one of us, no matter where we were from. In the developed world, infants and children are cared for by expert nurses, by nurses' aides, by paid attendants if family members are not available. In most hospitals in poor countries, family caregivers are simply admitted with the children. They feed and wash and tend their child patients, they sleep on or under the beds, and they stay until the child is discharged or, in the worst-case scenario, needs care no longer. Bottom line, though: a child is never alone in a hospital in most of the world.

This Ebola epidemic has been an entirely new and unimaginable circumstance. Family members who were Ebola positive were usually too sick at first to care for others, although when families presented together, the effort was always made to keep them together if possible. But family caregivers who were Ebola negative could not be allowed admission to the Ebola ward. The risk of cross-contamination was simply too great. It would almost surely have resulted in the infection, illness, and possibly the death of the caregiver. Our commitment, our medical and ethical duty, was never to risk that additional life. But in the face of the need for full PPE for our own survival, it was also not possible for us, professional caregivers, doctors, nurses, psychologists, and social workers, to accompany patients in the manner we had all been trained by profession and drawn by vocation to expect. We had neither the physical endurance nor the depth of human resources to do it. Our ability to endure the PPE—the "space suits"—was just too limited. One became faint and unable to function after a short time in the sweltering heat of the non-breathing plastic suits that were our protection against deadly infection. The masks became saturated with sweat and "insensible fluid loss"—the moisture of our own exhalations—and lost their protective filtration function, probably in less than an hour.

However it did not matter if you were from the United States or England, Belgium or Brazil, Guinea or Liberia or Sierra Leone: we all knew perfectly well we were supposed to be at the bedsides of our patients, and we were torn, heart and soul, when we could not save or even accompany these smallest among us as they lapsed, one by one, into the stunned silence of illness and isolation and death.

CONTAINMENT

9

Fear and Containment

Contact Follow-up Perceptions and Social Effects in Senegal and Guinea

ALICE DESCLAUX, MOUSTAPHA DIOP, AND STÉPHANE DOYON

Introduction

Fear and Ebola

The history of the social responses to epidemics shows that fear is a common mass reaction, not only accompanying the spread of disease outbreaks but very often occurring in advance of epidemiological events at the local level (Watts 1999). During the 2014-15 Ebola outbreak, fear of this highly lethal virus pervaded other West African countries' populations before cases had been declared outside Guinea. It spread with an increased intensity wherever national and local communities felt at risk for particular reasons (e.g., common borders with highly impacted countries, existing routine travel and migrations from these countries, uncontrolled exchanges by land or sea, common ecology with the same potential virus reservoir). The "epidemic of fear" was even considered worse than the Ebola epidemic itself by some analysts who focused on the magnitude of its economic and social consequences (Ropeik 2014).

In West Africa, fear was also spread by African and global media. This outbreak was treated at national and international levels as the first globalized African epidemic and it became a matter for breaking news, daily case-counting and alarmist coverage, and disruption in the usual prevention-driven institutional public communication about disease and health. Moreover, the first public health messages for community outreach and mobilization used fear as a pedagogic tool for communities as well as health workers, emphasizing the contagiousness and lethality of Ebola virus disease (EVD). Soon, the general population feared not just the Ebola virus but also the healthcare response, accusing health workers of introducing the disease and killing the people who died in Ebola treatment units

(ETUs). They became scapegoats, similar to doctors and other healers in prior episodes of Ebola or other epidemic diseases (Watts 1999; Epelboin 2007). Fear as a mass reaction to Ebola, driven by factors beyond this immediate outbreak, expressed itself in different ways as the result of interactions between communities, the healthcare response, and the political and cultural contexts in various countries. Especially in Guinea, where *réticences* (i.e., resistances[1]) were greater than in other countries, some analysts incriminated the role of the healthcare response in their emergence. Within the biomedical response, contact tracing, an encounter between public health actors and communities that involves a high number of people, could be critical in influencing fear of or trust in the Ebola response.

Contact Tracing and Containment

Contact follow-up includes a daily checkup of symptoms, including body temperature, for people who have been in direct or indirect contact with an EVD patient's body (alive or dead) or bodily fluids. This measure is based on a biosafety rationale: among the people infected by Ebola virus who will develop any symptoms, 95% will fall ill within 21 days after risk exposure and will be contagious when symptoms occur (Haas 2014). According to WHO, *contact tracing* (i.e., contact identification, assessment, and follow-up) prevents the spread of the virus and increases the chances of cure for infected people through their transfer to an ETU for best treatment as soon as symptoms occur (WHO 2014), after more or less strict social distancing and containment measures. During the West African epidemic, the total number of contacts was estimated at about 55,000 for Guinea alone in December 2015 (Migliani 2016b) and might have been more than 215,000 for all of the West African countries involved in the outbreak.

Measures applied to contacts have been named differently across countries and periods—for example, quarantine, surveillance, confinement, and social distancing. These words have inconsistent definitions and connotations according to institutions[2] (e.g., quarantine may cover or exclude aspects such as voluntary adherence or symptoms checking), to languages (e.g., the English word *quarantine* does not have the same connotation of rights infringement as the French word *quarantaine*), to institutional contexts (e.g., the word *surveillance* used by health institutions has a technical meaning related to data collection at the population level, while for the lay population it signifies individual control), and to fields of expertise (e.g., between epidemiologists and social workers). This semantic complexity is representative of the numerous approaches and issues about contact tracing, partly reflecting the multilevel dimensions of the Ebola response. In this chapter we will use the terms *contact* to refer to individuals who have recently been exposed to confirmed Ebola cases, *contact tracing* to refer to the overall intervention including both approaches based on voluntary adherence and on compliance and coercion, and *containment* for contact movement limitation to a defined space with or without separation from other people living in this space; otherwise terms used by the actors themselves are mentioned. When contact tracing relates to practices and using these terms avoids the unwanted connotations mentioned above, this chapter also engages with the concept of quarantine on the academic level and for more general social understandings of confinement in epidemics.

Regarding the biomedical and public health response to the Ebola epidemic, the definition and implementation of prevention and care measures should not have been driven by fear. As with any public health strategy and intervention, these measures were supposed to be carefully selected by WHO based on evidence (current knowledge in virology and biosafety rationale) and to be drafted into recommendations and guidelines, only later adapted to local contexts by national health authorities. However, during the Ebola epidemic, national authorities had considerable latitude to define the operating procedures for contact follow-up, for four main reasons. First, there was no guideline for implementation available from WHO when the epidemic began; the first guideline was published by the Brazzaville office of WHO only in late September 2014 (OMS 2014). U.S. Centers for Disease Control and Prevention guidelines published at the same period (2014) did not give definite recommendations, considering that "the required follow-up may vary depending on the policies of the ministry of health" and that "guidelines such as in-home quarantine of high-risk contact-persons can be used at the country's discretion." Second, the 2014-15 outbreak arose in a situation of lack of knowledge regarding public health prescriptions to be followed during an Ebola crisis, since previous epidemics of hemorrhagic fever had occurred on a smaller scale in different ecological and social situations and had produced limited knowledge that was largely based on pragmatic experience rather than controlled study. Third, the empirical approach to contact tracing followed two models: a model based on contacts' compliance with measures applied on the basis of medical, juridical, or political authority, and a model based on contacts' adherence to voluntary individual engagement driven by the understanding of the biosafety rationale under public health measures. Fourth, repeatedly interventions for contact tracing chosen by public health authorities came into conflict with other measures chosen by governments based on a political approach of public order and security that engaged the overall policy in favor of the "compliance" (rather than adherence) model. This confrontation between authoritarian interventions by government security decision makers and considerations for acceptability supported by health authorities blurred to some extent the rationale driving the methods implemented for contact tracing. This was the case in Liberia, where the violent containment of West Point district in Monrovia by the military short-circuited the health ministry response (Hilderbrand 2014), following political decisions that recalled recent armed conflicts as well as the martial global imagination for responses to epidemics (Benton 2014). In this context, intervention was not precisely defined on technical grounds through global recommendations. Like other social distancing measures such as border and school closures, bans on public gatherings, limited bus transportation, or restrictions on international travel, containment was inspired by the recent experience with the global epidemics of SARS (2003), H1N1 (2009), and MERS (2013), when it was widely used (Rothstein 2015b). In contrast to the EVD diagnosis and treatment protocols that were progressively studied and reinforced after analysis and publication during the Ebola crisis (Wojda et al. 2015), contact tracing, with or without containment, was defined and performed differently according to sites, countries, stakeholders, and contexts.

Recently, some analysts concerned about individual rights infringements under public health measures have raised controversy by suggesting that containment has been applied unnecessarily for Ebola, particularly in the United States (Rothstein 2015a). There, persons who were formerly considered as contacts filed lawsuits against state authorities over quarantine policy (Mataconis 2015; Fink 2016). Other analysts stated that, more generally, quarantine has relied on "coercion, persuasion (of contacts) or an appeal for self-sacrifice" rather than evidence for its efficacy (Calain and Poncin 2015). Concerned with ethical issues and interested in the "complexity of tensions between individual autonomy and the common good," these authors debate the acceptability of containment, a public health measure that may seem archaic in the 21st century, and question the basis for quarantine from a biosafety perspective (Calain and Poncin 2015, p. 126). Do the advantages of containment in terms of biosafety and contacts' need for treatment and isolation supersede its possible adverse effects, particularly at the social level? These interrogations on the rationale for containment in Ebola outbreaks join an ongoing reflection on its use in global transatlantic policies for security and health (Zylberman 2013).

Does Containment Reduce Fear?

As anthropologists and public health workers, we have observed that containment was interpreted in different ways at the field level, resulting in a variety of practices and experiences by the concerned parties. Analyzing first-line actors' perceptions (health workers, contacts, and communities) with a focus on local cultural readings and on the particularities of situations in their micro-social and material contexts may help give substance to debates on the global level.

An assessment of the capacity of contact tracing to prevent or engender fear, depending on confinement modalities (how it is implemented), will contribute to the critical analysis of this public health measure. We will analyze four case studies from Senegal and Guinea, collected at various stages during the outbreak, under different modalities of contact follow-up, to understand contacts' perceptions of fear and their experience of follow-up and the social consequences of containment. The settings of these case studies (two at the geographic fringes of the epidemic, two near the epicenter) do not result from a reasoned choice but depended on the ability to pursue anthropological inquiries with contacts during the outbreak. Showing varied settings and contact-tracing methods, they illustrate the range of social arrangements covered by this public health measure. Without developing an in-depth phenomenology, the analysis considers fear in a broad sense of the term, including expressions of anxiety or worry and actions dictated by fear such as escaping or hiding. Using an ethnographic perspective, we do not adopt a normative approach or interpret fear *a priori* as a negative or positive experience (Jeudy-Ballini and Voisenat 2004).

This chapter is based on ethnographic studies conducted in three research projects. In Senegal, data were collected within the EBSEN program ("Ebola outbreak and the social construction of trust in Senegal").[3] In Guinea, data were collected within two research contexts. The first case was observed within the POSTEBOGUI program ("Living again after EVD in Guinea: Clinical, immuno-virological, psychological and socio-anthropological consequence").[4] The second case was observed during a five-week field action-research intervention of a team of anthropologists.[5]

Case Studies in Senegal and Guinea

Case Study 1 (Dakar, Senegal): Patient Zero's Family Confined in the Family House

On August 29, 2014, an Ebola case was diagnosed for the first time in Senegal in a young Guinean (pseudonym Alpha) who arrived 10 days earlier in Dakar to visit his uncle in a working-class neighborhood of the capital. Before his Ebola diagnosis, he had sought care in two health facilities where, in the absence of hemorrhagic symptoms, he was treated at first for malaria or bacterial infection. After diagnosis, 74 people were then identified as "contacts": 34 members from the family of his uncle and their co-residents and 40 health agents from the two health facilities. After considering the use of police services to implement contact tracing, health authorities from the inter-ministerial committee in charge of response to epidemics, advised by WHO and MSF experts, opted for so-called voluntary home containment in the absence of guidelines or official procedures.

On August 30, a health team informed the "family members" that they must stay at home during 21 days; 11 of these "family members" were actually young men from Guinea who rented a room in the family compound. After disinfection of the compound by a team from hygiene services, the contacts were to be visited twice a day by the follow-up team made up of Senegalese Red Cross volunteers, under the supervision of the district medical team. The family house is composed of six rooms open on an internal courtyard with toilets and a water tap. One of the rooms is used as a shop, with its window open toward the street, where Alpha's uncle sells food and basic goods as his main income-generating activity. During containment, the residents were told that the shop should be closed and they should not leave the house, nor should people visit them.

Soon, the media broadcasted information about Alpha's stay in this street and a TV channel showed the house surrounded by people wearing personal protective equipment (PPE). In addition to criticism of Guineans by the media (particularly on the Internet and social networks), hostile demonstrations occurred in the neighborhood, and a police car was parked next to the compound; it would stay there until the end of the containment period. Some residents of the compound considered that the police were there to protect them from hostile passersby, but others believed that the police were present to prevent them from leaving the compound. During the first two days, inhabitants organized themselves to stay at home, something which the majority of them were unable to do immediately because they needed to get resources from outside of the compound for their daily food. Food support was set up so that collective containment would be effective, and the Ministry of Health with WHO soon considered providing stipends for the family house. Red Cross volunteers started their visits on the second day of containment and brought staple food and complementary goods that would be progressively adapted in quantity and quality according to the contacts' demands.

At first, relationships between volunteers and contacts were difficult because both sides were afraid of contagion. The house residents feared that they might have been contaminated when Alpha lived among them. Particularly the family members who helped him with cleaning, food, and transportation, such as his male cousin, his uncle, and his female cousin, shared this concern. Other residents in the compound also feared getting the virus through proximity with Alpha's relatives who had bodily contacts with him, or with the co-residents who shared his room, and they tried to keep some distance from them in the limited space of the compound. Volunteers feared that they might be contaminated when visiting the house; the rapid training they received had emphasized the seriousness of EVD and the contagiousness of the virus, illustrated mainly through PPE and ETUs, and conveyed alarmist messages. They were also taught that biosafety precautions with a contact subject should be the same as with a suspect or a confirmed case: volunteers should not only avoid any bodily contact with the people they visited, but should also keep a two-meter security distance, wear plastic gloves if they touched anything during the visit, never accept any food or drink, and avoid touching objects or sitting down in the compound. Volunteers were also anxious because their trainers did not seem to agree with each other on biosafety precautions, and several volunteers thought that doctors sent them to the frontline because they were too worried to do home visits themselves.

During the first three to four days, the situation was tense because the members of the confined unit felt stigmatized by this distance imposed by the volunteer visitors; contacts interpreted this behavior as a sign that they were infected and as a lack of respect to them. Progressively, volunteers found strategies to counteract these interpretations and gradually were able to get contacts to understand that they were compelled to comply with these biosafety constraints. Relationships improved as fear decreased on both sides: volunteers became better informed on the risks of infection through interactions with the medical team and were reassured by a medical authority who shook hands with a contact person without special precautions. Contacts appreciated when volunteers explained their actions and came to realize that these distancing behaviors were not due to moral judgments or social rejection. Volunteers also found practical ways to keep their distance without looking disrespectful or rude, and they were empathetic toward contacts when asking about their symptoms, giving health advice, answering their questions, and reassuring them. Increasingly, the twice-daily interactions resembled friendly visits, and contacts' anxieties and tension had largely disappeared by the time Alpha was recovering in the infectious disease ward of the main university hospital in Dakar (Bousso et al. 2015).

A small incident reveals the logics that drove containment, beyond the biosafety rationale. During the first week of confinement, a recently married cousin of Alpha who lived on a nearby street with her husband continued visiting her mother in the compound every day. When some neighbors saw her leaving the family house, they mistook her for a contact subject and complained to the police that a member of the family was escaping every night. The police and medical team subsequently confronted her, asking her to either stay in or out of the house, since she was not identified as a contact by the medical team. Since she preferred being with her family, she chose to be considered as a contact and confined to the compound. In this case the police and public health team favored a logic of convenience for contacts and community harmony over a strictly biomedical rationale.

As days passed, the family co-residents, among whom some had not even met Alpha, became increasingly worried about the loss of resources, especially the individuals who had continuing professional expenses. Moreover, several among them would not get their jobs back at the end of the containment period, because their employer wrongly feared contagion. The head of the family, Alpha's uncle, received funding assistance several times from the Ministry of Health, but he divided it inequitably, giving a larger share to his relatives. The cohesion of the community composed of the family and its co-residents became endangered, and power disputes arose, marked by unequal gender and age relationships. The end of the containment period found the community divided, as some of its members felt abusively detained, despoiled, or neglected by public health measures that had been applied indiscriminately.

Case Study 2 (Dakar, Senegal): Health Professionals Confined with Their Families

As soon as Alpha's Ebola diagnosis was announced, health authorities called the agents working in the two health services where he was treated: 20 people were identified in the health post nearby Alpha's family house and 20 more in the hospital service, where no particular precautions were taken at first because Alpha did not show the symptoms specific to hemorrhagic fevers. The health post was then closed and disinfected and all the staff were identified as contacts, including nonmedical employees such as security staff.

In the hospital, employees were asked to do a self-evaluation of their risk exposure; it was to be later completed and checked by epidemiologists. The proposed confinement methods would give them more autonomy than for Alpha's family: these contacts were confined at home and were asked to monitor their body temperatures. They would inform volunteers of their health status, according to modalities they would define together. This contact-tracing arrangement was applied immediately. For these health agents, no additional financial support was planned because they were to continue receiving a salary in spite of the suspension of their professional activity for three weeks. Health authorities were particularly concerned about the young doctors who were in contact with Alpha: these doctors felt that their level of risk was low or nonexistent, that they had applied strategies to protect themselves from this patient, and thus that they did not require confinement measures similar to all contacts whatever their exposure. Moreover, contacts who were medical doctors questioned the Red Cross volunteers' legitimacy to check their symptoms. For other hospital employees who did not have access to trainings about Ebola, the announcement of home containment caused panic. During confinement, many of them spoke about their anxiety and complained of insomnia. Everyone remembered the acts that might have transmitted the virus, as the Ebola patient was perfused and cleaned, and samples were taken from him because of his atypical and persistent pathology. Employees expressed their fear on three levels: (1) the fear of being already contaminated led them to self-monitor continuously, interpreting each bodily sign as a first symptom for EVD; (2) since they were not informed that the virus cannot be transmitted before symptom appearance, they were afraid of transmitting the virus, particularly to their children, and isolated themselves; and (3) they feared their relatives' reactions to the exposure to infectious risk.

This fear was even more difficult to live with as many health workers were forced to hide it, since they had not explained their exposure situation to their relatives. Their main reasons for this secrecy were to avoid the stigmatization associated with Ebola and to spare their relatives anxiety. Contacts' obligation to stay home drew questions from family members about their professional status, especially for women, who represented more than two thirds of the confined hospital contacts. These questions sometimes turned into arguments about the woman's decision to work outside, when her activity could "bring the virus back home." Thus, disclosing (or not disclosing) one's exposure to Ebola was a dilemma, and most of these contacts informed their relatives on a selective basis. This created circles of people who did and didn't know, and consequently they feared that a person who was not informed directly could be informed later indirectly, exacerbating preexisting tensions that were already common in polygamous and/or multigenerational households.

Contact identification also reveals the precarious status of health staff working on the frontline with patients. Among the 19 contacts for whom professional status was reported, only four were public officers, one was a contractual agent, eight were volunteer community health workers, five were trainees, and one was an intern. Thus, 14 already had an uncertain employment status, as their earnings were neither high nor guaranteed. While the Senegalese health system relies increasingly on community workers, the labor market leads more and more young graduates to work as volunteers for several years as a way of getting a coveted position in public services. Because the majority of identified contacts were living in insecure conditions, their limited resources did not permit them to lose paid work for long periods. Financial support was given to them by the Ministry of Health during their confinement, but the amount was less than the minimum wage. The Ebola outbreak revealed their uncertain and vulnerable situation along with the risks they faced in their work.

Case Study 3 (Conakry, Guinea): Confinement in a Urban Neighborhood

In Conakry, Coulara (a pseudonym) district was hit belatedly, in July 2015, when the epidemic curve at the national level was slowly decreasing and the number of new cases was declining after the November 2014–January 2015 peak. Actually, the epidemic in Guinea spread first in the forest zone in East Guinea from the village of Meliandou, reaching the coastal zone and the capital, Conakry, in a second phase beginning in September 2014 (Migliani 2016a). Coulara district, inhabited mainly by Peulh and Malinké traders and craftsmen with a very modest socioeconomic level, was hit when a sick pregnant woman visited her sister's home to request help for her delivery. Her sister's husband, a craftsman called Amadou (a pseudonym), helped her and accompanied her to the hospital, where the woman had a cesarean section but subsequently died, along with her baby. Ebola was diagnosed and contact tracing with containment was imposed on Amadou and his 10 cohabitants.

Ten days later, Amadou, who had avoided any physical contact with his family members, particularly his six children, started feeling fever and then an unbearable fatigue. After calling an acquaintance working in an ETU, he decided to go there without informing his relatives, worried that they would forbid him to go. At that time, the local population reacted in nearly all declared cases of Ebola by opposing health agents. A mapping of resistances reveals that this kind of reaction occurred in all districts hit by Ebola in Conakry. Rumors mentioned patients disappearing from ETUs, where they were being killed in order to sell their organs. A survivor who lived in another district and was hospitalized in an ETU in Conakry in September 2014, interviewed as part of the same research project, reported that when he returned to his neighborhood, he was accused of faking EVD and receiving money from MSF to say that he was ill and then cured of Ebola.

When Amadou was hospitalized, health authorities came to his district to extend contact tracing and confinement to all his contacts—that is, the people in 28 surrounding households: his nuclear family (his spouse and their six children), 21 households (147 people) living in the "concession" (a colonial term that refers to a compound belonging to an extended family), five neighboring households, and two households settled beside his workshop. The concession encompasses the living rooms and bedrooms of every household from its founder's extended family, and rented rooms occupied by Liberian refugees, among others, around common taps and toilets, and corridors that go through the concession. Overall, around 150 people live on about 100 square meters. One household only in the concession was not included among the contacts, since its members said they did not know Amadou and had not met him or his sister-in-law.

Because this occurred 15 months after the beginning of the epidemic, health authorities had had time to adjust their protocol in order to make confinement more acceptable for communities. Numerous actors arrived in the area to identify contact subjects (about 30 people from WHO), disinfect houses (communal hygiene services), set up follow-up (Red Cross volunteers), organize food distribution (World Food Program agents), and register the health status of contacts (agents from communal health services). Contacts were required to stay in the concession during 21 days, and people accustomed to frequent visiting had to suspend their visits. From the beginning of the containment period, health teams were a nearly permanently presence in the concession. Volunteers met contacts to check their health, symptoms, and temperature three times a day (6 a.m., noon, and 4 p.m.); between two of the checkups, they waited in their vehicles at the entrance to the concession. When epidemiologists left, agents called MOSO (*Mobilisateurs Sociaux* [Social Mobilizers]) would meet every household to educate them about various subjects in hygiene and prevention, including the WHO vaccine trial. All households received food, a limited amount of money for cooking expenses, and a hygiene kit (handwashing basin, soap, bleach, and individual sprayer).

At first, the precautions taken by WHO or Red Cross volunteers were surprising for the residents: they brought their own chairs to sit down in households. Many residents made negative comments and some threatened to resist the visits. However, the time spent by health actors talking to residents and the exchanges with volunteers when checking temperature and symptoms improved relationships. The president of the local youth organization recalls that when confinement ended, the health agents shared food with contacts, which showed that their relationships followed the West African norms of hospitality, volunteers being there as both invited guests by their hosts and as public health agents. Contact families were able to obtain information on EVD from MOSO, who were open to their questions and available to households for private discussions. Confined contacts welcomed Amadou when he left the ETU, showing solidarity. They did not criticize him for being the cause of a confinement that most of them experienced without too much hardship, owing to secondary support measures, and they did not show any fear of contagion toward him when he returned. Moreover, these families seem to have globally accepted confinement, especially as there were no secondary cases. Containment might have been so easily accepted because the concession was not physically isolated and its inhabitants could go on living as usual in their community, watching TV to pass the time. Because of their favorable perception of Ebola response teams, a high number of contacts volunteered to participate in the WHO vaccine trial, joined by other people from the neighborhood who were considered as potential "contacts' contacts" in the trial protocol.

However, interventions did not totally prevent negative attitudes toward confined contacts from neighbors or people from other areas, according to the president of a local youth organization. During the confinement period, neighbors were unfriendly when contacts wanted to buy goods in the local shops, and they asked contacts to make sure that their infants would not play with other children in the concession. Several contacts regretted that neighbors did not show empathy and solidarity as they would do in other cases of misfortune. On the other side, contacts' neighbors regretted that they did not receive assistance from health teams and were not provided as much information as Amadou's family.

The most striking difficulty was endured after the period of containment by craftsmen and merchants. Their clients did not return when confinement ended, either because they were afraid of Ebola or because they had taken their business to other providers who had not been constrained by confinement. Amadou was in this situation: seven months after he left the ETU he had not recovered any activity, and his family was totally dependent for their daily living on the material support provided by the World Food Program. Moreover, Amadou suffered losses due to disinfection: the television and a rice bag he kept in his workplace were destroyed by sprayings, and when he left the ETU, health agents soaked his cellphone in bleach, which destroyed it. Amadou was also affected by the social distance imposed by confinement. His trainees, who usually slept in his workplace, abandoned it when he was at the hospital, and his goods were stolen due to lack of surveillance. The only survivor in the neighborhood, Amadou suffered the greatest damage, particularly because the health system could not compensate him for the negative economic effects of the disease arising from stigma and follow-up health issues.

Case Study 4 (Kaliya, Guinea): *Cerclages* and *Ratissage* in a Rural District

The unexpected reemergence of EVD in October and November 2015 in the prefecture of Forécariah just as the epidemic seemed under control at the national level cast in doubt all the achievements of the local Ebola response platform. Two new EVD cases that were registered in Tana Marché, then Kindoya village, were shocking and engendered a vigorous reaction from authorities and partners, who decided to implement an exceptional surveillance and prevention apparatus. This apparatus included *cordon sanitaire* (consisting of checkpoints with vehicle control and passenger body temperature checkup, handwashing, inquiry, and eventually registration), *micro-cerclage* (defined as the ring containment of a small community with 21-day follow-up by daily visits) reinforced by *cantonnement* (defined as the encampment of all response teams and follow-up agents in the area beside the community during the 21-day period), and *ratissage* (defined as a sweep intervention based on door-to-door visits to locate contacts and provide information to every household).

Cordon sanitaire and *ratissage* were interventions adapted to a rural area with a particular geographic and economic situation that complemented the tracing strategies applied toward contacts. At the prefecture level, a *cordon sanitaire* was set at every entry point to the Forécariah area, performed by the police and the military. Anyone diagnosed with fever was isolated and referred for EVD biological testing, and co-travelers could be considered as possible contacts, depending on the individual situation. *Ratissage* was used for remote habitations, in a way adapted to the geographic configuration of Kaliya. The coastal Forécariah area, also called Moriya country[6] up to the border with Sierra Leone, contains rivers and sea inlets. This zone is occupied mainly by Soussou and Malinké populations and was historically dominated by human trafficking of "ebony wood" for the slave trade. Due to this land configuration of narrow ravines and impregnable hideaways, this is an area where people and weapons have long circulated and may still be circulating through hidden pathways; any surveillance is very difficult. Near the border with Sierra Leone, officially closed due to Ebola since August 2014, this area is not welcoming to visits by strangers, who might witness and disturb informal trafficking. Hence, visits from Ebola response teams here would be quite dangerous. Exacerbated by the socioeconomic effects of the Ebola outbreak at the frontier, the main problem faced by local populations, who live on fishing, survival farming, and trading, is poverty. The communities around Kindoya, as in other remote areas in coastal Guinea (or Maritime Guinea), consider themselves abandoned by the state; they lack quality public infrastructures such as schools and equipped health posts and have neither teachers nor health workers. The literacy rate is low and most children do not go to school. In this area, poverty has made the population distrustful about any government promises and any institutions representing the authorities.

A few weeks before, in September 2015, the Village Surveillance Committees in the Kaliya area, in charge of surveillance and alert for suspect cases, which formerly had received a stipend for this activity, had strongly reduced their engagement since the interruption of their remuneration and had stopped alerting authorities about suspect cases. EVD cases reappeared in Kaliya in this context of social demobilization. In addition, many traditional healers continued treating patients despite recommendations not to do so. EVD reached Tana Market through an Islamic healer who treated his infected sister-in-law, and later died, leaving his family in distress and the whole village under surveillance. Later, a second Ebola case was diagnosed in a young woman among this healer's contacts, and a new *cerclage* was implemented. *Cerclage* for the whole village of Kitérin and *micro-cerclage* for the healer's family in Tana Market (from October 3 to 18, 2015) and then for the woman's family in Kindoya (from October 14 to November 16) relaunched social mobilization and extended surveillance beyond *micro-cerclage* areas. *Cerclage* encompassed 53 contact subjects, including 23 high-risk contacts, a distinction recently introduced in contact assessment in 2015. These people were not allowed to leave their family home for 21 days, and visits by outsiders were suspended. A specific mark on the door signaled to visitors that they were not allowed to visit a household. Support including food (rice, fish) and kits (e.g., radios, lamps, mosquito nets) was provided to confined contacts to compensate for lost income.

Included for the first time in Guinea in the response measures in the Kaliya subprefecture, surveillance teams were encamped near *micro-cerclage* areas so they could be more efficient in controlling populations and could continue sensitization and social mobilization to favor acceptance of contact tracing. The camp was placed in Tana Market near the *cerclage* area of Kindoya. The response teams were each composed of an epidemiologist, a surveillance agent, a social mobilizer, and a socio-anthropologist. Within the teams, socio-anthropologists collected information on various kinds of resistances so they could understand barriers to community involvement and social mobilization. They also had to report information regarding missing contacts, dubbed fleeing contacts, and had to ensure the follow-up of high-risk contacts. The ethics of the socio-anthropologists' intervention, based on intense observation of the response teams and their relationships with local communities, emphasized respect toward community norms, listening to them, doing mediation between teams and communities, and performing negotiation and direct communication with affected communities. The teams worked every day from 6 to 9 a.m. and then 5 to 7 p.m., doing mainly contact follow-up, distribution of food and kits, door-to-door sensitization, and educational group talks with contacts and with the population. The tasks of follow-up and search for fleeing contacts were particularly difficult due to partly preexisting and partly induced community resistances.

On October 24, in order to find all dwellers either unaware of the event or fearing contact tracing, a new intervention was launched, called *active reinforced contact research*. *Ratissage* was conducted around remote zones, targeting populations who were suspected of hiding out inland or on nearby islands, in the expectation of finding sick people and high-risk contacts around the last active point in Kindoya. The existing teams were strengthened by community leaders, including the Kaliya mayor and prefect. At some point, teams and institutional representatives were more numerous than inhabitants of the targeted villages. Among the contacts under surveillance were traditional healers, corpse washers, EVD survivors, and health workers. Teams also performed community sensitization about individual and collective protective measures. This intervention involved 39 hamlets or villages around Kindoya zone under *cerclage* and within 5 km, including Kindoya, Sokhomakéléya, Sabouya, Saraboly, Tana village, Kalimodignabé, Dalonyah, Gbokoya, Kalakouré, Bendougou, and Gbéréka. These villages and hamlets were mapped using a geolocation system.

Ratissage beyond *micro-cerclage* areas engendered various kinds of resistances. People were absent from their villages when the health teams arrived, and many presumed contacts deliberately denied their relationship with the families of the EVD victims. Then contacts outside *cerclages*, who were visited twice a day for checkups without confinement because they lived in remote places and were low-risk contacts, wanted to receive the same support treatments as contacts who were under containment, even though, unlike those confined contacts, their ability to make a living had not been suspended. The villages where *ratissage* was performed threatened to refuse collaboration if they did not receive food support. Besides this clearly formulated threat, villagers also resisted with orchestrated lies, offering "red herrings" to social mobilizers, purposely providing false identities to hinder contact identification, failing to show up, and obfuscating the identity of leaders or elders while presenting in their place young people unable to engage the whole community. These attitudes, dictated by the fear of the stigma related to Ebola in a context of distrust in any state agent favorable to suspecting them of introducing the disease, changed after social outreach and mediation. The communities in these resistance areas later understood the cause of the outbreak, the intent and role of teams, and the purpose of contact tracing for EVD care, and then complied with Ebola surveillance. They also accepted that the sick should not be treated by traditional practitioners or at home, and agreed to declare every death that occurred outside of health facilities. These changes in attitudes were the result of social mobilization and may also have been related to the news from Tana Market and Kindoya where, after contacts ended their surveillance period without any new EVD case, friendly celebrations were organized with football games sponsored by the Ebola response teams. This experience was very different from their usual relationships with state agents, who seldom come to these villages, spend time there, or socialize with the local population.

Lastly, one individual lost to follow-up, Maimouna (a pseudonym), was the focus of all the teams' efforts. Maimouna was a former MOSO and a very good friend of the last EVD case. She was considered a high-risk contact subject and had escaped from Gbéréka village. Considerable pressure was placed on local teams, manifested by the presence of a large number of four-wheeled vehicles and agency or institutional representatives at the encampment, since this contact, called *la dame de Gbéréka*, was the last contact to follow up in order to declare the end of the epidemic in Guinea. The villagers were threatened and the local authorities were fired for letting the contact escape. Though several teams were trying to find her, Maimouna had still not been found by Ebola response teams in late November 2015. In a tragic move, and a context that drove extreme social pressure on her, she had transformed from a contact to be monitored and offered follow-up care to a fugitive escaping the Ebola response apparatus.

The last challenge for Ebola response teams was to convince hostile populations and escaped contacts in Kaliya that contact tracing and other public health measures should not be feared and were designed *for* them, rather than *against* them. This idea was contradictory to the local populations' history of exploitation and deception by the authorities, along with the absence of state-sponsored public services oriented toward equity (Fribault 2015). The anthropologists' team insisted on the need to set up basic public services in this area, where surveillance is particularly difficult and services are absent. A key intervention in that regard was the installation of a water-drilling rig in Kindoya, a village without any access to water, that was performed two days before the end of contacts' follow-up. In Kaliya, the implementation of contact tracing through a unique intervention strategy like in Coulara was not enough to challenge local issues related to the geographic repartition of domestic units and the population's distrust toward health teams. Besides, the local housing configuration in remote areas challenged the utility and interpretation of containment. These socio-geo-demographic conditions required complementary measures specific to EVD and of basic public services to complete the management of contacts. However, at last, the social pressure from national and international authorities for tracing the last contact subjects reached such a level that it provoked disruption in the social mobilization efforts and attempts to create bonds between communities and health teams.

Contacts' Fear: Topics and Dynamics

As well as contact-tracing practices, contacts' experiences have been poorly documented. These four case studies show that follow-up and containment were applied in different ways according to context, with differences in accompanying measures and social effects. Fear of EVD was intense among contacts in all contexts, but it was shaped differently according to contacts' individual concerns and contexts.

Specific Fears

Beyond the general fear spread in the population, the fear experienced by contacts was specifically attached to six main possibilities: (1) being already infected by the Ebola virus; (2) getting infected by other contacts; (3) transmitting Ebola virus; (4) being referred to an ETU; (5) being blamed for risk exposure; and (6) being stigmatized as an EVD contact.

In terms of the fear of being already infected, in the Senegalese case studies, follow-up interventions set up after contact identification started without providing information or "education" on Ebola to confined contacts. Thus, most contacts were very vulnerable to the fear of being already infected, since their knowledge about EVD derived from the alarmist public health messages spread by national sensitization campaigns or from sensationalistic outbreak reporting by the media and Internet that conveyed the idea of the high contagiousness of Ebola virus. In Guinea, where case studies 3 and 4 were collected one year later, interventions included social mobilizers who quickly after their identification gave contacts information about transmission modes and risks and about the possibility of recovery from EVD, which helped to reduce this particular fear. In Senegal contacts were scared when a fellow contact was declared suspect and the information was disseminated, but this was resolved a few hours later when the lab result was announced negative.

Second, contacts' fear of getting infected or transmitting Ebola virus during confinement was determined by the containment methods, as shown by the Senegalese case studies 1 and 2. On one hand, where contacts were contained together whatever the level of their risk exposure, they all feared getting infected by high-risk contacts, either those identified by epidemiologists or those perceived to be so. On the other hand, among health agent contacts who remained at home with their families, the fear of infecting their family members was acute. These observations underline the need to rapidly provide full information on transmission risk to contacts, conceptualized in a well-defined manner, including key notions such as the absence of virus transmission during the asymptomatic phase of the disease.

Contacts' fear of treatment in ETUs was highly differentiated between the two case countries: unlike those in Senegal, the contacts in Guinea considered treatment more dangerous than the disease itself. This fear, described at first encounters with follow-up agents and diminished after their interaction with response teams or treatment experience, derives from lay perceptions. In Conakry, a study done in early 2015 with 200 laypeople covering all municipalities showed that they generally agreed with the statement "Treating Ebola patients in hospital does not improve their chance of survival" with a mean score of 6.45 (on a 0-to-10 scale) and the statement "The purpose of quarantine measures is to hasten the death of Ebola patients" with a 6.24 mean score (Kpanake et al. 2016). Similar preconceived ideas and very low levels of comprehension about EVD were also found in other regions of Guinea (Buli et al. 2015) and in resistance areas (Anonymous 2015). In Senegal, while the absence of studies in the general population hinders comparisons, the contact subjects interviewed maintained trust in the Ebola response and in health services, even before the only Ebola case was cured. This divergence reflects the very different scales of the outbreak in the two countries, a very consistent communication strategy by the Senegalese Ministry of Health, and the contrast in relationships between these countries' populations and their unequally efficient health systems.[7] On another level, broader fear is also produced by a history of violence and neglect from the state and previous holders of power experienced by the Guinean population for several centuries; this favors an imaginary of the epidemic as a new political violence (Fribault 2015).

Regarding the fear of being blamed for risk exposure, in case study 2 health agents in Senegal did not fear that being identified as contacts would expose them to recriminations from their management for any failure to apply basic precautions in their work. Rather, they mentioned their worry that in case of Ebola infection, they might be left alone without support from the health system, since most of them already had an insecure employment status. Their fear highlights the status of trainees and volunteers employed as community health workers in Senegal and Guinea. Under various employment statuses, very often without any formal contract, these frontline agents do not have insurance or a protective regulation in case of a disease contracted at the worksite. Health agents' fear was also focused on reactions from their families, where there was the threat of blame or self-recrimination for introducing the Ebola risk in the home. In many households, this situation engendered questions about health agents' personal autonomy regarding their choice of professional activity, a very sensitive issue for women. Fear was also driven by economic, professional, and gender vulnerability among the contacts.

The fear of stigma related to being an EVD contact was a complex issue, depending on individual situations and contexts. In case study 1, since the Guinean family had been "outed" in the media as bringing Ebola to Senegal, health authorities set up a strategy for avoiding further stigma toward them and toward Guineans more generally. Besides transparency in information and messages against stigma spread by the media, measures were taken at the family level, based on the presence of police near the family house as a dissuasive force. With the health agent contacts in case study 2, follow-up volunteers engaged in adapting their approach to individual situations to keep confidentiality about their contact status (Desclaux and Sow 2015). Keeping contacts' status confidential was not possible in Guinea, where the number of people contained together was much higher, and where the follow-up interventions involved many stakeholders. There, case study 3 shows that the social mobilizers developed specific strategies to prevent stigmatization, such as interventions that targeted neighbors of contact households. In addition, in Guinea public celebrations to mark the end of containment periods and the provision of individual certificates to contacts may have helped prevent the exclusion from employment that some contacts in Senegal experienced. However, it did not prevent the stigmatization of Amadou, the Ebola survivor whose situation is described in case study 3.

Dynamics of Fear

The case studies in Senegal also show that fear could be either enhanced or reduced through interactions between contacts and health agents. During the first days of follow-up, contacts' fear was exacerbated by the fear expressed by volunteers. Sharing at first lay understandings of EVD, volunteers had received only a rapid training focused on the high-risk situations of the Ebola outbreak that emphasized the alleged high transmissibility and lethality of Ebola virus, and enhanced the fear they already felt. Created in an emergency situation in the absence of guidelines and not tailored to their specific role, this training did not give them confidence in their role in controlling transmission or in the knowledge that they were properly protected from contagion. Fear was also used as a pedagogical tool by some trainers in a belief that overstating risk would influence volunteers to comply with biosafety recommendations, a belief that was ultimately counterproductive. In a broader sense, the ambivalent use of fear in health information messages about EVD, either purposeful or incidental, should be questioned. Although it is difficult to define messages based on scientific knowledge that is still being worked out, accurate communication is essential to building trust; moreover, the EVD outbreak has illustrated that correcting misinformation is difficult (Chandler et al. 2015).

At first, contacts considered that the strict observance of biosafety recommendations by follow-up agents was disrespectful, suggesting their contamination or a sign of stigmatization. Case study 1 in Senegal shows that fear of the virus was a component of social relationships that subverted interactions toward distrust and conflict, but fear and its effects could also be overcome. The relief from the fear of contamination on follow-up agents' side, along with the provision of information to contacts, agents' caring attitudes, time spent together, and some familiarization to risk on both sides, was necessary to build friendly relationships. In Guinea, case study 3 shows that in a social context characterized by lay resistance and hostility toward Ebola responders, contacts' exchanges with WHO agents—made possible by the availability of 30 people staying permanently near the compound—defused harsh misconceptions among the population. Case study 4 shows that in late 2015, successful follow-up could be achieved, even in a context of hostility, with increased human resources, a better comprehension of social stakes through listening to populations, increased respect toward community values, and better focus on social mobilization. However, when social bonds were not established or were suspended, fear led contacts to flee, as shown in case study 4.

The variety of contacts' reasons for fear and fear dynamics show that fear is embedded in relationships between contacts, health agents, and communities and can be reshaped during the process of containment. Generally contacts did comply with containment out of fear of the Ebola virus rather than straight fear toward health agents or the police. Their fear was partly based on misinformation and overestimation of transmission risk that health agents did not challenge because many of them shared this perception that favored adherence over compliance to containment.

Containment: Social Logics and Effects

In the four case studies, containment for contacts was not an evidence-based intervention, neither in Guinea nor in Senegal. It was independent of any juridical decisions, unlike in the United States, and the intervention of militaries, unlike in Liberia. The choice for applying containment and the selected modalities arose from contextual factors and pragmatic decisions rather than planned and evaluated strategies, the application of WHO or Centers for Disease Control recommendations, or ethical considerations. In Senegal, some contacts were confined under police surveillance but others were not; the first ones had been considered a social unit on the basis of their common residency and Guinean origin, whereas the second ones were judged as capable of performing symptom surveillance and confinement alone because they were health agents. In Guinea, contacts were initially followed up mostly without confinement during the first months of the epidemic in 2014, particularly if they were health agents. Later, as the number of EVD cases increased and many contacts were lost to follow-up, contacts were more often confined together in family units, such as the compound described in case study 3. There, the ongoing vaccine trial that depended on reliable access to contacts (and to their own contacts) may have reinforced the option for confinement as a means of ensuring follow-up. Lastly, the *ratissage* strategy used from 2015 and the search for "fleeing contacts" occurred under high pressure from authorities and institutions, when contact containment had become an issue beyond the scope of technical advisers and the responsibility of Ebola response decision makers.

Confinement was accepted by contacts, provided that a number of accompanying measures were set up. First, material support needed to be guaranteed in acceptable ways (i.e., sufficient food and a stipend). On that matter, observations made in Senegal were consistent with recommendations defined during other outbreaks such as SARS (Holm 2009), in favor of a daily stipend for living expenses including phone calls, with online psychosocial support (Desclaux et al. 2016). A comparison of case studies 2 and 3 reveals that ongoing experience with the epidemic allowed support to be defined in a more equitable way in late 2015, as contacts in Coulara considered that their treatment was fair but felt that particular situations (contacts' dependents living out of the containment zone, polygamous households, professional expenses) were not sufficiently considered. Errors in health teams' understanding of the composition of the "family" in case study 1 were avoided in case studies 3 and 4, where teams spent considerable time in exchanges with the contacts' community to understand their needs and relationships. However, contacts who lost their jobs or their customers after the end of confinement in case studies 1 and 3 highlight a major ethical issue about the balance between personal benefits and risks related to containment.

Some statements by health authorities seemed focused on the objective of separation of EVD contacts to protect other people, at the expense of a careful consideration of the social dynamics and risk of infection among the confined. In case study 2, some contacts isolated with their families requested collective containment away from their homes for reasons similar to those mentioned by case study 3 contacts, to be confined elsewhere to protect their loved ones, and to be with placed with other contacts to face the experience together. These wishes, and more generally contacts' acceptance of social distancing and for some of them containment, are in agreement with the general public desire, shared also to some extent by health authorities, for segregation of potential, suspected, and confirmed Ebola cases. Such separation, along with measures such as border closures and isolation of the sick, has a symbolic value beyond its efficacy at a biological level (attested or discussed); it suggests an ideal order based on the visible distinction between the risky and the safe, a cultural process fundamental for the symbolic control of disorder (Douglas 2002). This separation simultaneously reassures populations inside and outside of protective barriers, when fear prevails. Besides the symbolic logic involved, separation encouraged contacts to develop a sense of solidarity in the face of adversity, and bonds were created or reinforced, making a transitory "contacts community" who developed collective coping strategies (prayers and games in case 1, discussions and common activities in case 3), particularly when this contained community was based on a preexisting one. However, each type of contained community had issues: where health authorities decided that individual confinement would be better accepted because it kept family organization unchanged, confidentiality issues arose and exacerbated tensions in the fragile balances between individual autonomy and family harmony.

The "contacts communities" created by containment had various identities and compositions. In case studies 1 and 3, containment relied on preexisting social and spatial frontiers and included households rather than individuals; some family members were contained although they had not been personally exposed to risk. In these cases, a pragmatic logic favoring acceptability and feasibility was applied, complemented at times by a social logic, for instance when the young woman married outside the house was confined together with the family to eliminate visits that might be misinterpreted by neighbors. In case studies 2 and 4 (where *ratissage* identified contacts in diverse households), containment could not be based on a preexisting or newly created spatial frontier since contacts were spread across an extensive area. In these cases, contacts created a sense of community in a different way, for instance through cellphone calls, as observed in case study 2. In Senegal, contacts were not treated differently according to their exposure to risk; all were confined at the same period with similar procedures. In Guinea, particularly in case study 4, levels and time of risk exposure were more differentiated, engendering an individualization of follow-up that was further adapted to every contact's compliance with more or less proactive interventions, leading to disruptive research for the last contact subjects.

Conclusion: Fear *of* Containment?

The four detailed case studies presented in this chapter show the variety of interpretations of contact tracing and containment in diverse contexts and at various times. However, the very different epidemiological and public health situations in Senegal and in Guinea do not fully explain the differences. The choice of containment methods was based on extreme caution against risk on the side of public health experts, in a context of lack of evidence about the efficacy of public health measures and uncertainty in the new eco-social context of the 2014-15 West African outbreak. Contact-tracing strategies were defined under tension between rationality and emotion, knowledge of virology and pragmatic experience, authoritative and deliberative approaches, and biosafety and social acceptability rationales.

All of the case studies show that contacts faced fear that was shaped, if not provoked, by containment. Beyond an individual emotion, fear was a social product attached to six particular issues related to the experience of "being an EVD contact" and influenced by contacts' individual economic, social, professional, gender, and family situation as well as the overall political, historical, and cultural context. Fear was enhanced or reduced by public health measures, including methods of confinement that could improve or worsen perceived security in matters of contagion, stigma, and social relationships. Minor social arrangements and side support measures considered negligible or self-evident from a global perspective were often very meaningful at the local level in a context of insecurity and acute psychological vulnerability. Last, fear and social pressure were used by agents of the Ebola response to maintain contacts' compliance to containment.

Social bonds that created a sense of solidarity between contacts in "contact communities" and with follow-up agents played a key role in reducing fear and reducing hostility engendered by misinterpretations or lack of information. These bonds were more effective when empathic approaches were used by follow-up agents, based on ethos (in the case of volunteers), method (in the case of health agents), or a social theory approach (in the case of anthropologists). Interventions such as contact follow-up and social mobilization necessitated human resources and skills that have been insufficiently acknowledged until present, as "social measures" are frequently considered collateral in public health interventions during a crisis. Although follow-up and containment were broadly accepted by the majority of contacts, some remained bitter about the imposed intervention, particularly the ones who lost their jobs and resources as a result of containment. Symbolic or material reparation for these losses should be considered in the critical analysis of containment and further preparedness measures.

Was containment the reason that some contacts fled follow-up? According to the anthropologists involved in the Kaliya intervention where contacts have been hiding or escaping, these contacts feared being ostracized due to their association with Ebola; they also feared the treatment from health workers, who were rumored to deliberately kill the sick. They also might have feared their followers since contact tracing under high social pressure resembled tracking, as also observed in Sierra Leone. In other contexts, like the urban district of Coulara or the Forécariah villages where *cerclage* was performed (regions described by health authorities as *a priori* resistant), the implementation of contact follow-up was accompanied by "education," secondary support measures, and interventions by social mobilizers and volunteers, creating conditions favorable to discussion with inhabitants and militating against hostile acts. But the flight of contacts and the exceptional pressure to locate them eliminated the chance for health agents and social mobilizers to inform, support, and protect them, or to open a dialogue to change misconceptions about authoritative measures. In Guinea, the only way to overcome escaped or hostile contacts' fear and to restore social links was to build confidence between local communities and public authorities and to fight against longstanding distrust of authorities from populations who until now had survived by defending themselves, often by escaping or bypassing public interventions. Only through effective local development of infrastructure and services by the state and its institutions can local populations overcome the *a priori* fear toward Ebola outbreak, response, and stigma and become part of the response. Otherwise, local cooperation in future cases will require a considerable input in communication, support, and mobilization at each instance, with likely limited results, as illustrated the case of the tragic loss of the Gbéréka contact. Besides, considering a public health measure with such dramatic social effects as containment, the transnational scientific community should engage rapidly in building evidence about the efficacy of containment in the Ebola outbreak and producing knowledge on epidemiological and virological aspects relevant for prevention.

Acknowledgments

To all participants in the studies. To research assistants Fatoumata Binta Dieng, Djénabou Diallo, Mohamed Diakité, Souleymane Diop, Maurice Camara (Guinea), Dioumel Badji, Albert Gautier Ndione, and Soukheye Diop (Senegal) and research partner Khoudia Sow. To Dr. B. Taverne, Dr. J. Anoko, C. Lanièce, Dr. M. Gastellu-Etchegorry, Dr. J. Loko Roka, and M. Fribault for their comments on a previous version of this chapter. Field studies were funded by IRD, AVIESAN, Expertise France (Senegal), INSERM, AVIESAN, and UNICEF (Guinea). The views expressed in this article are those of the authors and do not necessarily represent any institution with whom they have been affiliated.

Notes

1. The term *réticence* was used by the Ebola national committee to name the attitudes and acts showing a refusal, more or less asserted and in a more or less violent way.
2. Quarantine is defined by International Health Regulations (2005) as "the restriction of activities and/or separation from others of suspect persons who are not ill or of suspect baggage, containers, conveyances or goods in such a manner as to prevent the possible spread of infection or contamination" (WHO 2008, p.16), when other institutions such as the Presidential Commission for the Study of Bioethical Issues (U.S.) only consider separation (Calain and Poncin 2015).
3. EBSEN, "Epidémie d'Ebola et construction sociale de la confiance au Sénégal," co-directed by A. Desclaux and K. Sow, implemented by TransVIHMI (IRD) and CRCF (Centre Régional de Recherche et de Formation à la prise en charge de Fann) and funded by IRD, AVIESAN, and Expertise France.
4. POSTEBOGUI, "[Re] vivre après Ebola en Guinée: conséquences cliniques, immuno-virologiques, psychologiques et socio-anthropologiques," co-directed by E. Delaporte and M. Barry, implemented by TransVIHMI (IRD) and University of Conakry, and funded by INSERM and AVIESAN. The anthropological part of the research is directed by B. Taverne, A. Desclaux and M. Diop.
5. The team from Laboratoire d'Analyse Socio-Anthropologique de Guinée, Université Général Lansana Conté—Sonfonia à Conakry was under contract with UNICEF Guinea.
6. This means "the land of the marabout" in Malinké language.
7. The under-five mortality rate, considered an indicator for the population public health status, is 100.7 per 1,000 live births in Guinea and 55.3 in Senegal; their respective ranks according to the Human Development Index are 182 and 170 (UNDP 2015).

References

Anonymous. 2015. "Etude socio-anthropologique sur les réticences relatives à la prévention et au traitement médical de l'épidémie à virus Ebola." Conakry: UNICEF.

Benton, Adia. 2014. "The epidemic will be militarized: Watching outbreak as the West African Ebola epidemic unfolds—Cultural anthropology." *Fieldsights—Hot Spots, Cultural Anthropology Online.* October 7. http://www.culanth.org/fieldsights/599-the-epidemic-will-be-militarized-watching-outbreak-as-the-west-african-ebola-epidemic-unfolds. Accessed April 26, 2016.

Bousso, Abdoulaye, Moussa Seydi, Daye Ka, et al. 2015. "Experience on the management of the first imported Ebola virus disease case in Senegal." *Pan African Medical Journal* 22 (Supp 1). http://www.panafrican-med-journal.com/content/series/22/1/6/full/#.VoxDD_E4o2s. Accessed April 26, 2016.

Buli, Benti Geleta, Landry Ndriko Mayigane, Julius Facki Oketta, et al. 2015. "Misconceptions about Ebola seriously affect the prevention efforts: KAP related to Ebola prevention and treatment in Kouroussa Prefecture, Guinea." *Pan African Medical Journal.* http://www. panafrican-med-journal.com/content/series/22/1/11/full/#.Vo2Qd_E4o2t.   Accessed April 26, 2016.

Calain, Philippe, and Marc Poncin. 2015. "Reaching out to Ebola victims: Coercion, persuasion or an appeal for self-sacrifice?" *Social Science & Medicine* 147: 126–33. doi:10.1016/j.socscimed.2015.10.063.

Centers for Disease Control and Prevention. 2014. "CDC methods for implementing and managing contact tracing for Ebola virus disease in less-affected countries." CDC. http://www.cdc.gov/mmwr/preview/mmwrhtml/mm6404a10.htm. Accessed April 26, 2016.

Chandler, Clare, James Fairhead, Ann Kelly, et al. 2015. "Ebola: Limitations of correcting misinformation." *Lancet* 385(9975): 1275–77. doi:10.1016/S0140-6736(14)62382-5.

Desclaux, Alice, Albert Gautier. Ndione, Dioumel Badji, and Khoudia Sow. 2016. "La surveillance des personnes contacts pour Ébola : effets sociaux et enjeux éthiques au Sénégal." *Bulletin de la Société de pathologie exotique*, February, 1–7. doi:10.1007/s13149-016-0477-2.

Desclaux, Alice, and Khoudia Sow. 2015. "« Humaniser » les soins dans l'épidémie d'Ebola ? Les tensions dans la gestion du care et de la biosécurité dans le suivi des sujets contacts au Sénégal." *Anthropologie & Santé. Revue internationale francophone d'anthropologie de la santé*, November. doi:10.4000/anthropologiesante.1751 http://anthropologiesante.revues.org/1751. Accessed April 26, 2016.

Douglas, Professor Mary. 2002. *Risk and blame: Essays in cultural theory*. London: Routledge.

Epelboin, Alain. 2007. *Ébola, ce n'est pas une maladie pour rire*. Documentary film. https://www.canal-u.tv/video/smm/ebola_ce_n_est_pas_une_maladie_pour_rire.13710. Accessed April 26, 2016.

Fink, Sheri. 2016. "Connecticut faces lawsuit over Ebola quarantine policies." *New York Times*. February 7. http://www.nytimes.com/2016/02/08/nyregion/connecticut-faces-lawsuit-over-ebola-quarantine-policies.html. Accessed April 26, 2016.

Fribault, Mathieu. 2015. "Ebola en Guinée : violences historiques et régimes de doute." *Anthropologie & Santé. Revue internationale francophone d'anthropologie de la santé*, no. 11(November). doi:10.4000/anthropologiesante.1761. http://anthropologiesante.revues.org/1761 Accessed April 26, 2016.

Haas, Charles N. 2014. "On the quarantine period for Ebola virus." *PLoS Currents*. doi:10.1371/currents.outbreaks.2ab4b76ba7263ff0f084766e43abbd89.

Hilderbrand, Amber. 2014. "Ebola outbreak: Why Liberia's quarantine in West Point slum will fail." *CBCNews*. August 25. http://www.cbc.ca/news/world/ebola-outbreak-why-liberia-s-quarantine-in-west-point-slum-will-fail-1.2744292.

Holm, Søren. 2009. "Should persons detained during public health crises receive compensation?" *Journal of Bioethical Inquiry* 6(2): 197–205. doi:10.1007/s11673-009-9160-7.

Jeudy-Ballini, Monique, and Claudie Voisenat. 2004. "Ethnographier la peur." *Terrain* 43(September): 5–14. doi:10.4000/terrain.1803.

Kpanake, Lonzozou, Komlantsè Gossou, Paul Clay Sorum, and Etienne Mullet. 2016. "Misconceptions about Ebola virus disease among lay people in Guinea: Lessons for community education." *Journal of Public Health Policy*, February. doi:10.1057/jphp.2016.1.

Mataconis, Doug. 2015. "Nurse Kaci Hickcox sues Chris Christie for civil liberties violations during Ebola quarantine." October 23. http://www.outsidethebeltway.com/nurse-kaci-hickcox-sues-chris-christie-for-civil-liberties-violations-during-ebola-quarantine/. Accessed April 26, 2016.

Migliani, René. 2016a. "Evolution hebdomadaire de l'épidémie de maladie à virus Ebola (MVE) dans les sous-préfectures de Guinée de Décembre 2013 à Mars 2016." Diaporama, Paris.

Migliani, René. 2016b. "Situation de l'épidémie de maladie à virus Ébola (MVE) en Guinée. Bilan des données disponibles le 31 Janvier 2016." Paris.

OMS, Bureau Afrique. 2014. "Recherche des contacts pendant une flambée de maladie à virus Ebola." Brazzaville. http://www.who.int/csr/resources/publications/ebola/contact-tracing/fr/. Accessed April 26, 2016.

Ropeik, David. 2014. "Fear of Ebola. A greater risk than the disease itself." *Big Think*. October 21. http://bigthink.com/risk-reason-and-reality/criticism-of-ebola-mistakes-in-dallas-puts-us-at-greater-risk-than-the-disease-itself. Accessed April 26, 2016.

Rothstein, Mark A. 2015a. "Ebola, quarantine, and the law." *Hastings Center Report* 45(1): 5–6. doi:10.1002/hast.411.

Rothstein, Mark A. 2015b. "From SARS to Ebola: Legal and ethical considerations for modern quarantine." *Indiana Health Law Review* 12(1): 227–80. doi:10.2139/ssrn.2499701.

UNDP. 2015. "Human Development Report 2015." Washington: UNDP. http://www.undp.org/content/undp/en/home/librarypage/hdr/2015-human-development-report.html. Accessed April 26, 2016

Watts, Sheldon J. 1999. *Epidemics and history: Disease, power, and imperialism*. New Haven, CT: Yale University Press.

WHO. 2008. *International Health Regulations (2005)*. Geneva: WHO. http://www.who.int/ihr/publications/9789241596664/en/. Accessed April 26, 2016.

WHO. 2014. "Ebola and Marburg virus disease epidemics: Preparedness, alert, control, and evaluation. Interim manual version 1.2.". WHO/HSE/PED/CED/2014.05. http://www.who.int/csr/disease/ebola/manual_EVD/en/.

Wojda, Thomas R., Pamela L. Valenza, Kristine Cornejo, et al. 2015. "The Ebola outbreak of 2014-2015: From coordinated multilateral action to effective disease containment, vaccine development, and beyond." *Journal of Global Infectious Diseases* 7(4): 127. doi:10.4103/0974-777X.170495.

Zylberman, Patrick. 2013. *Tempêtes microbiennes: Essai sur la politique de sécurité sanitaire dans le monde transatlantique*. Paris: Gallimard.

Challenges of Instituting Effective Medevac Policies

DUNCAN MCLEAN

In Sierra Leone, during the fall of 2014, an innocuous open cut led to the high-risk exposure of an MSF international volunteer to the Ebola virus. This set in motion a series of procedures that resulted in the collective decision to remove the team member from the field. From the initial evaluation to eventual departure, extensive consultations were required with the individual concerned and among MSF medical staff, all undertaken with the pressure of a very short 48-hour timeframe. Once back in his own country, the staff member found that follow-up was no less complex. Along with managing the stress of potentially carrying a contagious and often fatal disease, he was subject to different emerging interpretations of post-exposure vaccination protocols, which is not surprising given that the science of Ebola vaccines was evolving at the same time as operations on the ground.[1]

This was hardly an isolated incident, as at the height of the West African Ebola epidemic teams of MSF medical referents were on call 24 hours a day. In addition to precautionary departures such as the one described, non–Ebola-related illnesses and basic procedural questions formed the basis of most inquiries.[2] It was however the relatively rare occurrence of full medical evacuation (medevac) for an Ebola-positive international volunteer that was the greatest source of stress for those responsible for staff health within MSF, with implications that went far beyond the individual concerned.

The medevac of a Norwegian doctor from Freetown to Oslo in October 2014 provides an apt illustration. In this case the private air ambulance service Medic' Air International was hired by MSF to undertake the evacuation. The same process of internal consultation took place after the onset of initial symptoms, with the plane departing from Paris to Dakar 48 hours later. Following an obligatory 10-hour rest for the flight crew, the plane continued to Sierra Leone. The return flight took roughly 10 hours to reach Oslo, including two 45-minute refueling stops in the Canary Islands and then Paris, both conducted under "high-level police surveillance with the opening of the airplane door prohibited." During this period the Norwegian authorities organized reception at the military airport in Oslo and the hospital isolation unit.[3]

In addition to delays while ensuring that the evacuation was technically feasible in medical terms for the patient but also in terms of securing the aircraft, political delays rose to the fore. With the flight plan requiring overflight and landing permission in the Canary Islands, the Spanish government closed its airspace, effectively canceling the medevac. Only after MSF lobbying and high-level political intervention was the evacuation able to proceed.[4] In the words of one observer, "Spain became hysterical, almost certainly linked to a recent experience of an unrelated secondary infection, and wanted full medevac even for non-contagious high-risk exposure." When refueling the pilot "couldn't leave the cockpit, although medically and scientifically this was completely ridiculous."[5]

The Norwegian doctor recovered 12 days after repatriation, fortunate in the care provided after international medical evacuation.[6] Nevertheless, despite this harrowing experience, the risk of infection for international staff (and the number infected) was insignificant compared to the number of local health workers affected. In addition to "threats, intimidations, and sometimes even violence at the hands of the populations they have come to help," there existed the obvious danger of death from infection. According to a WHO report from May 2015, this translated to 815 confirmed or probable Ebola cases out of a total 20,955 infections in West Africa, including 28 MSF employees—half of whom died. In other words, health workers were 21 to 32 times more likely than the general population of affected West African countries to become sick with Ebola.[7]

However, if the number of international staff infected was minute compared to total staff numbers on the ground, the process involved in managing these cases—both in the specific cases and in the broader attempt at finding a medevac solution—would prove to be one of the more significant hurdles to overcome in the Ebola response. The summer and fall of 2014 was a key period and will be a focus in this chapter. As the crisis escalated in Guinea, Liberia, and Sierra Leone, the need for a functioning system became obvious. Unable to guarantee the evacuation of sick staff members, recruitment difficulties for an already unprecedented number of staff recruited for the epidemic response could only worsen. And while technical logistic problems were far from insignificant, the lack of "political will" stood out, indicative of a broader fear that succeeded only in further isolating the stricken countries.

Medevac as Duty of Care

The medical evacuation of ill international staff can be considered a basic responsibility of a humanitarian organization, falling broadly under "duty of care." In the context of Ebola in West Africa it was necessary in order for the individual to "benefit from an intensive care unit and access to family members."[8] Three particular situations needed to be taken into account: the medevac of non-Ebola cases; the exit of a person "at risk post-incident of exposure to Ebola virus"; and finally the medical evacuation of a person confirmed Ebola positive.[9]

In the first category, severe illnesses unrelated to Ebola were already difficult to evacuate given the limited number of transport options. By the summer of 2014 only Brussels Air lines and Air Maroc were maintaining a small number of regional flights, and even those required "regular visits [by MSF representatives] in order to reassure them."[10] Given the "stigma around Sierra Leone, Liberia, Guinea and even Nigeria," an "abnormal delay" was to be expected between the "request and the realization of the medevac."[11] Indeed, MSF's main medevac provider, International SOS (ISOS), warned of "possible major delays" in the evacuation of patients suffering from "an urgent medical condition" other than Ebola, mainly arising from air ambulance providers and receiving medical facilities due to "reluctance to take in charge patients coming from Ebola-affected countries."[12]

In both the second and third categories, time is of the essence. In a "high-risk exposure, you need to get staff out in less than 48 hours as they are not contagious—no symptoms have yet developed."[13] Consequently, the legal requirement to disclose the health situation of a patient "requiring urgent transfer by air" can be avoided so long as the flight takes place "within a safe window of opportunity or 2 days after exposure to a high-risk VHF (viral hemorrhagic fever) contact."[14] This includes commercial flights, given the "incubation period is from day 2 to day 21."[15]

The medevac of a patient confirmed with Ebola is certainly the most complex. Again, time is a key issue. Organizational responsibility includes ensuring the best possible care for those recruited internationally but also proximity to family members. The objective is to "get the patient back to a high-level hospital within 24 hours post confirmation of the positivity" because there is a better chance for the patient with an early start to treatment, and to "discharge the field and the colleagues."[16] At a very basic level this requires ensuring primary extraction to the local capital, helicopter eventually becoming the preferred option for MSF.[17]

After extraction of the patient to the capital, three further aspects need to be taken into account. First a well-equipped plane that accepts transporting a patient from West Africa to Europe must be located, further complicated by the need to find a crew prepared both to fly and to accept a lengthy decontamination process that includes destroying all material that might have been in contact with the patient.[18] Overflights are likewise a problem, requiring "explicit permission."[19] As seen with the Oslo–Freetown example, international aviation regulations "may interdict trespassing in national air space, or deny landing rights in case refueling is needed."[20] Finally a "green light" from the national authorities of the country and hospital where the patient will be received is necessary.[21]

Early Lessons and Limited Options

Stated quite simply, medevacs in the context of viral hemorrhagic fevers such as Ebola require "planes, airspace (and landing) permission, and hospitals" if they are to be conducted successfully.[22] We must also keep in mind the almost unquantifiable equation that during the transport of an Ebola case, the potential benefits to the patient become "inversely proportional to the risks faced by the caregivers."[23] Two early attempts at medical evacuation in July 2014 highlighted the problems faced. In both cases MSF was only tangentially involved, but important lessons could be taken from those first experiences that allowed "a real improvement after them." This included a practical demonstration as to workable options, in addition to identifying key problems so as to "lobby for the necessary improvements."[24]

In the first case, the director of Kenema Hospital in Sierra Leone was cared for in the MSF isolation center in Kailahun while the WHO attempted to coordinate his medical evacuation, as he was a prominent figure in the fight against Ebola. ISOS eventually refused the medevac because the patient was symptomatic, and it was likewise difficult to find an accepting medical facility in Europe, particularly as he was not a European Union citizen. Eventually a hospital in Hamburg agreed to receive him, although the patient died before he could be evacuated. The second instance concerned an American doctor who tested positive for Ebola in Foya, Liberia. Because the Foya center was a former MSF project run by Samaritan's Purse, MSF was consulted regarding evacuation procedures and options. Again ISOS refused because the patient was demonstrating symptoms. Medic' Air then attempted to organize the medevac but additional problems of discretion and overflight permissions blocked the process. Ultimately, Phoenix Air conducted a successful evacuation to the United States, where the patient recovered.[25]

General conclusions reached by MSF at time included the lack of reliability of ISOS, including delays and eventual refusal to take a patient, general difficulties in finding planes for both ISOS and Medic' Air, and difficulties in locating a receiving hospital.[26] Lack of discretion also stood out. As Medic' Air noted shortly afterwards, "the evacuation must stay confidential from the beginning to the end, mainly with diagnosis and patient's identity."[27] In the second case, Samaritan's Purse published a press release while the evacuation was still being negotiated, including details of the case, the patient's name and profession, and confirmation of his medical status.[28] This presents particular problems for over-flights and was partly responsible for the initial failed medical evacuation.[29]

In fact, ISOS had long said it "couldn't assure medevacs during the Ebola crisis,"[30] as it considered the medical evacuation of Ebola patients "highly complex and extremely difficult to achieve."[31] Officially there was reference to patients demonstrating "active clinical symptoms" with "uncontrolled body fluids, such as vomiting, diarrhea or bleeding."[32] This in turn led to unwillingness on the part of aircraft operators; reluctance from "health authorities and other governmental bodies" in receiving countries; difficulties in overflight and landing permission; and further deterioration of the patient's condition.[33] Undoubtedly all these reasons presented valid obstacles to a successful medical evacuation. However, as the company itself pointed out, even if the management politely agreed to do "all they could," the pilots themselves refused.[34]

The lack of pilots and air crews prepared to undertake Ebola evacuations was not a problem restricted to ISOS but was "a major problem in Europe for everyone."[35] Indeed, individual pilots are bound to international aviation regulations and are "entitled to refuse to fly a plan arranged for the medevac of a suspected VHF contact."[36] Medic' Air International faced an identical problem, along with a limited number of aircraft.[37] However, with most medevac service providers "refusing due to fear," Medic' Air was contacted as it at least presented a viable option for MSF. Smaller than ISOS, it actually "suited [MSF's] needs in terms of flexibility."[38]

MSF also had previously worked with Medic' Air, having used its services to successfully organize the medical evacuation of a Lassa fever case from Sierra Leone in 2011.[39] Although there have only been a small number of hemorrhagic fever cases touching Europe, meaning relatively limited research in medical evacuation possibilities for the West African crisis, MSF had been encouraged by this positive experience.[40] At the time it was possible to operate "under the radar," a far more difficult prospect in 2014 given the scale of the West African epidemic along with the associated media attention. As Medic' Air noted, "during the Lassa evacuation on 2011 there was no collective psychosis," it was possible to operate more discreetly.[41]

Publicity aside, there were other drawbacks to the services provided by Medic' Air. In a press release during the summer of 2014 it warned of "restricted aircraft availability" for medevacs from West Africa to Europe. Even a successful medevac could take between 36 and 42 hours, "assuming no specific mitigating factors causing delay along the way."[42] Not only did Medic' Air have few planes at its disposition, those it did have were small, meaning refueling stops were necessary when traveling between West Africa and Europe.[43] Further, although it could transport patients openly displaying some Ebola symptoms, there were limits; if a patient's "clinical condition is decreasing with diarrhea, vomiting, shock, neurologic disorders, pulmonary distress," the evacuation would be "immediately cancelled."[44]

So for all its advantages of flexibility, Medic' Air was clearly insufficient as a sole medevac option for the reasons described. In the words of MSF's Staff Health Unit, "we realized that discretion would no longer work, the situation was too large, too mediatized." An alternative solution was that used by Samaritan's Purse in July. The U.S.-based ambulance service Phoenix Air, described as the "Rolls Royce of 'medevacs,'" had the unique advantage of being able fly if a patient is in an "advanced state."[45] However, its two medevac-equipped Gulfstream jets were based on the other side of the Atlantic. And in terms of availability, Ebola in West Africa was only one of its priorities, as Phoenix Air was already under contract to the U.S. State Department.[46]

Considering the possible scenarios for Ebola medical evacuations, MSF would only launch the process once "the case was confirmed," and even in that instance, none of the existing options in the summer of 2014 provided guarantees of a successful extraction. In practice this lack of certitude meant "launching all medevac transport options at once" while trying to locate a "receiving hospital" and juggling the necessary authorizations.[47] This was hardly a reassuring situation in which to send an increasing number of international volunteers to West Africa as the Ebola crisis escalated.

Recruitment Implications

Recruiting experienced international volunteers for humanitarian missions can be challenging irrespective of the circumstances. In the context of hemorrhagic fevers, this was particularly problematic given the "fear and stigma associated with the Ebola virus."[48] The lack of a functioning system for medical evacuations has direct and obvious implications for activities on the ground. In the words of MSF's director of operations, "we will not be able to convince volunteers to go to these countries to help tackle the epidemic if we don't have a good evacuation system."[49]

Consequently it was necessary to inform international staff prior to departure that there "was no certitude of medical evacuation, irrespective of the illness." This meant of course that no effort would be spared to ensure a medevac but there was "no 100% guarantee."[50] Indeed this is still the case today, including internal briefing documents that state MSF cannot ensure the evacuation of Ebola-positive patients or "even a medevac for a non-Ebola medical problem," which could take "much more time than usual."[51] The potential inability for international staff to be transferred to "hospitals in Europe or the United States where experimental drugs and modern facilities raise the chances of survival" was a serious obstacle to recruitment. This was a problem that was expected to compound as the demand for more staff increased with the scaling up of the Ebola response.[52]

An additional problem presented itself with MSF international staff with non-European nationalities, "especially when treatment in their own countries was difficult or impossible."[53] MSF would eventually have upwards of "70 different nationalities" in Guinea, Liberia, and Sierra Leone.[54] Even without guaranteed medevac, the medicalized repatriation of European or North American citizens to their own countries "generally seemed OK." However, non-EU staff presented particular risks over which politicians had "understandable public relations concerns." Even within MSF there had been internal debate and hesitation as to whether to take all nationalities in the field, but with "so many needs in terms of staffing" a decision was taken to pose no limits.[55]

In practice, there was an uneasy assumption of there being "little chance that an MSF patient would be refused." The real risk was in losing precious time, "especially if an extra administrative day was necessary for non-European patients."[56] The staffing decision would have direct implications on the position MSF would take in its medevac lobbying activities, the demand for an "effective system for medical evacuation of international staff—whatever their nationality."[57] This would become one of many priorities for the organization as the scale of the crisis unfolded.

Deterioration and Urgency

By the beginning of August 2014, over 1,000 Ebola deaths had been recorded in West Africa and the crisis was receiving considerable international coverage, particularly after the WHO finally declared a "public health emergency of international concern."[58] As the situation on the ground deteriorated, the need for a medevac solution became more pressing. Although MSF had been aware of the medevac problem since the initial cases appeared in March, this urgency "followed the epidemiological curve, meaning the need for a system quickly got larger."[59]

Certainly the infection, evacuation, and successful recovery of several American aid workers, including the Samaritan's Purse employee described, raised the issue of medical evacuations more publicly—along with provoking greater interest in the response.[60] Nevertheless in mid-August very real questions were being asked internally over the ability for MSF to "maintain operations in case of incident." This essentially meant that response capacity was being "jeopardized" by the lack of a system for medical evacuation. Duty of care remained central but also the "need to preserve the trust of the teams that all will be done to provide them with the best possible care."[61]

The period in question was "extremely stressful" for those responsible for staff health, given the lack of certainty over evacuation possibilities.[62] The potential availability of Phoenix Air in August provided partial reassurance as an additional option.[63] Indeed, when Medic' Air was unavailable in September, Phoenix successfully evacuated a French national from Liberia to Paris, although the entire process took close to 50 hours after the individual tested positive for Ebola.[64] This was the first case of an international medical evacuation in the crisis for MSF and was qualified internally as "burdensome" in addition to confirming the "urgency of receiving the guarantee that a fast and effective medevac system be made available."[65]

It was the subsequent unavailability of Phoenix Air in October that led MSF to return to Medic' Air to manage the Norwegian evacuation.[66] It was during this operation that the need for political support, notably around implicated states to "facilitate the opening airspace for stopovers (refueling)," assumed special importance.[67] In the words of the general director of Medic' Air, "basically after the Oslo evacuation, the realization that you need strong collaboration with states rather than small structures" became obvious.[68]

The fact that MSF eventually managed to successfully evacuate two international staff who had tested positive for Ebola should not mask the challenges in securing such state cooperation.[69] An MSF operations director has likened the organization of medevacs to "begging door-to-door." With the European Union in particular lacking "collective means," individual states "gave what they wanted to or could, everyone had a different piece of the puzzle."[70] MSF was not alone in this predicament, of course: during the summer of 2014, medevac blockages were likewise affecting the attempted scale-up of operations by other organizations.

Implications for Partners

Over the course of the Ebola epidemic, external communication by MSF shifted with the scale of the crisis and the lack of international response. As early as July 2014, states were being asked to "deploy extra capacity" as nongovernmental organizations (NGOs) could not handle the burden alone. Calls for international support culminated in a September 2 address to United Nations member states to "deploy civilian and military assets with expertise in biohazard containment."[71] From MSF's perspective, calls for greater involvement in scaling up the response required a medevac option for all because "treatment centers are useless without trained workers to manage and operate them."[72]

The involvement of other international organizations is essential in understanding MSF's demands for a functioning medevac system. Internal prerogatives included issues of recruitment and duty of care to its own staff; however, "we needed options for partners as well."[73] If it was apparent that other actors were needed, it would have been "irresponsible" to call for their presence without the means for medevacs. In other words, it was simply not enough to demand financial support, ensure training, and so on.[74] Medevacs were an "absolute necessity to preserve the capacity of the actors involved in the response."[75]

Of course MSF was far from alone in grappling with this issue, including duty of care to staff. A WHO staff health official noted that "simply saying 'good luck' to colleagues was not acceptable."[76] Neither was MSF alone in attempting to ensure medevac services for all its international staff, as the EU also expressed frustration at resolving the "problem presented by non-European citizens" involved in the response.[77] Outside the EU, the Americans were likewise well aware of the difficulties when evacuating their own citizens, their recent experience having demonstrated the "limits of existing capabilities."[78]

An additional factor that organizations smaller than MSF faced was that of cost. With insurance waivers that "limit coverage of Ebola-related evacuations" and even the cheaper companies such as Medic' Air costing "between $100,000 to $150,000 per patient," the costs could be prohibitive.[79] This had a direct impact on the decision for an organization to expand its field operations, or indeed for international staff to be posted. [80]

Quiet and Not-So-Quiet Diplomacy

For all the described reasons, the need for action on the medevac issue was clear, although the way in which the message was passed carried attendant risks. The distinction between public communication and advocacy through lobbying activities in this regard is crucial. Too much external communication risked shifting the focus away from the crisis and "people suffering in West Africa" while giving the impression of being overly focused on expatriates and less concerned about national staff. There was also the danger of unintended consequences, such as creating panic among international staff and their families. Finally, it was also necessary to consider the potential negative impact on relations with "governments with whom we will have to liaise in case of medevac."[81]

Nevertheless, in choosing the means with which to demand action, MSF had multiple "political levers at its disposition as it was at the heart of the operations."[82] Internally, MSF's network was mobilized, with diverse national MSF offices asked to contact their foreign ministries on the need to facilitate medical evacuation, including the 16 European MSF offices. Yet while the science and logistics of medevacs remains complex, "the main problem was political rather than technical."[83] Further, given the overall deterioration of the epidemic, it was necessary to move beyond awareness raising to highlighting inappropriate reactions such as the "reduction of international flights and restrictions of movement."[84] Medevac blockages and the necessity of state support needed to be addressed directly with the governments concerned.

During the second week of August, the number of meetings between MSF and various government ministries increased throughout Europe as the decision to make more noise was translated into action.[85] The key message passed orally concerned the "unprecedented nature of the outbreak," the fact that it went beyond "regular humanitarian means," and the need for state assets—the latter eventually culminating in the call for military biohazard means in early September. The typical response from external interlocutors was, "What do you need?" The means for medical evacuation came to the fore as the "first minimum step" that needed to be taken. "Medevacs are necessary for us to keep working."[86]

More specifically, MSF asked for the "organization of a medical evacuation system that will guarantee" the following: a "one-stop centralized set-up that can be called upon when needed"; an appropriately equipped airplane "ready to leave at all times, to be made available to the region"; and the repatriation of any international staff member to Europe "within a maximum of 24 hours" to a hospital with Ebola management capacity.[87] This essentially translated to "planes, hospitals and political agreement" with the authorities concerned.[88]

Support often manifested itself in promises for financial support along the lines of "we are doing everything we can" for yet another African crisis far from European shores. The point relayed by MSF in these meetings was that Ebola "is not a foreign problem, it is everybody's problem, and beyond the reach of humanitarian workers, there needs to be a reaction." And as the frontline agency, MSF was "at its limit . . . we need this medevac and also for others to scale up."[89] Similar messages were echoed by WHO in European forums, noting at the end of August that the "situation is critical and there is a real threat that current activities will have to be downscaled due to the transportation problem." More specifically, the "immediate need is to solve the problem with medical evacuations, landing rights and long-range capacity/air bridge to move personnel and equipment in and out of Europe."[90]

The situation remained dramatic with "little reaction other than the Americans with Phoenix Air, but this was not enough."[91] Indeed the

U.S. ambassador to NATO had noted that a standby aircraft would be "challenging" given that the U.S. government does not "own this capability." And as we have seen, the U.S. State Department's commercial contract with Phoenix was only an option "provided that the aircraft in question were not urgently needed for other critical missions."[92] In practical terms, MSF wanted to increase medevac options by having the EU "pool resources and place military or civilian planes on standby in West Africa or Europe." However, even with general agreement on the objective among all interlocutors, disputes persisted over the supply of the aircraft, who would pay what, and most importantly who would have overall responsibility.[93]

In a letter to the European Commission's High Representative for Foreign Affairs and Security Policy at the end of August, MSF formalized its request. In noting that the organization finds itself "at the very core of the response," MSF would be able to continue operations only "if it can ensure duty of care to its personnel." Highly problematic was the absence of a guaranteed medevac "for MSF international personnel, being exposed to the virus, diagnosed as infected, or showing symptoms of the infection." Specific requests to the Commission included medicalized aircraft, permission to fly over and land during an evacuation, and "specific hospitals capable to host any MSF international volunteer, European or non-European citizen."[94] Once again the nationality question was repeatedly emphasized in that "we need 100% coverage for all our staff." And once again the noncommittal "probably ok was the insufficient response."[95]

The main medevac requests were repeated in "different fora, at different levels and in different countries" without success. By mid-September MSF's tone was "gaining in urgency and irritation."[96] At this point the "need for ensuring 'medevac' capacities and transport solutions" was pushed more strongly in public fora.[97] As an MSF representative noted, "we need other options than Phoenix, we need rapid mobilization" in what is really a "structural problem" with the European Union.[98] A stronger approach included an editorial in the *New York Times* that claimed Europe's inability to establish a functioning medevac system had become "a serious hurdle impeding the battle against Ebola in West Africa." The political angle was likewise given greater prominence, with the MSF director of operations finding it "amazing that everyone we talk to says that we are right, that there is enough money, but nothing is happening."[99]

It is difficult to measure the final impact of MSF's medevac lobbying on the eventual European Commission decision to formally support an evacuation system at the end of October.[100] Indeed, there had been general agreement on the need for such a system since August, but with no European country actually stepping forward "to provide the aircraft, personnel or other resources needed to make it work," progress was slow.[101] The "enormous pressure from MSF to establish a structured system" quite likely influenced the political reticence from key state actors.[102] However, overcoming the generalized fear of the epidemic was far more difficult.

Between Reluctance and Fear

In discussions on the challenges of instituting a medevac system in the context of Ebola, invariably the conversation included words such as "fear" or "panic."[103] However, beyond the structural and political constraints described, there were other reasons why "everyone was so scared to make a decision."[104] In the face of the epidemic, hostile perceptions were even understandable as Ebola "generates reactions which are often irrational and driven by the universal fear of epidemics."[105] The lack of effective treatment and "the painful and distressing symptoms and the high mortality rate cause extreme public anxiety."[106]

One of the most obvious manifestations of this anxiety can be seen in the security-oriented response, both in the countries most affected and internationally. Borders were closed and flights were canceled amid broader attempts at containment. As alarmingly, Ebola's dangers were explicitly framed in "national and international security terms," especially after aid workers returned to Europe and the United States for treatment.[107] MSF's own attempts at raising awareness risked being counterproductive, as more "awareness has triggered more fear (hindering the response) than response capacities." This included not only the reduction in commercial flights but also difficulties in organizing medevacs.[108]

WHO noted that although the medevac situation was "particularly difficult early on, we don't necessarily realize the problems for countries—meaning political challenges rather than technical."[109] And such reluctance is not entirely without foundation. If secondary infections can occur in the field, they can also occur in Europe. The delayed Norwegian medevac due to the closure of Spanish airspace was a case in point, "specifically linked to a secondary (but unrelated) infection in Spain."[110] There is also a valid point concerning the quality of medevac services themselves. Medic' Air has described air ambulances that can be up to "thirty years old, generally recycled, and requiring heavy maintenance with frequent stops."[111]

Fortunately, not all states went to the extremes of the Australian government in altogether refusing to send doctors or nurses to West Africa because, in the words of Foreign Minister Julie Bishop, there was no guarantee that if Ebola was contracted "they would be able to be transported or treated in a hospital either in the region or in Europe."[112] Indeed, while Bishop's official statement of policy gets to the heart of the medevac predicament, Australian nationals did actively take part in the response on their own initiative, including with MSF. Other well-documented reactions included "mandatory quarantines" for returning aid workers in some U.S. states despite the complete absence of symptoms. Indeed, in such cases where restrictions were considered unreasonable, "MSF offered its staff the ability to stay in more 'friendly' countries in Europe for 21 days to avoid potential problems."[113]

Toward a Decision

In the absence of a formal medevac system, several stopgap measures were enacted. American plans to "strengthen services on the ground were better than nothing but clearly not enough for aid workers."[114] Referred to as "centers of excellence," these medical facilities had additional resources to treat "national staff, along with expatriates awaiting evacuation." While certainly helpful, such gestures could not replace the timely medical evacuation of international staff.[115] The lack of progress at the EU became even more apparent with the successful Phoenix Air medevacs in August and September. Prior to the European Commission decision at the end of October, those outside MSF were left equally frustrated at the "amazing situation, where we had to ask a private American company to fly to Africa to evacuate to Europe."[116]

This successful evacuation by a U.S. company could also be seen as having a positive effect. The general director at Medic' Air noted that he spent "three months running around Europe" trying to locate pilots and aviation companies willing to fly Ebola patients in the summer of 2014. He considers the American use of Phoenix more than symbolic, "provoking something akin to European pride." The day after the Oslo evacuation, "offers began arriving from European aviation companies." This included support through state contracts, once again necessary to "unblock political obstacles such as overflights and stopovers."[117]

September also saw limited advances on the political front, even if this remained more in the sphere of fine words rather the concrete change. On September 17, the European Parliament resolution on the EU's response to the Ebola outbreak called "on the Member States to coordinate flights and establish dedicated air bridges to move health personnel and equipment to the affected countries and to provide medical evacuation if necessary."[118]

More dramatically, on September 18, United Nations Security Council Resolution 2177 declared the epidemic "a threat to international peace and security." While expressing concern about the "detrimental effect of the isolation of the affected countries as a result of trade and travel restrictions," there was specific mention of the "necessary repatriation and financial arrangements, including medical evacuation capacities and treatment and transport provisions, to facilitate their immediate and unhindered deployment to the affected countries."[119]

Reaction, however, continued to focus on individual states rather than broader system, with little interest shown in coordinating under the auspices of the EU. At best, member states "organize for their own citizens first and help others if they are not busy."[120] This included failed French and Swiss initiatives, the latter having received initial enthusiasm but eventually being reserved for "Swiss nationals or possibly international health workers under Swiss contracts."[121] Italy had "good possibilities" but acted alone, the lack of coherence compounded by the "problem of delay" with each state having a "different time-frame for medical evacuation."[122] In the words of MSF's Ebola task force, by the end of September the "different initiatives and processes" in various countries were "too slow too late."[123]

It is also misleading to compare Europe and the United States in this regard. There is no European air force and certainly no centralized management; use of such resources was at the discretion of individual states.[124] The earlier description that likened securing assets for medical evacuation in Europe as "begging door-to-door" remained appropriate.[125] As the European External Action Service (EEAS) stated at an earlier meeting end of August, "EU Military Staff does not have their own assets and thus they have to rely on member states to provide the assets." At the time "only one responded positively."[126]

By mid-October, members of the Global Ebola Response Coalition were still stressing the "remaining gap in Medevac provision" and the "importance of establishing a systematic process for medical evacuation or best-quality in situ care for responders."[127] In the intervening period, the European Commission and others likewise turned to the private sector, with both Medic' Air and Phoenix Air figuring prominently.[128] In the original EU plan, the Commission used the "same options as MSF, meaning ISOS, then Phoenix, then Medic' Air."[129] WHO had likewise concluded an agreement with the U.S. State Department for accessing Phoenix Air services, even though the evacuation of American citizens was prioritized.[130]

With the emerging paper agreement at the end of October 2014, which was essentially a "practical solution," MSF decided "to put further pro-active advocacy on this issue on hold."[131] The EU system as such had the Emergency Response Coordination Center of the European Commission coordinating requests, the actual medevac decision made by WHO, and the use of rotating member state planes in the event that a private plane was unavailable.[132] A high-risk exposure debate took place internally as these preemptive departures were "extremely expensive" to operate, although no patients evacuated under these circumstances would eventually test positive for Ebola. This would include a "black week" in March 2015 when multiple American and British personnel were evacuated due to potential exposure.[133] The EU was eventually involved directly in medevacs of 16 patients, four of whom tested positive for Ebola, all of whom survived.[134]

The entire process was formally based on the European Council conclusions of October 23 and 24, 2014. A key component was that "it applies to international health/humanitarian aid workers—of any nationality" so long as they are directly involved in the West African Ebola crisis. This includes personnel with "suspected or confirmed infection." Overall responsibility was under the Emergency Response Coordination Center of the European Commission: the WHO approves the request and the European Commission then "determines the medevac provider" (DG-ECHO) and the "accepting hospital" (DG-SANTE). (DG-ECHO: "Directorate-General for European Civil Protection and Humanitarian Aid Operations". DG-SANTE: "Directorate-General for Health and Food Safety"). "If the insurance does not, or only partially, cover the costs, the EC will cover the bill/the rest."[135]

Smaller Was Easier; Bigger Was Necessary

Over the course of the summer of 2014, the need for a formal medevac system gained in urgency. From the perspective of MSF at the time, the delays were hugely problematic even if in the final analysis internal opinions differed. For some the 10 weeks it took for the political solution proposed by the European Commission to emerge "did not seem that long," especially when taking into account the myriad of technical and contextual factors involved in international medevacs even at the best of times.[136] For others the EU was "catastrophic in terms of leadership" in this regard, with "the 10 weeks between the initial August lobbying of EU leaders and the formal decision at the end of October" far too long.[137]

Even the resulting decision left considerable leeway to individual states. Appropriately equipped hospitals were generally receptive, but there was never an official political "yes" regarding nationalities, despite this essential inclusion being part of the European Council's remarks.[138] Meanwhile the unspoken possibility of evacuating local health staff was not broached, even if they were likewise voluntarily putting themselves in danger, and the shortage of health workers was long identified as a key issue.[139] Indeed, the "difference in treatment was striking" knowing that enlarging the evacuation criteria was neither logistically nor financially feasible.[140]

Those external to MSF have identified obvious risks for the future—namely, now that the crisis is over, what limited "political will" existed will disappear.[141] This is all the more striking given that "the overall problem of medical evacuations is still not resolved." Only Phoenix Air can guarantee an evacuation irrespective of the state of the patient, even if it cannot guarantee the availability of an aircraft. As WHO notes, "it is important to ask questions about the future, to prepare and do better."[142] Certainly this comment is as relevant to the overall Ebola response as it is to the specifics of medevacs.

Looking back at MSF's medevac lobbying, one observer highlighted a seeming contradiction in actions and results, as "MSF demanded a system but never used it."[143] In practice, MSF actually preferred to use smaller companies such as Medic' Air as it was easier if "we operated under the radar." The real problem was the limited number of options for medevacs. When the Ebola crisis became dramatic, "everybody was watching us, it was impossible to be small and discreet, but at least we had more options."[144] Even then, having a system "may not solve all the problems" and MSF would always want to make "its own choices for medevac if we think it will be better for the staff."[145] Resort to the system when established was not so much the point given the means at MSF's disposal.[146] Efforts to reform the medevac system were about establishing the maximum number of options for all organizations fighting Ebola while trying to ensure the best possible care for its own staff. It was also about highlighting broader weaknesses in the Ebola response, relevant to all concerned as help belatedly arrived.

Notes

1. Dr. Estrella Lasry, Tropical Medicine Advisor, MSF, interview by the author, March 14, 2016.
2. Ibid.
3. Hervé Raffin. 2015. "Evacuation aérienne d'une patiente Ebola: critères de décisions et modalités de transport." *Journal Européen des Urgences et de Réanimation* 27: 9–13.
4. Brice de le Vingne, Director of Operations, MSF, interview by the author, February 23, 2016.
5. "Non-contagious high-risk exposure" refers to patients who display no symptoms and are not at risk of spreading the disease, despite having been potentially exposed. Dr. Françoise Saive, Staff Health Unit Manager, MSF, interview by the author, March 1, 2016.
6. Raffin, "Evacuation aérienne d'une patiente Ebola."
7. Risks faced MSF numbers taken from Marc Poncin, "Ebola healthcare workers: A hazardous and isolating job," *Humanitarian Practice Network*, June 8, 2015; general health worker data from "Health worker infections in Guinea, Liberia and Sierra Leone, a preliminary report," WHO, May 21, 2015.
8. Internal MSF document, "Advocacy—Main Lines/Ebola," August 14, 2014.
9. Internal MSF document, "Implementation & Impact of Ebola Staff Health Policy on HR Management (updated)," September 2014.
10. Rosa Crestani, Emergency Coordinator, MSF, interview by the author, February 16, 2016.
11. Internal MSF document, "Implementation & Impact of Ebola Staff Health Policy on HR Management (updated)," September 2014.
12. Email, ISOS to MSF, August 29, 2014.
13. Saive interview.
14. Internal MSF document, "Medevac Liberia—Ebola Intervention 2014," September 12, 2014.
15. Internal MSF document, "Implementation & Impact of Ebola Staff Health Policy on HR Management (updated)," September 2014.
16. Ibid.
17. Crestani and Saive interviews.
18. Andrew Higgins, "Ebola fight in Africa is hurt by limits on ways to get out," *New York Times*, October 14, 2014.
19. Crestani interview.
20. Internal MSF document, "Medevac Liberia—Ebola Intervention 2014," September 12, 2014.

21. Internal MSF document, "Implementation & Impact of Ebola Staff Health Policy on HR Management (updated)," September 2014.
22. Saive interview.
23. Raffin, "Evacuation aérienne d'une patiente Ebola."
24. Françoise Saive, email message to author, March 21, 2016.
25. Internal MSF document: "Medevac Process for Ebola + Case," July 20, 2014.
26. Ibid.
27. Medic' Air International, press release, August 14, 2014.
28. "Samaritan's Purse doctor serving in Liberia, West Africa, tests positive for Ebola." Press release, Samaritan's Purse, July 26, 2014.
29. Dr. Hervé Raffin, Medic' Air International, interview by the author. March 21, 2016.
30. Interviews with Brice de le Vingne, Director of Operations, MSF, February 23, 2016, and Edouard Rodier, Representative to the European Union, MSF, February 26, 2016.
31. "International SOS Evacuation Capability Statement," ISOS, undated.
32. Quoted in "Medevac policy gaps slow volunteer recruitment," *IRIN*, November 7, 2014.
33. "International SOS Evacuation Capability Statement," ISOS, undated.
34. Crestani and Saive interviews.
35. Raffin interview.
36. Internal MSF document, "Medevac Liberia—Ebola Intervention 2014," September 12, 2014.
37. Higgins, "Ebola fight."
38. Saive interview.
39. Crestani interview.
40. Saive interview. Medevacs for viral hemorrhagic fevers were rare, and initially concerned Lassa fever, dating back to 1969. See Abe M. Macher and Martin S. Wolfe. 2006. "Historical Lassa fever reports and 30-year clinical update." *Emerging Infectious Diseases* 12(5): pp. 835–37. It should also be noted that some medevac specialists have noted improvements, notably in the use of negative air pressure units and hygiene management. See Raffin, "Evacuation aérienne d'une patiente Ebola."
41. Raffin interview.
42. Medic' Air International, press release, August 14, 2014.
43. de le Vingne interview.
44. Medic' Air International, press release, August 14, 2014.
45. Saive interview.
46. Higgins, "Ebola fight."
47. Saive interview.
48. Nick Cumming-Bruce, "Global response to Ebola highlights challenges in delivering aid," *New York Times*, October 10, 2014. The same article goes on to compare the 151 aid agencies active following Typhoon Haiyan in the Philippines, compared with four medical organizations responding to Ebola in West Africa by October 2014.
49. Quoted in Higgins, "Ebola fight."
50. Crestani, de le Vingne, and Saive interviews.
51. Internal MSF document, "Implementation & Impact of Ebola Staff Health Policy on HR Management (updated)," September 2014.
52. Higgins, "Ebola fight."
53. Note that MSF "international staff" refers to staff from outside the three affected countries. Crestani interview.
54. Internal MSF document, "MSF Ebola Task Force Advocacy Info 2," September 22, 2014.
55. Saive interview.
56. Ibid.
57. Internal MSF document, "MSF Ebola Task Force Advocacy Info 2," September 22, 2014.
58. "Statement of the 1st meeting of the IHR Emergency Committee on the 2014 Ebola outbreak in West Africa," WHO, August 8, 2014.
59. Saive interview.
60. Eric A. Friedman, "Medical evacuations for West African Ebola patients: The unspoken possibility," O'Neill Institute for National and Global Health Law, October 6, 2014.
61. Internal MSF document, "Advocacy—Main Lines/Ebola," August 14, 2014.

62. Crestani interview.
63. Saive interview.
64. Cumming-Bruce, "Global response"; Higgins, "Ebola fight."
65. Internal MSF document, "MSF Ebola Task Force Advocacy Info 2," September 22, 2014.
66. Crestani interview.
67. Raffin, "Evacuation aérienne d'une patiente Ebola."
68. Raffin interview.
69. Poncin, "Ebola healthcare workers."
70. de le Vingne interview.
71. Internal MSF document, "MSF Ebola desk meeting: Brief review on advocacy messages (Aug.-Nov.)," November 2014.
72. Cumming-Bruce, "Global response."
73. Saive interview.
74. de le Vingne interview.
75. Internal MSF document, "Advocacy—Main Lines/Ebola," August 14, 2014.
76. Dr. Caroline Cross, Director, Staff Health and Wellbeing Services, WHO, interview by the author, February 26, 2016.
77. Didier Merckx, Air Transport and Logistic, ECHO Flight, European Commission, interview by the author, February 19, 2016.
78. Letter from U.S. Permanent Representative on the North Atlantic Council to MSF, August 28, 2014.
79. Higgins, "Ebola fight."
80. "Medevac policy gaps slow volunteer recruitment," IRIN, November 7, 2014.
81. Internal MSF document, "Ebola: Medevac External Communication," October 16, 2014.
82. de le Vingne interview.
83. Crestani interview.
84. Internal MSF document, "MSF Ebola Task Force Advocacy Info 6," November 20, 2014.
85. de le Vingne interview.
86. Edouard Rodier, Representative to the European Union, MSF, interview by the author, February 26, 2016.
87. Internal MSF document, "MSF Ebola Task Force Advocacy Info 2," September 22, 2014.
88. Rodier interview.
89. Ibid.
90. "12th EU Coordination Meeting on the Response to the Ebola Epidemic in West Africa," European Commission, August 26, 2014.
91. Rodier interview.
92. Letter from U.S. Permanent Representative on the North Atlantic Council to MSF, August 28, 2014.
93. Higgins, "Ebola fight."
94. Internal MSF document, "Letter to H.E. Catherine Ashton, High Representative of the Union for Foreign Affairs and Security Policy/Vice-President of the European Commission," August 24, 2014.
95. Rodier interview.
96. Internal MSF document, "MSF Ebola Task Force Advocacy Info 2," September 22, 2014.
97. Internal MSF document, "MSF Ebola Task Force Advocacy Info 6," November 20, 2014.
98. Rodier interview.
99. Higgins, "Ebola fight."
100. de le Vingne interview.
101. Cumming-Bruce, "Global response."
102. Didier Merckx, Air Transport and Logistic, ECHO Flight, European Commission, interview by the author, February 19, 2016.
103. Saive and Raffin interviews.
104. de le Vingne interview.
105. Poncin, "Ebola healthcare workers."
106. "Pushed to the Limit and Beyond," MSF, March 23, 2015.

107. "The Politics Behind the Ebola Crisis," International Crisis Group, Africa Report Number 232, October 28, 2015.
108. Internal MSF document, "Advocacy—Main Lines/Ebola," August 14, 2014.
109. Cross interview.
110. Raffin interview.
111. Ibid.
112. Adam Withnall, "Ebola outbreak: Tony Abbott says Australia will not 'send health workers into harm's way' to combat the deadly disease in West Africa," *Independent*, October 12, 2014.
113. Poncin, "Ebola healthcare workers."
114. Internal MSF document, "Advocacy—Main Lines/Ebola," August 14, 2014.
115. Crestani interview.
116. Cross interview.
117. Raffin interview.
118. "European Parliament resolution on the EU's response to the Ebola outbreak," 2814/2842(RSP), September 17, 2014.
119. Resolution 2177, United Nations Security Council, S/RES/2177, September 18, 2014.
120. Higgins, "Ebola fight."
121. Saive interview.
122. Merckx interview.
123. Internal MSF document, "MSF Ebola Task Force Advocacy Info 2," September 22, 2014.
124. Higgins, "Ebola fight."
125. de le Vingne interview.
126. "12th EU Coordination Meeting on the Response to the Ebola Epidemic in West Africa," European Commission, August 26, 2014.
127. Global Ebola Response Coalition Call, October 10, 2014.
128. Higgins, "Ebola fight."
129. Saive interview.
130. Merckx and Cross interviews.
131. Internal MSF document, "MSF Ebola Task Force Advocacy Info 5," November 1, 2014.
132. Internal MSF document, "MSF Ebola Task Force Advocacy Info 6," November 20, 2014.
133. Merckx interview.
134. "Overview Ebola Medevacs to Europe," European Commission, May 13, 2016.
135. European Commission Ebola MEDEVAC Standard Operating Procedures for the Field with the Cooperation of the World Health Organization (WHO), European Commission, (updated) July 1, 2015.
136. Saive interview.
137. de le Vingne interview.
138. Crestani interview.
139. Friedman, "Medical evacuations."
140. Lasry interview.
141. Merckx interview.
142. Cross interview.
143. Merckx interview.
144. Saive interview.
145. Internal MSF document, "Ebola: Medevac External Communication," October 16, 2014.
146. Saive interview.

Returning to the "Ebola World"

MAUD SANTANTONIO

Six months after my first Ebola mission in Sierra Leone, I prepared myself to leave again, this time to Guinea, for a two-month mission in the Ebola Treatment Center (ETC) in the capital city of Conakry. My feelings were mixed. The five weeks I spent in the ETC in Sierra Leone had been stressful, both psychologically and physically, and I was apprehensive to find myself again submerged in "the world of Ebola." At that same time, I very much wanted this. If, in my previous mission, the violence of this disease—decimating families without warning, torturing both the body and the soul—profoundly affected me, there were also positive, magical moments that touched me as deeply. These moments in time, when a man or woman or child returned almost from the dead, provided me with unspoken encouragement to continue fighting for such invaluable gains. I had fought with them against the disease in Sierra Leone and I wanted to take up the fight again in Guinea.

In early February 2015, the Ebola epidemic seemed to be in decline. While too many people continued to fall ill and die of Ebola, we no longer felt overwhelmed by its malignance. We even dared to believe that the epidemic would be coming to an end in the near future. The ETC in Conakry was like an island—made essentially of tents—in the heart of the national hospital. This was quite a different setup than that on the outskirts of Kailahun, a village in eastern Sierra Leone. The incorporation of the ETC in the hospital environment allowed patients presenting at the general emergency area suspected of having Ebola to be processed more quickly, but it also allowed easier referrals to necessary services for those whose blood test ruled out the disease. On the other hand, it was more inconvenient, as the entrance to the center was much more visible. Ebola caused fear;

thus, a patient seen entering or exiting risked becoming a subject of malicious gossip, even becoming a pariah among his neighbors.

During my two months in Guinea, I discovered that the Ebola epidemic creates havoc not only by leaving sickness and death in its wake, but also by its perversity; when it seemed to be in decline, new flare-ups would spring up to extend its life. After having reached a peak in Conakry at the end of 2014, the epidemic had progressively diminished from January 2015 onward until it fell below 20 patients, suspect or confirmed, under care in the high-risk zone (the zone where the famous yellow spacesuits, or PPEs, were required). When I arrived, this new calmness could be felt in the mood of the staff. The Guinean staff, who had struggled against this epidemic for almost a year, seemed to be awakening from a long nightmare—a nightmare during which most of them had lost at least one close acquaintance, sometimes a colleague working in another health service. Tension was no longer etched onto their faces and staff were organizing among themselves to take their long-deferred vacations. Work days passed discussing the party that would be organized to celebrate the end of this cursed epidemic. Everyone hoped that it would be over at the end of March 2015, a year after the first case had been declared.

But Ebola decided otherwise. In one day at the end of February, 10 new patients were admitted, eight of whom tested positive. The next day, three new patients arrived, one of them a pregnant woman, all positive. These new cases meant that others were most likely contaminated and the flame of the epidemic was reviving. For three weeks, the entire ETC operated to the rhythm imposed by fluctuating numbers of incoming patients. While the number remained moderate, it was enough to make us nervous. Then another wave would break upon us: the number of confirmed cases exploded, forcing us to reopen a part of the treatment center that had been closed two months earlier. The silence was deafening—a stony, tearful, angry silence.

A few days after this reopening, a young man was brought to the ETC by his family. He had fever, vomiting, and a level of fatigue so extreme that he could hardly sit up. The interviewer did not obtain a clear history of any contacts with someone sick with Ebola, although he could not exclude the possibility. Considering the symptomology, we decided to admit the young man as a suspect case. I was part of the team that entered in the high-risk zone to welcome and examine him. He was particularly weak; two of us had to help him over to his bed. His vital signs were very troubling. We placed him on an intravenous perfusion as quickly as possible for rehydration and began the standard treatment. Consisting of antibiotics and an antimalarial drug, this treatment was administered on a practical basis to all new patients, orally or intravenously depending on their general state. In effect, clinical signs of severe sepsis or malaria are similar and easily confused with those of Ebola. Each time someone is admitted in the high-risk zone on suspicion of Ebola, the patient must await the result of a blood test to be released from the ETC. At the same time, if this blood test is performed in the four days following the onset of symptoms and is negative, a second test has to be performed later to confirm the first result. The young man was admitted in the morning and his blood test was performed shortly after admission. He remained in critical condition, despite the rehydration and intravenous treatments. A few hours later, we received his test results: negative. Accompanied by a Guinean colleague, I went to announce the results to his family, who had been waiting since the morning. In this case, I was not all smiles as I announced the news, because I was still quite worried about his very poor health. While he did not have Ebola, he was clearly at risk of dying of something else, and quite rapidly. The family consented to have him transferred to intensive care and thanked us for the care given. A little while later, the ambulance arrived. I was finishing the transfer paperwork when I was notified on the walkie-talkie that the young man had just passed away on the gurney. Everyone was shocked. My colleague agreed to accompany me to inform the family. The short distance that separated our work space from the visitors' tent became a psychological gauntlet to traverse. How would I explain that their child, brother, cousin, just died on the gurney, when he hadn't even reached adulthood and he did not have Ebola? We had hardly finished announcing the terrible news when their anger began to explode. The head of the family, who had only an hour earlier thanked us profoundly, screamed now of his sadness and his incomprehension, laying the blame on me. It was I, the white doctor, who killed his son, with the complicity of the ETC. Words had no effect. We returned to our office as the shouts of the family grew. We saw them circling the ETC with rocks in their hands. A few seconds later, they faced us from a few meters away, separated behind the orange plastic barrier marking the borders of the ETC. The head of the family glared at me, screaming words I couldn't understand. The first rock flew. Instinctively, we ran for cover under the tents, where I contacted the coordinator of the center to inform him of the situation. The atmosphere was tense. The uproar grew as some spectators who were watching the drama from the upper floors of the surrounding hospital joined in. I was far from reassured. I acutely felt every gesture and hostile word flung at us from this family, distraught and angry. After a few moments that nonetheless seemed like an eternity, hospital security arrived, followed by the military. A level of calm slowly returned to the center, allowing workers to leave safely.

This was not the only violent incident since the beginning of the epidemic, but it was the first time that I found myself at the center of the storm. The violence of the family's reaction relayed their incomprehension in the face of the death of a loved one. When he was admitted, he was not strong but he was at least still able to talk and move. Once he was moved into the high-risk zone, he was unable to move around on his own and to see his family due to his weakened condition. And as he was being transferred 12 hours later, he died. Should we have immediately sent him to another service, since we had found no evidence of a history of contact with an Ebola case? It is the question that each health worker must ask each time he or she decides to admit somebody among the suspected Ebola cases. For a healthcare worker, making a first probable diagnosis and beginning treatment before definitive test results are available is common practice. With Ebola, not only must healthcare providers make a decision before a biological test result, but they must also do so without a real clinical examination because of the "no-touch policy." For the first time as a doctor, with this epidemic I found myself evaluating patients from two meters away. The exam was based on several pre-established questions, a temperature reading, and a visual assessment of the patient: Does she look tired? Are his eyes red? Can she manage to eat the small biscuit offered? Does he seem nauseous or on the verge of vomiting? This system of triage puts us in a difficult situation, because if we decide that the patient is likely suffering from this hemorrhagic fever, he or she must be admitted with "suspects" in the high-risk zone. But placing someone in the high-risk zone who is ultimately negative means putting him or her at risk of contamination for Ebola while at the ETC. On the other hand, allowing someone to leave who is a short while later confirmed positive places everyone around that person at risk. Sometimes the choice is clear, but often—because Ebola symptoms are nonspecific and some of those afflicted are afraid to admit contact with a positive case—the decision is arduous. How many times did I cross my fingers and hope that I was not wrong?

Triage is a crucial moment of terrible responsibility, as it has life-and-death consequences for the patient and, sometimes, his or her community. With our limited diagnostic tools, we have no other choice but to render a verdict, a sword of Damocles: those not suspected of having Ebola may return to "real" life, and suspect cases must accept entry into "the Ebola world," the high-risk zone. Patients placed in the suspect area are advised not to interact with the other sick patients, not to share their blankets, and to wash their hands thoroughly after going to the bathroom, before eating, and if they should come in contact with another patient. A major problem is that often a person is admitted simultaneously with one or more members of his family or community. How are such people persuaded once they are "inside" that they should not take care of their loved ones as a measure to protect each other? How is a mother made to accept that she cannot help feed her child who is so weak he can hardly feed himself? How does a brother ignore his sister as she stumbles walking to the toilet? How does one convince a human being that acts of kindness and tenderness can spread death? There are no words to effectively illuminate this absurd cruelty.

Today, we have no alternative but to separate the afflicted and the suspected cases from their communities to stem the flow of Ebola. The fight to save lives creates the alienation of victims. Based on a set of criteria, a strange doctor decides that some sick people are suspect cases, and they are cajoled to enter a place of which they know little except that many don't come out alive. Until they receive the result of their blood tests, they are urged to avoid all contact with other sick patients. Other sick patients may be loved ones who have a high likelihood of dying in the coming days or even hours. And yet they are still told to stay away, abandoning them in their final hours. When some patients finally have the chance to return home, not only will many be in mourning but they will also face stigma from their communities. Where does their dehumanization end? The measures put in place to combat this epidemic may have been indispensable, but their application remains, nonetheless, against human nature.

INDEX